Handbook of Antimicrobial Therapy

Selected Articles from *Treatment Guidelines*
with updates from *The Medical Letter*®

Published by

The Medical Letter, Inc.
145 Huguenot St.
New Rochelle, New York 10801-7537

800-211-2769
914-235-0500
Fax 914-632-1733
www.medicalletter.org

D1563687

19th Edition

Contents

Introduction

The Medical Letter, Inc. is a nonprofit company founded in 1958 by Arthur Kallet, the co-founder of Consumers Union, and Dr. Harold Aaron, with the goal of providing healthcare professionals with objective, independent analyses of both prescription and over-the-counter drugs. In addition to its newsletters, *The Medical Letter on Drugs and Therapeutics* and *Treatment Guidelines from The Medical Letter*, the company also publishes handbooks and software on topics such as antimicrobial therapy and adverse drug interactions. It is supported solely by subscription fees and accepts no advertising, grants or donations.

The Medical Letter on Drugs and Therapeutics offers comprehensive drug evaluations of virtually all new drugs and reviews of older drugs when important new information becomes available on their usefulness or adverse effects. Occasionally, *The Medical Letter* publishes an article on a new non-drug treatment or a diagnostic aid. *Treatment Guidelines from The Medical Letter* consists of review articles of drug classes for treatment of major indications. A typical issue contains recommendations for first choice and alternative drugs with assessments of the drugs' effectiveness and safety. *The Medical Letter* is published every other week and *Treatment Guidelines* is published once a month. Both are intended to meet the needs of the busy healthcare professional who wants unbiased, reliable and timely information on new drugs and comprehensive reviews of treatments of choice for major indications. Both publications help healthcare professionals make decisions based on the best interests of their patients, rather than the commercial interests of the pharmaceutical industry.

The editorial process used for Medical Letter publications relies on a consensus of experts to develop prescribing recommendations. An expert consultant, one of our editors or a contributing editor prepares the preliminary report on a drug (for *The Medical Letter*) or drugs for common disorders (for *Treatment Guidelines*) in terms of their effectiveness, adverse effects and possible alternatives. Both published and available unpublished studies are carefully examined, paying special attention to the results of controlled clinical trials. The preliminary draft is edited and sent to our contributing editors, to 10-20 other reviewers who have clinical and experimental experience with the drug or type of drug or disease under review, to the FDA and CDC, and to the first authors of all the articles cited in the text.

Many critical observations, suggestions and questions are received from the reviewers and are incorporated into the article during the revision process. Further communication as needed is followed by checking and editing to make sure the final appraisal is not only accurate, but also easy to read.

The Medical Letter, Inc., is based in New Rochelle, NY. For more information go to www.medicalletter.org or call (800) 211-2769.

ANTIBACTERIAL DRUGS:
A BRIEF SUMMARY FOR QUICK REFERENCE

AMINOGLYCOSIDES — Aminoglycosides are effective against many gram-negative bacteria and mycobacteria. They may be ototoxic and nephrotoxic, especially in patients with diminished renal function. They are often used together with penicillin or ampicillin in treatment of enterococcal endocarditis in order to achieve synergy. They are sometimes used empirically in septic patients or in those with serious gram-negative pneumonia together with ß-lactam antibiotics. When there is resistance to other safer antibiotics they are sometimes used to treat urinary tract infections.

Amikacin (*Amikin*, and others) — Amikacin is often effective for treatment of infections caused by gram-negative strains resistant to gentamicin and tobramycin, including some strains of *Pseudomonas aeruginosa* and *Acinetobacter*. It is generally reserved for treatment of serious infections caused by amikacin-susceptible gram-negative bacteria known or suspected to be resistant to the other aminoglycosides. Like other aminoglycosides, its distribution to the lungs is limited and when used to treat gram-negative bacilli that cause pneumonia it should be combined with another agent to which the organism is susceptible, such as a ß-lactam. It has also been used concurrently with other drugs for treatment of some mycobacterial infections.

Gentamicin (*Garamycin*, and others) — Gentamicin is useful for treatment of many hospital-acquired infections caused by gram-negative bacteria. Strains of gram-negative bacilli resistant to gentamicin are often susceptible to amikacin or to one of the third-generation cephalosporins, cefepime, or imipenem or meropenem. Gentamicin is also used with penicillin G, ampicillin or vancomycin for treatment of endocarditis caused by susceptible enterococci.

1

Kanamycin (*Kantrex*, and others) — Active against some gram-negative bacilli (except *Pseudomonas* or anaerobes), but most centers now use gentamicin, tobramycin or amikacin instead. Kanamycin can be useful concurrently with other drugs for treatment of tuberculosis.

Neomycin — A drug that can cause severe damage to hearing and renal function and has the same antibacterial spectrum as kanamycin. Parenteral formulations have no rationale for use because of their toxicity. Deafness has also followed topical use over large areas of skin, injection into cavities such as joints, and oral administration, especially in patients with renal insufficiency.

Streptomycin — Streptomycin has been displaced by gentamicin for treatment of gram-negative infections, but it is still sometimes used concurrently with other drugs for treatment of tuberculosis, tularemia and plague and is occasionally used with penicillin, ampicillin or vancomycin to treat enterococcal endocarditis.

Tobramycin (*Nebcin*, and others) — Similar to gentamicin but with greater activity *in vitro* against *Pseudomonas aeruginosa* and less activity against *Serratia*. In clinical use, it is not certain that it is significantly less nephrotoxic than gentamicin.

AMINOSALICYLIC ACID (PAS) — Used in antituberculosis regimens for many years, its distressing gastrointestinal effects caused many patients to stop taking it prematurely. An enteric-coated oral formulation *(Paser)* is more tolerable, and is used occasionally in combination with other drugs in treating tuberculosis due to organisms resistant to first-line drugs.

AMOXICILLIN (*Amoxil*, and others) — See Penicillins

AMOXICILLIN/CLAVULANIC ACID (*Augmentin*, and others) — See Penicillins

AMPICILLIN (*Principen*, and others) — See Penicillins

AMPICILLIN /SULBACTAM (*Unasyn*, and others) — See Penicillins

AZITHROMYCIN (*Zithromax*, and others) — See Macrolides

AZTREONAM (*Azactam*, and others) — A parenteral monobactam (ß-lactam) antibiotic active against most aerobic gram-negative bacilli, including *Pseudomonas aeruginosa*, but not against gram-positive organisms or anaerobes. Aztreonam has little cross-allergenicity with penicillins and cephalosporins. Aztreonam is also available in a solution for inhalation *(Cayston)* for use in patients with cystic fibrosis who are colonized with *Pseudomonas aeruginosa*.

BACITRACIN — A nephrotoxic drug used in the past to treat severe systemic infections caused by staphylococci resistant to penicillin G. Its use is now restricted mainly to topical application.

CAPREOMYCIN *(Capastat)* — A second-line antituberculosis drug.

CARBAPENEMS — There has been an emergence of gram-negative bacteria, especially in hospitalized patients that can produce carbapene-mase enzymes enabling them to be resistant to the carbapenems, penicillins and cephalosporins.

Imipenem/Cilastatin *(Primaxin)* — The first carbapenem, imipenem, has an especially broad antibacterial spectrum. Cilastatin sodium inhibits renal tubular metabolism of imipenem. This combination may be especially useful for treatment of serious infections in which aerobic gram-negative bacilli, anaerobes, and *Staphylococcus aureus* (but not methicillin-resistant strains) might all be involved. It is active against many gram-negative bacilli that are resistant to third- and fourth-generation cephalosporins, aztreonam and aminoglycosides. Resistance to imipenem in *Pseudomonas aeruginosa* occasionally develops during therapy. It has been rarely associated with seizures particularly with high doses in elderly patients.

Meropenem (*Merrem*, and others) — A carbapenem for parenteral use similar to imipenem/cilastatin. It may have less potential than imipenem for causing seizures.

Doripenem *(Doribax)* — Doripenem has a spectrum of activity similar to imipenem/cilastatin. *In vitro*, it is more active than imipenem and meropenem against *Pseudomonas aeruginosa* and is active against some pseudomonal isolates resistant to the other carbapenems; the clinical significance of this *in vitro* activity is unknown. It may have less potential than imipenem for causing seizures.

Ertapenem (*Invanz*) — Ertapenem has a longer half-life, but narrower antibacterial spectrum than imipenem, meropenem and doripenem. It is more active against some extended-spectrum ß-lactamase-producing gram-negative bacilli, but less active against gram-positive cocci, *Pseudomonas aeruginosa* and *Acinetobacter* spp. For empiric treatment of intra-abdominal, pelvic and urinary tract infections and community-acquired pneumonia, it offers no advantage over older drugs other than once-daily dosing.

CARBENICILLIN — See Penicillins

CEPHALOSPORINS — All cephalosporins except ceftazidime have good activity against most gram-positive cocci, and all cephalosporins are active against many strains of gram-negative bacilli. All currently FDA-approved cephalosporins are inactive against enterococci and all but ceftaroline are not active against methicillin-resistant staphylococci. These drugs are often prescribed for patients allergic to penicillin, but such patients may also have allergic reactions to cephalosporins. Rare, potentially fatal immune-mediated hemolysis has been reported, particularly with ceftriaxone and cefotetan.

The cephalosporins can be classified into four "generations" based on their activity against gram-negative organisms. All first-generation drugs have a similar spectrum, including many gram-positive cocci (but not enterococci or methicillin-resistant *Staphylococcus aureus*), *Escherichia coli*, *Klebsiella pneumoniae* and *Proteus mirabilis*. Among the first-generation parenteral cephalosporins, **cefazolin** (*Ancef*, and others) is less painful on intramuscular injection than **cephapirin** (*Cefadyl*; no longer available in the US). The first-generation parenteral cephalosporins are usually given intravenously, and cefazolin is most frequently used because of its longer half-life.

The second-generation cephalosporins have broader *in vitro* activity against gram-negative bacteria. **Cefamandole** (*Mandol*; no longer available in the US) has increased activity against *Haemophilus influenzae* and some gram-negative bacilli, but is occasionally associated with prothrombin deficiency and bleeding. **Cefoxitin** (*Mefoxin*, and others) has improved activity against *Bacteroides fragilis*, *Neisseria gonorrhoeae* and some aerobic gram-negative bacilli. **Cefotetan** (*Cefotan*, and others) has a spectrum of activity similar to that of cefoxitin; it has a side chain that has rarely been associated with prothrombin deficiency and bleeding. **Cefuroxime** (*Zinacef*, and others), another second-generation cephalosporin, has a spectrum of activity similar to cefamandole. Cefuroxime and cefamandole are less active than third-generation cephalosporins against penicillin-resistant strains of *Streptococcus pneumoniae*. **Cefonicid** (*Monocid*; no longer available in the US) has a longer half-life than the other second-generation cephalosporins, but is less active against gram-positive organisms and less active than cefoxitin against anaerobes.

The third-generation cephalosporins, **cefotaxime** (*Claforan*, and others), **cefoperazone** (*Cefobid*; no longer available in the US), **ceftizoxime**

(*Cefizox*; no longer available in the US), **ceftriaxone** (*Rocephin*, and others) and **ceftazidime** (*Fortaz*, and others), and the fourth-generation cephalosporin, **cefepime** (*Maxipime*, and others), are more active than the second-generation cephalosporins against enteric gram-negative bacilli, including nosocomially acquired strains resistant to multiple antibiotics. These agents are highly active against *Haemophilus influenzae* and *Neisseria gonorrhoeae*, including penicillinase-producing strains. Except for ceftazidime, they are moderately active against anaerobes, but often less so than metronidazole, chloramphenicol, clindamycin, cefoxitin, cefotetan, ampicillin/sulbactram, piperacillin/tazobactam, ticarcillin/ clavulanic acid, or carbapenems. Ceftazidime has poor activity against gram-positive organisms and anaerobes. Cefotaxime, ceftizoxime, ceftriaxone and cefepime are the most active *in vitro* against gram-positive organisms, but ceftizoxime has poor activity against *Streptococcus pneumoniae* that are intermediate or highly resistant to penicillin. Cefoperazone, which can cause bleeding, is less active than other third-generation cephalosporins against many gram-negative bacilli, but more active than cefotaxime, ceftizoxime or ceftriaxone against *Pseudomonas aeruginosa*. Ceftazidime and cefepime have the greatest activity among the cephalosporins against *Pseudomonas aeruginosa*. Cefepime has somewhat greater activity against enteric gram-negative bacilli than the third-generation cephalosporins. The third-generation cephalosporins and cefepime are expensive, but are useful for treatment of serious hospital-associated gram-negative infections when used alone or in combination with aminoglycosides such as gentamicin, tobramycin or amikacin. Gram-negative bacteria that produce "broad spectrum" ß-lactamases are resistant to first-generation cephalosporins, but are usually sensitive to second and third generation cephalosporins. However, gram-negative bacilli that produce "extended spectrum ß-lactamases", particularly some *Klebsiella* strains and those that produce chromosomally-encoded ß-lactamases, are usually resistant to first, second and third-generation cephalosporins. These organisms are often hospital-associated. Cefipime may be more active than the third-generation cephalosporin against these strains, but imipenem and meropenem are most consistently active against them. Gram-negative bacilli that produce carbapenemase enzymes are resistant to all cephalosporins. Cefotaxime and ceftriaxone are often used for treatment of meningitis. Ceftriaxone has been widely used for single-dose treatment of gonorrhea, but resistance to it has increased.

Cephalexin (*Keflex*, and others), **cephradine** (*Velosef*; no longer available in the US), and **cefadroxil** (*Duricef*, and others) are well-absorbed oral cephalosporins with first-generation antimicrobial activity; cephradine is also available for parenteral use. **Cefaclor** (*Ceclor*, *Raniclor*, and others), **cefuroxime axetil** (*Ceftin*, and others), **cefprozil** (*Cefzil*, and others) and **loracarbef** (*Lorabid*; no longer available in the US) are oral second-generation agents with increased activity against *Haemophilus influenzae* and *Moraxella catarrhalis*. **Cefixime** *(Suprax),* an oral cephalosporin with activity against gram-positive organisms similar to that of first-generation cephalosporins except for its poor activity against staphylococci; against gram-negative bacteria, it has greater activity than second-generation cephalosporins. It is useful for single-dose oral treatment of gonorrhea. **Cefpodoxime proxetil** (*Vantin*, and others), **cefdinir** (*Omnicef*, and others) and **cefditoren pivoxil** (*Spectracef*) are oral cephalosporins similar to cefixime, but with greater activity against methicillin-susceptible staphylococci. **Ceftibuten** *(Cedax)* is an oral cephalosporin similar to cefixime in its gram-negative activity and poor activity against staphylococci, but it has only inconsistent activity against *Streptococcus pneumoniae*.

Ceftaroline *(Teflaro)* is an intravenous cephalosporin FDA-approved in 2010. It is similar to ceftriaxone in its gram-negative activity, but its gram-positive activity is better than that of ceftriaxone and includes methicillin-resistant *Staphylococcus aureus*. It has some anerobic activity, but not against *Bacteroides*.

Ceftobiprole is an investigational broad-spectrum parenterally administrated cephalosporin with activity against MRSA. It may soon become available.

CHLORAMPHENICOL (*Chloromycetin*, and others) — An effective drug for treatment of meningitis, epiglottitis, or other serious infections caused by *Haemophilus influenzae*, severe infections with *Salmonella typhi*, for some severe infections caused by *Bacteroides* (especially those in the central nervous system), and for treatment of vancomycin-resistant *Enterococcus*. Chloramphenicol is often an effective alternative for treatment of pneumococcal or meningococcal meningitis in patients allergic to penicillin, but some strains of *Streptococcus pneumoniae* are resistant to it. Because it can cause fatal blood dyscrasias, chloramphenicol should be used only for serious infections caused by susceptible bacteria that cannot be treated effectively with less toxic agents.

CINOXACIN (*Cinobac*, and others) — See Quinolones

CIPROFLOXACIN (*Cipro*, and others) — See Fluoroquinolones

CLARITHROMYCIN (*Biaxin,* and others) — See Macrolides

CLINDAMYCIN (*Cleocin*, and others) — A derivative of lincomycin with a similar antibacterial spectrum, clindamycin can cause severe diarrhea and pseudomembranous colitis caused by *Clostidium difficile*. It is one of the alternative drugs for anaerobic infections outside the central nervous system, and can also be used as an alternative for treatment of some staphylococcal infections in patients allergic to penicillins. Strains of *S. aureus* that are sensitive to clindamycin, but resistant to erythromycin become rapidly resistant to clindamycin when it is used. Clindamycin is also used concurrently with other drugs to treat *Pneumocystis carinii* pneumonia and toxoplasmosis. Clindamycin may be beneficial in treatment of necrotizing fasciitis due to Group A streptococcus but, because of the possibility of resistance to clindamycin, it should be used in combination with penicillin G.

CLOFAZIMINE (*Lamprene*) — An oral agent used with other drugs for treatment of leprosy.

COLISTIMETHATE (*Coly-Mycin M*, and others) — See Polymyxins

CYCLOSERINE (*Seromycin*) — A second-line antituberculosis drug.

DAPTOMYCIN (*Cubicin*) — A cyclic lipopeptide antibiotic that is effective for treating complicated skin and soft tissue infections and methicillin-sensitive and methicillin-resistant *S. aureus* bacteremia, including right-sided endocarditis. It is rapidly bactericidal against gram-positive bacteria by causing membrane depolarization. Its anti-bacterial activity includes methicillin-sensitive and -resistant, and van-comycin-sensitive and -resistant *S. aureus* and coagulase-negative staphylococci, streptococci and vancomycin-sensitive and -resistant enterococci. Rarely, *S. aureus* strains with decreased susceptibility to daptomycin have emerged during treatment of *S. aureus* endocarditis with daptomycin. Some strains of *S. aureus* that have emerged with reduced susceptibility to vancomycin during treament with vancomycin, have shown reduced susceptibility to daptomycin. It is administered intravenously once daily and is excreted unchanged in urine; dose adjustments are required when given to individuals with severe renal insufficiency. Adverse effects include the potential for skeletal muscle damage, with rare reversible CPK elevations. More severe muscle effects, which were seen in preclinical studies, do not seem to occur with the currently approved doses; higher doses may increase the potential for rhabdomyolysis. Daptomycin should not be used to treat pneumonia because it is inactivated by surfactant.

DEMECLOCYCLINE (*Declomycin*, and others) — See Tetracyclines

DICLOXACILLIN (*Dycill*, and others) — See Penicillinase-resistant Penicillins

DORIPENEM (*Doribax*) — See Carbapenems

DOXYCYCLINE (*Vibramycin*, and others) — See Tetracyclines

ERTAPENEM *(Invanz)* — See Carbapenems

ERYTHROMYCIN (*Erythrocin*, and others) — See Macrolides

ERYTHROMYCIN-SULFISOXAZOLE *(Pediazole*, and others) — See Macrolides

ETHIONAMIDE *(Trecator)* — A second-line antituberculosis drug.

ETHAMBUTOL (*Myambutol*, and others) — Often used in antituberculosis regimens, it can cause optic neuritis.

FLUOROQUINOLONES — Fluoroquinolones are synthetic anti-bacterial agents with activity against gram-positive and gram-negative organisms. With the increased use of fluoroquinolones, resistant organisms have become more frequent, especially among strains of *Staphylococcus aureus* and *Pseudomonas aeruginosa*. Resistance among *Streptococcus pneumoniae* strains has begun to emerge but is still rare, especially in the US. None of these agents is recommended for use in children or pregnant women. All can cause gastrointestinal disturbances and, less commonly central nervous system toxicity. Tendon effects and hypersensitivity reactions, including vasculitis, serum sickness-like reactions and anaphylaxis, occur rarely. Hypo- and hyperglycemia can also occur rarely.

   Ciprofloxacin (*Cipro*, and others) — Used for oral or intravenous treatment of a wide variety of gram-positive and gram-negative bacterial infections in adults, including those due to methicillin-susceptible and resistant staphylococci, *Haemophilus influenzae*, *Neisseria*, enteric pathogens and other aerobic gram-negative bacilli, and *Pseudomonas aeruginosa*, but not anaerobes. Newer fluoroquinolones such as levofloxacin, gemifloxacin and moxifloxacin are preferred for treatment of gram-positive coccal infections such as those caused by *S. pneumoniae* and *S. aureus*. Ciprofloxacin is useful for treatment of urinary tract infections caused by enteric gram-negative bacilli or *Pseudomonas aeruginosa*. Oral ciprofloxacin has been effective in treating patients with neutropenia and fever who are at low risk for mortality. Ciprofloxacin is now one of the preferred prophylactic agents for contacts of patients with meningococcal disease. It is also used for prophylaxis after *Bacillus anthracis* (Anthrax) exposure. Emergence of resistance in staphylococcal and *Pseudomonas* strains and other gram-negative organisms is increasingly encountered.

Levofloxacin *(Levaquin)*, **moxifloxacin** *(Avelox)* and **gemifloxacin** *(Factive)* — More active than ciprofloxacin or ofloxacin against gram-positive organisms, such as *Streptococcus pneumoniae*, including strains highly resistant to penicillin, and *Staphylococcus aureus*. Like other fluoroquinolones, they are active against *Legionella pneumophila, Chlamydia spp., Mycoplasma pneumoniae, Haemophilus influenzae* and *Moraxella catarrhalis*. All are effective for many community-acquired respiratory infections. Levofloxacin and moxifloxacin are less active than ciprofloxacin *in vitro* against enteric gram-negative bacilli and *Pseudomonas aeruginosa*, but have been effective in treating urinary tract infections and other systemic infections caused by these organisms. Levofloxacin and moxifloxacin have been used to treat some methicillin-sensitive and methicillin-resistant *S. aureus* infections, although resistance is increasing. Levofloxacin, moxifloxacin, ofloxacin or ciprofloxacin are sometimes used as second-line anti-tuberculous drugs in combination with other agents. Moxifloxacin has been used more frequently for treatment of tuberculosis than the other fluoroquinolones. Levofloxacin is more effective for treatment of *Legionella pneumophila* than azithromycin. The use of fluoroquinolones has been associated with the recent increase in severe cases of *C. difficile* infection. Levofloxacin and moxifloxacin are available for both oral and parenteral use. Gemifloxacin is only available for oral use. Levofloxacin and moxifloxacin have rarely been associated with torsades de pointes arrhythmia. Gemifloxacin has produced more rashes than other fluoroquinolones.

Gatifloxacin — Gatifloxacin has been associated with hypergylcemia and hypoglycemia more often than the other fluoroquinolones and it is no longer available for systemic use.

Norfloxacin *(Noroxin)* — An oral fluoroquinolone for treatment of urinary tract infections due to Enterobacteriaceae, *Enterococcus* or *Pseudomonas aeruginosa.*

Ofloxacin (*Floxin,* and others) — An oral and intravenous fluoroquinolone similar to ciprofloxacin, but less active against *Pseudomonas.* Ofloxacin can be used for single-dose treatment of gonorrhea and for seven-day treatment of chlamydial infections. It is sometimes used as a second-line anti-tuberculous drug in combination with other agents.

FOSFOMYCIN *(Monurol)* — Can be used as a single-dose oral agent with moderate effectiveness for treatment of uncomplicated urinary tract infections caused by many strains of enteric gram-negative bacilli, enterococci and some strains of *Staphylococcus saphrophyticus*, but generally not *Pseudomonas.* It is much more expensive than trimethoprim/sulfamethoxazole.

FURAZOLIDONE *(Furoxone)* — An oral nonabsorbable antimicrobial agent of the nitrofuran group that inhibits monoamine oxidase (MAO). The manufacturer recommends it for treatment of bacterial diarrhea. Its safety has been questioned (oral administration induces mammary tumors in rats) and other more effective drugs are available. It is no longer available in the US.

GATIFLOXACIN *(Tequin)* — See Fluoroquinolones (has been withdrawn)

GEMIFLOXACIN *(Factive)* — See Fluoroquinolones

GENTAMICIN *(Garamycin*, and others) — See Aminoglycosides

IMIPENEM/CILASTATIN *(Primaxin)* — See Carbapenems

ISONIAZID (*Nydrazid*, and others) — A major antituberculosis drug that can cause fatal hepatitis. **Rifampin-isoniazid-pyrazinamide** *(Rifater)* and **rifampin-isoniazid** (*Rifamate*, and others) are fixed-dose combinations for treatment of tuberculosis.

KANAMYCIN (*Kantrex***, and others)** — See Aminoglycosides

LEVOFLOXACIN *(Levaquin)* — See Fluoroquinolones

LINCOMYCIN *(Lincocin)* — Similar to clindamycin in antibacterial activity and adverse effects. Rarely indicated for treatment of any infection because it is less active than clindamycin.

LINEZOLID *(Zyvox)* — An oxazolidinone bacteriostatic antibiotic available in both an oral and intravenous formulation. It is active against *Enterococcus faecium* and *E. faecalis* including vancomycin-resistant enterococcal infections. Linezolid is also active against methicillin-resistant *Staphylococcus aureus*, *S. epidermidis* and penicillin-resistant *Streptococcus pneumoniae*. Reversible thrombocytopenia has occurred, especially with therapy for more than 2 weeks. Peripheral and optic neuropathy may occur with long-term use. A serotonin syndrome has been observed in patients taking linezolid together with a selective serotonin reuptake inhibitor. Emergence of resistance has been observed with enterococcal and *S. aureus* strains.

MACROLIDES — These antibiotics have anti-inflammatory activities that may be clinically relevant as well as their anti-bacterial effects.

 Azithromycin (*Zithromax*, and others) — A macrolide antibiotic that has much less gastrointestinal toxicity than erythromycin and is not associated with drug interactions with the CYP3A cytochrome P-450 enzyme systems. A single dose has been effective for treatment of urethritis and cervicitis caused by *Chlamydia* and for treatment of trachoma. Azithromycin is useful in treating *Mycoplasma pneumoniae, Chlamydia* *pneumoniae* and *Legionella pneumophila* pneumonias, as well as some respiratory infections due to *Streptococcus pneumoniae, Haemophilus influenzae* or *Moraxella catarrhalis*. However, an increasing number of *S. pneumoniae* strains have become resistant to the macrolides and azithromycin should not be used alone to treat pneumococcal pneumonia unless the causative strain is known to be sensitive to the macrolides. Azithromycin alone is effective for prevention of *Mycobacterium avium* infections, and combined with other drugs, such as ethambutol, rifabutin or ciprofloxacin, it is effective for treatment. Azithromycin has been shown to improve pulmonary function in patients with cystic fibrosis when used over long periods.

Clarithromycin (*Biaxin*, and others) — A macrolide antibiotic similar to azithromycin, but with a shorter half-life. It is somewhat more active than azithromycin against gram-positive organisms and less active against gram-negative organisms. Clarithromycin is effective for prevention of *Mycobacterium avium* infections and, combined with other drugs, for treatment of both *M. avium* and *Helicobacter pylori*. It has more adverse drug interactions than azithromycin. Clarithromycin is a strong inhibitor of CYP3A4 and can increase the serum concentrations of many drugs. It prolongs the QT interval and may rarely be associated with torsades de pointes, a potentially fatal arrhythmia. The risk is increased with concurrent use of other drugs that prolong the QT interval.

Erythromycin (*Erythrocin*, and others) — Used especially for respiratory tract infections due to pneumococci or Group A streptococci in patients allergic to penicillin, for pneumonia due to *Mycoplasma pneumoniae* or *Chlamydia spp.*, and for treatment of infection caused by *Legionella pneumophila*, erythromycin has few adverse effects except for frequent gastrointestinal disturbances but many drug interactions involving the CYP3A cytochrome P-450 system. Erythromycin given orally or intravenously may rarely be associated with torsades de pointes, a potentially fatal arrhythmia; risk of torsades is increased by concurrent use of CYP3A inhibitors and other drugs that prolong the QT inverval. Use in young infants has rarely been associated with hypertrophic pyloric stenosis. The estolate formulation *(Ilosone)* can cause cholestatic jaundice. Erythromycin is not recommended for treatment of serious staphylococcal infections, even when the organisms are susceptible to the drug *in vitro*, because of potential for rapid development of resistance. Strains of *Streptococcus pneumoniae* and Group A streptococci resistant to erythromycin have become more frequent and the drug should not be used alone to treat community-acquired pneumonia when pneumococcus is likely, unless susceptibility of the organism has been established.

Erythromycin/Sulfisoxazole (*Pediazole*, and others) — A combination of 100 mg of erythromycin ethylsuccinate and 300 mg sulfisoxazole acetyl per half-teaspoon for oral treatment of acute otitis media.

MEROPENEM (*Merrem*, and others) — See Carbapenems

METHENAMINES (*Mandelamine* [no longer available in the US], and others) — Methenamines are oral drugs that can sterilize an acid urine. They are used for prophylaxis of chronic or recurrent urinary tract infections, but trimethoprim/sulfamethoxazole is more effective.

METHICILLIN — See Penicillinase-resistant Penicillins

METRONIDAZOLE (*Flagyl*, and others) — Available in oral form for treatment of trichomoniasis, amebiasis, giardiasis and *Gardnerella vaginalis* vaginitis, metronidazole is also available for intravenous treatment of anaerobic bacterial infections. Good penetration of the blood-brain barrier may be an advantage in treating central nervous system infections due to *Bacteroides fragilis*. Metronidazole is frequently used for treatment of pseudomembranous enterocolitis due to *Clostridium difficile*. However, vancomycin given orally is more effective in serious cases. It is sometimes used in combination with other drugs to treat *H. pylori* infection.

MINOCYCLINE (*Minocin*, and others) — See Tetracyclines

MOXIFLOXACIN (*Avelox*) — See Fluoroquinolones

NAFCILLIN (*Nallpen*, and others) — See Penicillinase-resistant Penicillins

NALIDIXIC ACID (*NegGram*, and others) — See Quinolones

NEOMYCIN — See Aminoglycosides

NITROFURANTOIN (*Macrodantin*, and others) — This oral agent is used for prophylaxis or treatment of urinary tract infections, especially those resistant to other agents. Because of its potential toxicity, nitrofurantoin should not be used when renal function is markedly diminished. Nausea and vomiting are often troublesome, and peripheral neuropathy, pulmonary reactions and severe hepatotoxicity may occur.

NORFLOXACIN (*Noroxin*) — See Fluoroquinolones

OFLOXACIN (*Floxin*, and others) — See Fluoroquinolones

OXACILLIN — See Penicillinase-resistant Penicillins

PENICILLINS
Natural Penicillins
Penicillin remains the drug of choice for Group A streptococcal infections and for treatment of syphilis and some other infections. Clindamycin may be beneficial for treatment of Group A streptococcal necrotizing fasciitis, but it should be combined with penicillin G because of increasing resistance to clindamycin in Group A streptococcus. *Streptococcus pneumoniae* strains frequently show intermediate- or high-level resistance to penicillin. Penicillin is effective for fully sensitive strains, and high doses of penicillin, cefotaxime or ceftriaxone are effec-

tive for pneumonia due to strains with intermediate sensitivity; vancomycin is added for highly resistant strains, especially for meningitis.

Aminopenicillins

Amoxicillin (*Amoxil,* and others) — An oral semisynthetic penicillin similar to ampicillin, it is better absorbed and may cause less diarrhea. Amoxicillin is at least as effective as oral ampicillin for the treatment of most infections, with the exception of shigellosis. High doses (at least 3000 mg/day) have been successful in treating pneumococcal respiratory infections caused by strains with reduced susceptibility to penicillin.

Amoxicillin/Clavulanic Acid (*Augmentin,* and others) — The ß-lactamase inhibitor, potassium clavulanate, extends amoxicillin's spectrum of activity to include ß-lactamase-producing strains of *Staphylococcus aureus*, *Haemophilus influenzae*, *Moraxella catarrhalis* and many strains of enteric gram-negative bacilli, including anaerobes such as *Bacteroides* spp. This combination may be useful for oral treatment of bite wounds, otitis media, sinusitis and some lower respiratory tract and urinary tract infections, but it can cause a higher incidence of diarrhea and other gastrointestinal symptoms than amoxicillin alone, and less costly alternatives are available. An oral extended-release form of *Augmentin (Augmentin XR)* containing a higher content of amoxicillin in each tablet (1000 mg) has been successful in treating acute bacterial sinusitis and community-acquired pneumonia caused by strains of pneumococci with reduced susceptibility to penicillin, but high dose amoxicillin which costs much less can also be used.

Ampicillin (*Principen,* and others) — This semisynthetic penicillin is as effective as penicillin G in pneumococcal, streptococcal and meningococcal infections, and is also active against some strains of *Salmonella*, *Shigella*, *Escherichia coli* and *Haemophilus influenzae* and many strains of *Proteus mirabilis*. The drug is not effective against penicillinase-producing staphylococci or ß-lactamase-producing gram-negative bacteria. Rashes are more frequent with ampicillin than with other penicillins. Taken orally, ampicillin is less well absorbed than amoxicillin.

Ampicillin/Sulbactam (*Unasyn*, and others) — A parenteral combination of ampicillin with the ß-lactamase inhibitor sulbactam, which extends the antibacterial spectrum of ampicillin to include ß-lactamase-producing strains of *Staphylococcus aureus* (but not those resistant to methicillin)*, Haemophilus influenzae, Moraxella catarrhalis, Neisseria* and many gram-negative bacilli, including *Bacteroides fragilis*, but not *Pseudomonas aeruginosa, Enterobacter* or *Serratia*. It may be useful for treatment of gynecological and intra-abdominal infections. Some strains of *Acinetobacter* resistant to all other antibiotics may respond to high doses of ampicillin/sulbactam in combination with polymyxins.

Penicillinase-Resistant Penicillins

The drugs of choice for treatment of infections caused by penicillinase-producing staphylococci that are methicillin-sensitive, they are also effective against penicillin-sensitive pneumococci and Group A streptococci. For oral use for methicillin-sensitive *S. aureus* infections, **dicloxacillin** is preferred; for severe infections, a parenteral formulation of **nafcillin** or **oxacillin** should be used. **Methicillin** is no longer marketed in the US. Strains of *Staphylococcus aureus* or *epidermidis* that are resistant to these penicillins ("methicillin-resistant") are also resistant to cephalosporins, and carbapenems. Infections caused by these strains should be treated with vancomycin, or with linezolid or daptomycin. Neither ampicillin, amoxicillin, carbenicillin, piperacillin nor ticarcillin is effective against penicillinase-producing staphylococci.

Extended-Spectrum Penicillins

Carbenicillin (*Geocillin*; no longer available in the US) — The oral indanyl ester of carbenicillin; it does not produce therapeutic blood levels, but can be used for treatment of urinary tract infections, including those due to susceptible gram-negative bacilli such as *Pseudomonas aeruginosa* that may be resistant to other drugs.

Piperacillin (*Pipracil*, and others) — A penicillin for parenteral treatment of gram-negative bacillary infections. It is similar to ticarcillin in antibacterial activity, but covers a wider spectrum, particularly against *Klebsiella pneumoniae* and *Bacteroides fragilis*. Its *in vitro* activity against *Pseudomonas* is greater than that of ticarcillin, but increased clinical effectiveness in *Pseudomonas* infections has not been demonstrated. Piperacillin is also active against some gram-positive cocci, including streptococci and some strains of *Enterococcus*. For treatment of serious gram-negative infections, it should generally be used in combination with an aminoglycoside such as gentamicin, tobramycin or amikacin.

Piperacillin/Tazobactam (*Zosyn*, and others) — A parenteral formulation combining piperacillin with tazobactam, a ß-lactamase-inhibitor. The addition of the ß-lactamase inhibitor extends the spectrum of piperacillin to include ß-lactamase producing strains of staphylococci and some gram-negative bacilli, including *Bacteroides fragilis*. Infections caused by gram-negative bacilli that produce "extended spectrum" ß-lactamase are often resistant to piperacillin/tazobactam, those that produce chromosomal ß-lactamase or carbapenemase are always resistant. The combination of the two drugs is usually no more active against *Pseudomonas aeruginosa* than piperacillin alone.

Ticarcillin (*Ticar*; no longer marketed in the US) — A penicillin similar to carbenicillin. Large parenteral doses of this semisynthetic penicillin can cure serious infections caused by susceptible strains of *Pseudomonas*, *Proteus* and some other gram-negative organisms. *Klebsiella* are generally resistant. Ticarcillin is also active against some gram-positive cocci, including streptococci and some strains of *Enterococcus*. It is often given together with another drug such as gentamicin, tobramycin or amikacin for treatment of serious systemic infections. It is less active than ampicillin, amoxicillin or piperacillin against strains of *Streptococcus pneumoniae* with reduced susceptibility to penicillin and against enterococci.

Ticarcillin/Clavulanic Acid *(Timentin)* — A parenteral preparation combining ticarcillin with potassium clavulanate, a ß-lactamase inhibitor. The addition of the ß-lactamase inhibitor extends the antibacterial spectrum of ticarcillin to include ß-lactamase producing strains of *Staphylococcus aureus*, *Haemophilus influenzae*, and some enteric gram-negative bacilli, including *Bacteroides fragilis*. The combination is usually no more active against *Pseudomonas aeruginosa* than ticarcillin alone.

POLYMYXINS B AND E (polymyxin B – various generics; polymyxin E – *Coly-Mycin*; colistimethate; colistin sulfate) — The polymyxins are used topically in combination with other antibiotics for treatment of infected wounds and otitis externa. Some strains of gram-negative bacilli (particularly *Klebsiella*, *Pseudumonas aeruginosa* and *Acinetobacter)* resistant to all other available antibiotics have been treated with one of the polymyxins; for infections caused by *Acinetobacter,* sulbactam (in the form of ampicillin/sulbactam) is often added, though some strains are resistant to it. The polymyxins used systemically are often nephrotoxic.

PYRAZINAMIDE — An antituberculosis drug now often used in the initial treatment regimen. Rifampin-isoniazid-pyrazinamide *(Rifater)* is a fixed-dose combination for treatment of tuberculosis.

QUINOLONES
Nalidixic Acid *(NegGram*, and others) — An oral drug active *in vitro* against many gram-negative organisms that commonly cause urinary tract infections. Development of resistance by initially susceptible strains is rapid, however, and clinical results are much less favorable than would be expected from sensitivity testing alone. Nalidixic acid can cause severe adverse effects, including visual disturbances, intracranial hypertension, and convulsions. Other drugs are generally preferred for treatment of urinary tract infections.

Cinoxacin *(Cinobac*; no longer available in the US) — An oral drug similar to nalidixic acid for treatment of urinary tract infections.

QUINUPRISTIN/DALFOPRISTIN *(Synercid)* — Two streptogramin antibacterials marketed in a fixed-dose combination for parenteral use. The combination is active against vancomycin-resistant *Enterococcus faecium* (but not *E. faecalis*) as well as *Staphylococcus aureus*, *Streptococcus pneumoniae* and *S. pyogenes*. Adverse effects include frequent thrombophlebitis at the infusion site (it is best given through a central venous catheter) and arthralgias and myalgias. It has a number of drug interactions. The availability of linezolid and daptomycin as alternates have lead to infrequent use of quinupristin/dalfopristin.

RETAPAMULIN *(Altabax)* — A topical pleuromutilin antibiotic approved for treatment of impetigo caused by methicillin-susceptible *S. aureus* and Group A streptococci *(S. pyogenes)*.

RIFABUTIN *(Mycobutin)* — Similar to rifampin, rifabutin is used to prevent and treat tuberculosis and disseminated *Mycobacterium avium* infections in patients with AIDS. It has fewer drug interactions than rifampin.

RIFAMPIN *(Rifadin, Rimactane,* and others*)* — A major drug for treatment of tuberculosis. To prevent emergence of resistant organisms, it should be used together with other antituberculosis drugs. It is sometimes used concurrently with other drugs for treatment of *Mycobacterium avium* infections in AIDS patients. Rifampin is also useful for prophylaxis in close contacts of patients with sulfonamide-resistant meningococcal disease and for prophylaxis in children who are close contacts of patients with *Haemophilus influenzae* meningitis. Rifampin is a potent inducer of CYP3A enzymes and may increase the metabolism of the many drugs, particularly some protease inhibitors. **Rifampin-isoniazid-pyrazinamide** *(Rifater)* and **rifampin-isoniazid** *(Rifamate,* and others*)* are fixed-dose combinations for treatment of tuberculosis. Rifampin has been used in combination with other antibiotics in treatment of staphylococcal or gram-negative bacterial infections to increase effectiveness, but some studies have shown diminished effectiveness with such use, except for treatment of methicillin-resistant prosthetic valve endocarditis in which it is used with vancomycin and gentamicin. It is also recommended for use in combination with other antibiotics in treatment of other infections of prosthetic devices.

RIFAPENTINE *(Priftin)* — A long-acting analog of rifampin used in the treatment of tuberculosis. Studies of its effectiveness are limited. Until more data become available, rifampin is preferred.

RIFAXIMIN *(Xifaxan)* — A non-absorbed oral antibiotic derived from rifampin, it is about as effective as ciprofloxacin for treatment of traveler's diarrhea, which is mostly caused by *E. coli*. It is not effective against gastrointestinal infections associated with fever or blood in the stool or those caused by *Campylobacter jejuni*. It has fewer adverse effects and drug interactions than systemic antibiotics, but should not be taken during pregnancy. Hypersensitivity reactions have been reported.

SPECTINOMYCIN *(Trobicin)* — A single-dose alternative for treatment of urogenital or anal gonorrhea. It is effective for penicillin-resistant infections and for patients who are allergic to penicillin. Spectinomycin is not effective against syphilis.

STREPTOMYCIN — See Aminoglycosides

SULFONAMIDES — Previously used for acute, uncomplicated urinary tract infections sulfonamides are now rarely used because of the increasing frequency of sulfonamide-resistance among gram-negative bacilli and the availability of fluoroquinolone and trimethoprim/sulfamethoxazole. When used, a soluble oral sulfonamide such as sulfisoxazole (*Gantrisin*, and others) is preferred.

TELAVANCIN *(Vibativ)* — Telavancin is a lipoglycopeptide derivative of vancomycin that is active against gram-positive cocci, including methicillin-sensitive (MSSA) and -resistant *Staphylococcus aureus* (MRSA), *Staphylococcus pyogenes*, *Staphylococcus agalactiae*, *Staphylococcus* *pneumoniae* (including penicillin-resistant isolates) and *Enterococcus fecalis* (vancomycin-susceptible isolates only). It has a long half-life and can be given intravenously once every 24 hours. There is no evidence as yet that it is more effective than vancomycin and it has more adverse effects, including taste disturbances and increased nephrotoxicity. Like vancomycin it may cause the "red man syndrome" when administered too rapidly.

TELITHROMYCIN *(Ketek)* — A ketolide antibiotic, derived from erythromycin, it is only approved for oral treatment of mild to moderate community-acquired pneumonia in adults. Telithromycin is often active against most strains of *S. pneumoniae* that are resistant to penicillin and macrolides (erythromycin, clarithromycin and azithromycin). It can cause serious, even fatal, hepatotoxicity, exacerbation of myasthenia gravis, visual disturbances, and it is expensive. It is a strong inhibitor of CYP3A enzymes and can cause potentially dangerous increases in serum concentrations of substrates, including simvastatin (*Zocor*, and others), lovastatin (*Mevacor*, and others), atorvastatin *(Lipitor)* and midazolam (*Versed*, and others). Like clarithromycin and erythromycin, it may prolong the QT inverval and should not be taken concurrently with other drugs that prolong the QT interval. Medical Letter consultants advise against its use.

TETRACYCLINES — **Doxycycline** (*Vibramycin*, and others), **oxytet-racycline** (*Terramycin*; no longer available in the US), and **minocycline** (*Minocin*, and others) are available in both oral and parenteral formulations; **tetracycline** and **demeclocycline** (*Declomycin*, and others) are available only for oral use. Parenteral tetracyclines can cause severe liver damage, especially when given to patients with diminished renal function or in pregnancy. Doxycycline requires fewer doses and causes less gastrointestinal disturbance than other tetracyclines. It can be used for prophylaxis after *Bacillus anthracis* (anthrax) exposure. Doxycycline and other tetracyclines are effective in treating pneumonia caused by *Mycoplasma pneumoniae*, *Chlamydia pneumoniae* and *Legionella* species and are commonly used to treat Lyme disease in adults and urethritis, cervicitis, proctitis or pelvic inflammatory disease when caused by *Chlamydial* species. **Minocycline** may be useful for prophylactic treatment of close contacts of patients with meningococcal infection, but it frequently causes vomiting and vertigo.

TIGECYCLINE (*Tygacil*) — The first glycylcycline, tigecycline is FDA-approved for parenteral treatment of complicated intra-abdominal infections and complicated skin and skin structure infections in adults. It has a broad spectrum of antimicrobial activity, including activity against methicillin-resistant *S. aureus* (MRSA) and some multiply resistant gram-negative bacilli. Its effectiveness may be limited by the limited blood and tissue levels that it achieves.

TOBRAMYCIN (*Nebcin*, and others) — See Aminoglycosides

TRIMETHOPRIM (*Proloprim*, and others) — An agent marketed only for oral treatment of uncomplicated urinary tract infections caused by gram-negative bacilli. Frequent use has the potential for producing organisms resistant not only to this drug but also to trimethoprim/sulfamethoxazole.

TRIMETHOPRIM/SULFAMETHOXAZOLE (*Bactrim, Septra*, and others) — A combination of a folic acid antagonist and a sulfonamide, useful especially for oral treatment of urinary tract infections, shigellosis, otitis media, traveler's diarrhea, bronchitis, *Pneumocystis carinii* pneumonia and methicillin-resistant *S. aureus* (MRSA) infections. An intravenous preparation is available for treatment of serious infections. Allergic reactions are common, especially in HIV-infected patients. It may occasionally produce elevation of serum creatinine, hyperkalemia and renal insufficiency.

VANCOMYCIN (*Vancocin*, and others) — An effective alternative to the penicillins for endocarditis caused by *Streptococcus viridans* or

Enterococcus, for severe staphylococcal infections, and for penicillin-resistant *S. pneumoniae* infections. An increasing number of strains of enterococci (especially *E. faecium*), however, are resistant to vancomycin. Some strains of *S. aureus* have reduced susceptibility to vancomycin or rarely are highly resistant. Linezolid or daptomycin may be used to treat infections caused by these strains of enterococci or *S. aureus*. Vancomycin is widely used for treatment of infections caused by methicillin-resistant *Staphylococcus aureus* and *epidermidis*, but for strains that are methicillin-sensitive, nafcillin or oxacillin are more effective. For serious infections caused by *S. aureus* or enterococci, higher than the traditional doses of 15 mg/kg every 12 hours IV for adults with normal renal function are being advocated by some consultants, but improved efficacy of such regimens has not yet been demonstrated and such higher dose regimens increase the incidence of nephrotoxicity, especially when combined with the use of aminoglycosides.

Oral treatment with vancomycin is more effective than metronidazole in treating severe antibiotic-associated colitis due to *Clostridium difficile*.

PATHOGENS MOST LIKELY TO CAUSE INFECTIONS
IN SPECIFIC ORGANS AND TISSUES

In many acute and most chronic infections, the choice of antimicrobial therapy can await the results of appropriate cultures and antimicrobial susceptibility tests. In acute life-threatening infections such as meningitis, pneumonia or bacteremia, however, and in other infections that have reached a serious stage, waiting 24 to 48 hours can be dangerous, and the choice of an antimicrobial agent for initial use must be based on tentative identification of the pathogen. Knowing the organisms most likely to cause infection in specific tissues, together with evaluation of gram-stained smears and familiarity with the antimicrobial susceptibility patterns of organisms prevalent in the hospital or community, permits a rational choice of initial treatment.

In the table below, bacteria, fungi, viruses and other pathogens are listed in estimated order of the frequency with which they cause acute infection, but these frequencies are subject to annual, seasonal and geographical variation. The order of pathogens may also vary depending on whether the infections are community or hospital-acquired, and whether or not the patient is immunosuppressed. This listing is based both on published reports and on the experience of Medical Letter consultants. Organisms not listed here may also be important causes of infection.

TABLE OF BACTERIA, FUNGI, AND SOME VIRUSES
MOST LIKELY TO CAUSE ACUTE INFECTIONS

BLOOD (SEPTICEMIA)
Newborn Infants
1. *Streptococcus* Group B
2. *Escherichia coli* (or other gram-negative bacilli)
3. *Listeria monocytogenes*
4. *Staphylococcus aureus*
5. *Streptococcus pyogenes* (Group A)

6. Enterococcal spp.
7. *Streptococcus pneumoniae*

Children
1. *Streptococcus pneumoniae*
2. *Neisseria meningitidis*
3. *Staphylococcus aureus*
4. *Streptococcus pyogenes* (Group A)
5. *Haemophilus influenzae*
6. *Escherichia coli* (or other gram-negative bacilli)

Adults
1. *Staphylococcus aureus*
2. *Escherichia coli* (or other enteric gram negative bacilli)
3. *Streptococcus pneumoniae*
4. Enterococcal spp.
5. Non-enteric gram-negative bacilli
   (Pseudomonas, Acinetobacter, Aeromonas)
6. *Candida* spp. and other fungi
7. *Staphylococcus epidermidis*
8. *Streptococcus pyogenes* (Group A)
9. Other streptococci (non-Group A and not Lancefield-groupable)
10. *Bacteroides* spp.
11. *Neisseria meningitidis*
12. *Neisseria gonorrhoeae*
13. *Fusobacterium* spp.
14. Mycobacteria
15. *Rickettsia* spp.
16. *Ehrlichia* spp.
17. *Brucella* spp.
18. *Leptospira* spp.

MENINGES
1. Viruses (enterovirus, herpes simplex, HIV, arbovirus, lymphocytic choriomeningitis [LCM] virus, mumps and others)

2. *Neisseria meningitidis*
3. *Streptococcus pneumoniae*
4. *Streptococcus* Group B (infants less than two months old)
5. *Escherichia coli* (or other gram-negative bacilli)
6. *Haemophilus influenzae* (in children)
7. *Streptococcus pyogenes* (Group A)
8. *Staphylococcus aureus* (with endocarditis or after neurosurgery, brain abscess)
9. *Mycobacterium tuberculosis*
10. *Cryptococcus neoformans* and other fungi
11. *Listeria monocytogenes*
12. Enterococcal spp. (neonatal period)
13. *Treponema pallidum*
14. *Leptospira* spp.
15. *Borrelia burgdorferi*
16. *Toxoplasma gondii*

BRAIN AND PARAMENINGEAL SPACES
1. Herpes simplex (encephalitis)
2. Anaerobic streptococci and/or *Bacteroides* spp. (cerebritis, brain abscess, and subdural empyema)
3. *Staphylococcus aureus* (cerebritis, brain abscess, epidural abscess)
4. *Haemophilus influenzae* (subdural empyema)
5. Arbovirus (encephalitis)
6. Mumps (encephalitis)
7. *Toxoplasma gondii* (encephalitis)
8. Human immunodeficiency virus (HIV)
9. *Mycobacterium tuberculosis*
10. *Nocardia* (brain abscess)
11. *Listeria monocytogenes* (encephalitis)
12. *Treponema pallidum*
13. *Cryptococcus neoformans* and other fungi
14. *Borrelia burgdorferi*
15. Other viruses (varicella-zoster [VZV], cytomegalovirus [CMV], Ebstein-Barr [EBV] and rabies)

16. *Mycoplasma pneumoniae*
17. *Taenia solium* (neurocysticercosis)
18. *Echinococcus* spp. (echinococcosis)
19. *Strongyloides stercoralis* hyperinfection
20. *Angiostrongylus cantonensis*
21. Free-living amoeba (*Naegleria, Acanthameoba* and *Balamuthia* spp.)

ENDOCARDIUM
1. *Staphylococcus aureus*
2. Viridans group of *Streptococcus*
3. Enterococcal spp.
4. *Streptococcus bovis*
5. *Staphylococcus epidermidis*
6. *Candida albicans* and other fungi
7. Gram-negative bacilli
8. *Streptococcus pneumoniae*
9. *Streptococcus pyogenes* (Group A)
10. *Corynebacterium* spp. (especially with prosthetic valves)
11. *Haemophilus, Actinobacillus, Cardiobacterium hominis* or *Eikenella* spp.

BONES (OSTEOMYELITIS)
1. *Staphylococcus aureus*
2. *Salmonella* spp. (or other gram-negative bacilli)
3. *Streptococcus pyogenes* (Group A)
4. *Mycobacterium tuberculosis*
5. Anaerobic streptococci (chronic)
6. *Bacteroides* spp. (chronic)

JOINTS
1. *Staphylococcus aureus*
2. *Streptococcus pyogenes* (Group A)
3. *Neisseria gonorrhoeae*
4. Gram-negative bacilli
5. *Streptococcus pneumoniae*

6. *Neisseria meningitidis*
7. *Haemophilus influenzae* (in children)
8. *Mycobacterium tuberculosis* and other *Mycobacteria*
9. Fungi
10. *Borrelia burgdorferi*

SKIN AND SUBCUTANEOUS TISSUES
Burns
1. *Staphylococcus aureus*
2. *Streptococcus pyogenes* (Group A)
3. *Pseudomonas aeruginosa* (or other gram-negative bacilli)

Skin infections
1. *Staphylococcus aureus*
2. *Streptococcus pyogenes* (Group A)
3. Dermatophytes
4. *Candida* spp. and other fungi
5. Herpes simplex or zoster
6. Gram-negative bacilli
7. *Treponema pallidum*
8. *Borrelia burgdorferi*
9. *Bartonella henselae* or *quintana*
10. *Bacillus anthracis*

Decubitus Wound infections
1. *Staphylococcus aureus*
2. *Escherichia coli* (or other gram-negative bacilli)
3. *Streptococcus pyogenes* (Group A)
4. Anaerobic streptococci
5. *Clostridia* spp.
6. Enterococcal spp.
7. *Bacteroides* spp.

Traumatic and Surgical Wounds
1. *Staphylococcus aureus*

2. Anaerobic streptococci
3. Gram-negative bacilli
4. *Clostridia* spp.
5. *Streptococcus pyogenes* (Group A)
6. Enterococcal spp.

EYES (Cornea and Conjunctiva)
1. Herpes and other viruses
2. *Neisseria gonorrhoeae* (in newborn)
3. *Staphylococcus aureus*
4. *Streptococcus pneumoniae*
5. *Haemophilus influenzae* (in children), including biotype *aegyptius* (Koch-Weeks bacillus)
6. *Moraxella lacunata*
7. *Pseudomonas aeruginosa*
8. Other gram-negative bacilli
9. *Chlamydia trachomatis* (trachoma and inclusion conjunctivitis)
10. Fungi

EARS
Auditory Canal
1. *Pseudomonas aeruginosa* (or other gram-negative bacilli)
2. *Staphylococcus aureus*
3. *Streptococcus pyogenes* (Group A)
4. *Streptococcus pneumoniae*
5. *Haemophilus influenzae* (in children)
6. Fungi

Middle Ear
1. *Streptococcus pneumoniae*
2. *Haemophilus influenzae* (in children)
3. *Moraxella catarrhalis*
4. *Streptococcus pyogenes* (Group A)
5. *Staphylococcus aureus*
6. Anaerobic streptococci (chronic)

7. *Bacteroides* spp. (chronic)
8. Other gram-negative bacilli (chronic)
9. *Mycobacterium tuberculosis*

PARANASAL SINUSES
1. *Streptococcus pneumoniae*
2. *Haemophilus influenzae*
3. *Moraxella catarrhalis*
4. *Streptococcus pyogenes* (Group A)
5. Anaerobic streptococci (chronic sinusitis)
6. *Staphylococcus aureus* (chronic sinusitis)
7. *Klebsiella* spp. (or other gram-negative bacilli)
8. *Mucor* spp., *Aspergillus* spp. (especially in diabetics and immunosuppressed patients)

MOUTH
1. Herpes viruses
2. *Candida* spp.
3. *Leptotrichia buccalis* (Vincent's infection)
4. *Bacteroides* spp.
5. Mixed anaerobes
6. *Treponema pallidum*
7. *Actinomyces*

THROAT
1. Respiratory viruses
2. *Streptococcus pyogenes* (Group A)
3. *Neisseria meningitidis* or *gonorrhoeae*
4. *Leptotrichia buccalis*
5. *Candida* spp.
6. *Corynebacterium diphtheriae*
7. *Bordetella pertussis*
8. *Haemophilus influenzae*
9. *Fusobacterium necrophorum*

LARYNX, TRACHEA, AND BRONCHI
1. Respiratory viruses
2. *Streptococcus pneumoniae*
3. *Haemophilus influenzae*
4. *Streptococcus pyogenes* (Group A)
5. *Corynebacterium diphtheriae*
6. *Staphylococcus aureus*
7. Gram-negative bacilli
8. *Fusobacterium necrophorum*

PLEURA
1. *Streptococcus pneumoniae*
2. *Staphylococcus aureus*
3. *Haemophilus influenzae*
4. Gram-negative bacilli
5. Anaerobic streptococci
6. *Bacteroides* spp.
7. *Streptococcus pyogenes* (Group A)
8. *Mycobacterium tuberculosis*
9. *Actinomyces, Nocardia* spp.
10. Fungi
11. *Fusobacterium necrophorum*

LUNGS
Pneumonia
1. Respiratory viruses (influenza virus A and B, adenovirus, respiratory syncytial virus, parainfluenza virus, rhinovirus, enteroviruses, cytomegalovirus, Epstein-Barr virus, varicella-zoster virus, measles virus, herpes simplex virus, hantavirus and coronavirus [SARS])
2. *Mycoplasma pneumoniae*
3. *Streptococcus pneumoniae*
4. *Haemophilus influenzae*
5. Anaerobic streptococci, fusospirochetes
6. *Bacteroides* spp.

7. *Staphylococcus aureus*
8. *Klebsiella* spp. (or other gram-negative bacilli)
9. *Legionella pneumophila*
10. *Chlamydia pneumoniae* (TWAR strain)
11. *Streptococcus pyogenes* (Group A)
12. *Rickettsia* spp.
13. *Mycobacterium tuberculosis*
14. *Pneumocystis carinii*
15. Fungi (especially *Aspergillus* species in immunosuppressed patients)
16. *Moraxella catarrhalis*
17. *Legionella micdadei (L. pittsburgensis)*
18. *Chlamydia psittaci*
19. *Fusobacterium necrophorum*
20. *Actinomyces* spp.
21. *Nocardia* spp.
22. *Rhodococcus equi*
23. *Bacillus anthracis* (mediastinitis)
24. *Yersinia pestis*

Abscess
1. Anaerobic streptococci
2. *Bacteroides* spp.
3. *Staphylococcus aureus*
4. *Klebsiella* spp. (or other gram-negative bacilli)
5. *Streptococcus pneumoniae*
6. Fungi
7. *Actinomyces, Nocardia* spp.

GASTROINTESTINAL TRACT
1. Gastrointestinal viruses
2. *Campylobacter jejuni*
3. *Salmonella* spp.
4. *Escherichia coli*
5. *Shigella* spp.

6. *Yersinia enterocolitica*
7. *Entamoeba histolytica*
8. *Giardia lamblia*
9. *Staphylococcus aureus*
10. *Vibrio cholerae*
11. *Vibrio parahaemolyticus*
12. Herpes simplex (anus)
13. *Treponema pallidum* (rectum)
14. *Neisseria gonorrhoeae* (rectum)
15. *Candida* spp.
16. *Clostridium difficile*
17. *Cryptosporidium parvum*
18. Cytomegalovirus (CMV)
19. Human immunodeficiency virus (HIV)
20. *Mycobacterium avium* complex
21. *Helicobacter pylori*
22. *Tropheryma whippelii*

URINARY TRACT
1. *Escherichia coli* (or other gram-negative bacilli)
2. *Staphylococcus aureus* and *epidermidis*
3. *Neisseria gonorrhoeae* (urethra)
4. Enterococcal spp.
5. *Candida* spp.
6. *Chlamydia* spp. (urethra)
7. *Treponema pallidum* (urethra)
8. *Trichomonas vaginalis* (urethra)
9. *Ureaplasma urealyticum*

FEMALE GENITAL TRACT
Vagina
1. *Trichomonas vaginalis*
2. *Candida* spp.
3. *Neisseria gonorrhoeae*
4. *Streptococcus pyogenes* (Group A)

5. *Gardnerella vaginalis* and associated anaerobes
6. *Treponema pallidum*

Uterus
1. Anaerobic streptococci
2. *Bacteroides* spp.
3. *Neisseria gonorrhoeae* (cervix)
4. *Clostridia* spp.
5. *Escherichia coli* (or other gram-negative bacilli)
6. Herpes simplex virus, type II (cervix)
7. *Streptococcus pyogenes* (Group A)
8. *Streptococcus,* Groups B and C
9. *Treponema pallidum*
10. *Actinomyces* spp. (most common infection of intrauterine devices)
11. *Staphylococcus aureus*
12. Enterococcal spp.
13. *Chlamydia trachomatis*
14. *Mycoplasma hominis*

Fallopian Tubes
1. *Neisseria gonorrhoeae*
2. *Escherichia coli* (or other gram-negative bacilli)
3. Anaerobic streptococci
4. *Bacteroides* spp.
5. *Chlamydia trachomatis*

MALE GENITAL TRACT
Seminal Vesicles
1. Gram-negative bacilli
2. *Neisseria gonorrhoeae*

Epididymis
1. *Chlamydia*
2. Gram-negative bacilli

3. *Neisseria gonorrhoeae*
4. *Mycobacterium tuberculosis*

Prostate Gland
1. Gram-negative bacilli
2. *Neisseria gonorrhoeae*

PERITONEUM
1. Gram-negative bacilli
2. Enterococcal spp.
3. *Bacteroides* spp.
4. Anaerobic streptococci
5. *Clostridia* spp.
6. *Streptococcus pneumoniae*
7. *Streptococcus* Group

DRUGS FOR
Bacterial Infections

Original publication date – June 2010

The text below reviews some common bacterial infections and their treatment. The recommendations made here are based on the results of susceptibility studies, clinical trials and the opinions of Medical Letter consultants. A table listing the drugs of choice and alternatives for all bacterial pathogens begins on page 56. A table listing oral antibacterial drug dosages begins on page 76. Parenteral drug dosages can be found on page 397.

INFECTIONS OF SKIN, SOFT TISSUE AND BONE

SKIN AND SOFT TISSUE — Uncomplicated skin and skin structure infections in immunocompetent patients are most commonly due to *Staphylococcus aureus, Streptococcus pyogenes* (group A streptococci) or *Streptococcus agalactiae* (group B streptococci). Complicated skin and skin structure infections, such as those that occur in patients with burns, diabetes mellitus, infected pressure ulcers and traumatic or surgical wound infections, are more commonly polymicrobial and often include gram-negative bacilli such as *Escherichia coli* and *Pseudomonas aeruginosa*. Group A streptococci, *S. aureus* or *Clostridium* spp., with or without other anaerobes, can cause fulminant soft tissue infection and necrosis, particularly in patients with diabetes mellitus.[1]

Methicillin-resistant *S. aureus* (MRSA) – In the past few years, methicillin-resistant *S. aureus* strains (MRSA) have become the predominant cause of suppurative skin infection in many parts of the US.[2-4] Community-acquired MRSA (CA-MRSA) usually causes furunculosis and abscesses, but necrotizing fasciitis and sepsis can occur.[5,6]

MRSA should be considered a likely cause of infection if the patient was recently treated with antibiotics, is known to be colonized, has a history of recent hospitalization, or is in a geographic area of high prevalence.[7,8]

Treatment of MRSA – Treatment should be guided by the severity of infection and susceptibility tests. Patients with serious skin and soft tissue infections suspected to be caused by CA-MRSA should be treated empirically with vancomycin, linczolid or daptomycin. Tigecycline can be used, but because it has a very broad spectrum of activity, it is best reserved for patients unable to take other drugs or those with documented polymicrobial coinfection.[9]

CA-MRSA strains often are susceptible to trimethoprim/sulfamethoxazole, clindamycin and tetracyclines; nosocomial strains often are not. For small abscesses and less serious CA-MRSA skin or soft tissue infections, drainage or local therapy alone may be effective. When it is not, oral trimethoprim/sulfamethoxazole, minocycline, doxycycline, clindamycin or linezolid could be tried.[10] Fluoroquinolones should not be used empirically to treat MRSA infections because resistance is common and increasing in both nosocomial and community settings.

Treatment of Non-MRSA Infections – For **uncomplicated** infections unlikely to be due to MRSA (no recent hospitalizations, etc.), an antistaphylococcal penicillin such as dicloxacillin or a first-generation cephalosporin such as cephalexin would be a reasonable choice. If the patient requires hospitalization, the same classes of drugs (nafcillin, cefazolin) can be given intravenously (IV). Clindamycin or vancomycin would be a reasonable choice for patients who are allergic to a beta-lactam.

For **complicated** infections that could be polymicrobial and are unlikely to be MRSA, ampicillin/sulbactam, piperacillin/tazobactam, ticarcillin/clavulanate, imipenem or meropenem would be reasonable empiric monotherapy. If group A streptococcus or *Clostridium* spp. is the likely cause, a combination of clindamycin and a penicillin is recommended.[11] In severely ill patients, vancomycin or linezolid should be added until MRSA is ruled out. Surgical debridement is essential to the management of necrotizing skin and skin structure infections.[6]

BONE AND JOINT — *Staphylococcus aureus* is the most common cause of **osteomyelitis**. *Streptococcus pyogenes* and *S. agalactiae* are less common pathogens. *Salmonella* spp. can cause osteomyelitis in patients with sickle cell disease, as can other gram-negative bacteria (*Escherichia coli, Pseudomonas* spp.), particularly in patients who have had orthopedic procedures or have open fractures or vertebral infection. Infections of the feet are common in diabetic patients, often involve both bone and soft tissue, and may be polymicrobial, including both aerobic and anaerobic bacteria.[12]

Septic arthritis may be due to *S. aureus*, *S. pyogenes* or *Streptococcus pneumoniae*, gram-negative bacteria or, in sexually active patients, *Neisseria gonorrhoeae*.[13] Coagulase-negative staphylococci and *S. aureus* are the most common causes of prosthetic joint infection.

For empiric treatment of acute osteomyelitis unlikely to be caused by MRSA, IV administration of an antistaphylococcal penicillin such as nafcillin or a first-generation cephalosporin such as cefazolin would be appropriate. Many Medical Letter consultants would use vancomycin until culture results are available. Ceftriaxone would be a reasonable first choice for empiric treatment of a joint infection to include coverage for *S. aureus* and *N. gonorrhoeae*. For both bone and joint infections, IV penicillin or ceftriaxone can be used to treat *Streptococcus* spp.. If MRSA or methicillin-resistant coagulase-negative staphylococci are the pathogens, vancomycin, daptomycin or linezolid should be used. Ceftriaxone, ceftazidime or cefepime would be a good option for empiric treatment of bone and joint infections with gram-negative bacteria; ciprofloxacin would be an alternative.

For prosthetic joint infections, rifampin is often added to antistaphylococcal therapy because of its effect on staphylococcal isolates that are adherent to the prosthesis.[14]

Chronic osteomyelitis, common in complicated diabetic foot infection, usually requires surgical debridement of involved bone followed by 4-8 weeks of antibacterial therapy. Well-absorbed oral antibacterials such as trimethoprim/sulfamethoxazole, metronidazole, linezolid or moxifloxacin can be used for chronic osteomyelitis depending on the susceptibility of the pathogen.[15]

MENINGITIS

The organisms most commonly responsible for community-acquired bacterial meningitis in children and adults are *Streptococcus pneumoniae* (pneumococcus) and *Neisseria meningitidis*, which cause about 80% of all cases.[16] As a result of childhood immunization, meningitis due to *Haemophilus influenzae* type b has decreased markedly in adults and children and pneumococcal meningitis has declined in children.[17] Enteric gram-negative bacteria cause meningitis in neonates, the elderly, and in patients who have had recent nosocomial infections or neurosurgery, or are immunosuppressed.[18] Group B streptococcus often causes meningitis in neonates or in the elderly. *Listeria monocytogenes* may be the cause in pregnant women, neonates, patients >50 years old and in immunosuppressed patients.[19]

For empiric treatment of meningitis in **adults and children more than two months old,** high-dose ceftriaxone or cefotaxime plus vancomycin is generally recommended; vancomycin is given at a dosage of 15-20 mg/kg every 8-12 hours to reach a serum trough level of 15-20 mcg/mL to cover highly penicillin- or cephalosporin-resistant pneumococci.[20] Vancomycin should be stopped if the etiologic agent proves to be susceptible to ceftriaxone or cefotaxime. Ampicillin, sometimes in combination with gentamicin for severely ill patients, is added in patients in whom *L. monocytogenes* is a consideration.

Neonatal meningitis is most often caused by group B streptococci, gram-negative enteric organisms or *L. monocytogenes.* For meningitis in the first two months of life, while waiting for the results of cultures and susceptibility tests, many Medical Letter consultants use ampicillin plus ceftriaxone or cefotaxime, with or without gentamicin.

For treatment of **nosocomial** meningitis, vancomycin and a cephalosporin with good activity against *Pseudomonas* such as ceftazidime are appropriate. In hospitals where gram-negative bacilli that produce extended-spectrum ß-lactamases are common, use of meropenem or doripenem should be considered instead of a cephalosporin.

Ceftriaxone or cefotaxime can often be used safely to treat meningitis in **penicillin-allergic** patients. When allergy truly prevents the use of a cephalosporin, chloramphenicol can be given for initial treatment, but may not be effective if the infecting pathogen is an enteric gram-negative bacillus or *L. monocytogenes*, or in some patients with penicillin-resistant pneumococcal meningitis. For coverage of enteric gram-negative bacilli and *P. aeruginosa* in patients with penicillin and cephalosporin allergy, aztreonam could be used. Trimethoprim/sulfamethoxazole can be used for treatment of *Listeria* meningitis in patients allergic to penicillin. As with nonallergic patients, vancomycin should be added to cover resistant pneumococci.

A **corticosteroid**, usually parenteral dexamethasone (*Decadron*, and others), given in a dose of 0.15 mg/kg IV q6h starting before or at the same time as the first dose of antibiotics and continued every 6 hours for 4 days, has been reported to decrease the incidence of hearing loss in children, particularly with *Haemophilus influenzae* meningitis, and to decrease mortality rates and other neurological complications in adults.[21,22] The benefits in adults have been most striking in those with pneumococcal meningitis. Since the incidence of adverse effects has been low, the potential benefits of such treatment would appear to outweigh the risks.

INFECTIONS OF THE UPPER RESPIRATORY TRACT

Acute sinusitis in adults is often due to viral infections. When acute sinusitis is bacterial, it is usually caused by pneumococci, *H. influenzae* and *Moraxella catarrhalis* and can generally be treated with an oral antibacterial such as amoxicillin or amoxicillin/clavulanate, cefuroxime axetil or cefpodoxime, or a fluoroquinolone with good antipneumococcal activity such as levofloxacin or moxifloxacin. Monotherapy with a macrolide (erythromycin, clarithromycin or azithromycin) is generally not recommended because of increasing resistance among pneumococci. Doxycycline or trimethoprim/sulfamethoxazole may be considered for patients with mild acute bacterial sinusitis who are allergic to penicillins and cephalosporins.[23] In patients with moderate acute bacterial sinusitis or with risk factors for infection with drug-resistant *S. pneumoniae*, such as recent antibiotic use, amoxicillin/clavulanate or an antipneumococcal fluoroquinolone could be used. Addition of intranasal corticosteroids may improve symptoms and decrease the need for pain medications.[24]

Acute exacerbation of chronic bronchitis (AECB) is also often viral. When it is bacterial, it may be caused by *H. influenzae, S. pneumoniae* or *M. catarrhalis* and can be treated with the same antimicrobials used to treat acute bacterial sinusitis.[25] In patients with severe COPD, *Pseudomonas* can be a cause of AECB and addition of an antipseudomonal agent such as ciprofloxacin or ceftazidime should be considered.

The most common bacterial cause of **acute pharyngitis** in adults and children is group A streptococci. Penicillin, amoxicillin or a macrolide is usually given for 10 days.[26] In the US, about 5% of pharyngeal isolates of group A streptococci are resistant to macrolides.[27] In some areas, much higher rates of resistance can occur.

PNEUMONIA

The pathogen responsible for **community-acquired bacterial pneumonia (CAP)** is often not confirmed, but *S. pneumoniae* and the "atypical" pathogens *Mycoplasma pneumoniae, Chlamydophila pneumoniae* (formerly *Chlamydia pneumoniae*) and *Legionella* spp. are frequent pathogens. Among **hospitalized patients with community-acquired bacterial pneumonia,** *S. pneumoniae* is still probably the most common cause. Other bacterial pathogens include *H. influenzae, S. aureus* and occasionally other gram-negative bacilli and anaerobic mouth organisms.

In **ambulatory** patients, an oral macrolide (erythromycin, azithromycin or clarithromycin) or doxycycline is generally used in otherwise healthy adults. Pneumococci may, however, be resistant to macrolides and to doxycycline, especially if they are resistant to penicillin.[28] For older patients or those with comorbid illness, a fluoroquinolone may be a better choice. A fluoroquinolone with good antipneumococcal activity such as levofloxacin or moxifloxacin is generally used for adults with comorbidities or antibiotic exposure during the past 90 days.[29] Nationally, about 1% of pneumococcal isolates are resistant to fluoroquinolones, but in some areas the percentage is higher.[30]

In **community-acquired pneumonia requiring hospitalization,** an IV beta-lactam (such as ceftriaxone or cefotaxime) plus a macrolide (erythromycin, azithromycin or clarithromycin), or a fluoroquinolone with good activity against *S. pneumoniae* (levofloxacin or moxifloxacin) alone, is recommended pending culture results.[29] If aspiration pneumonia is suspected, metronidazole or clindamycin can be added; moxifloxacin or ampicillin/sulbactam, which also have anaerobic activity, are reasonable alternatives. In severe cases, CA-MRSA should be considered as a possible pathogen and addition of vancomycin, trimethoprim/sulfamethoxazole or linezolid as possible therapy.

In treating pneumococcal pneumonia due to strains with an intermediate degree of penicillin resistance (minimal inhibitory concentration [MIC] 4 mcg/mL), ceftriaxone, cefotaxime, or high doses of either IV penicillin (12 million units daily for adults) or oral amoxicillin (1-3 g daily) can be used. For highly resistant strains (MIC $\geq$8 mcg/mL), a fluoroquinolone (levofloxacin or moxifloxacin), vancomycin or linezolid should be used in severely ill patients (such as those requiring admission to an ICU) and those not responding to a beta-lactam.

Hospital-acquired or ventilator-associated pneumonia is often caused by gram-negative bacilli, especially *P. aeruginosa*, *Klebsiella* spp., *E. coli*, *Enterobacter* spp., *Serratia* spp., and *Acinetobacter* spp.; it can also be caused by *S. aureus*, usually MRSA. Many of these bacteria are multidrug resistant, particularly when disease onset is after a long hospital admission with prior antibacterial therapy, and further resistance can emerge on treatment. Pneumonia with *S. aureus*, particularly methicillin-resistant strains, is also more common in patients with diabetes mellitus, head trauma, or intensive care unit admission. Hospital-acquired pneumonia due to *Legionella* species can also occur, usually in immunocompromised patients.[31]

In the absence of risk factors for multi-drug resistant organisms, initial empiric therapy for hospital-acquired pneumonia can be limited to one antibiotic, such as ceftriaxone, a fluoroquinolone (levo-floxacin or moxifloxacin) or piperacillin/tazobactam. In other patients, however, particularly those who are severely ill or in an ICU, broader-spectrum coverage with a beta-lactam with antipseudomonal activity such as piperacillin/tazobactam, cefepime, imipenem, doripenem or meropenem, combined with a fluoroquinolone with antipseudomonal activity (ciprofloxacin or levofloxacin) would be a reasonable choice. Addition of vancomycin or linezolid should be considered in hospitals where MRSA are common. Multi-drug resistant gram-negative bacteria, particularly *Acinetobacter* spp., *Pseudomonas* spp. and *Klebsiella* spp., are increasingly common. Treatment options are often limited, but isolates may be susceptible to polymyxin B, colistin (polymyxin E) or tigecycline; some *Acinetobacter* strains are also sensitive to sulbactam.

INFECTIONS OF THE GENITOURINARY TRACT

URINARY TRACT INFECTION (UTI) — *E. coli* causes most uncomplicated cystitis. *Staphylococcus saprophyticus* is the second most common pathogen, and the remaining cases are due to *Proteus* spp., other gram-negative rods and enterococci.[32]

Although fluoroquinolones (especially ciprofloxacin) have become the most common class of antibiotic prescribed for UTI, other drugs are generally preferred for uncomplicated infection due to concerns about cost-effectiveness and emerging fluoroquinolone resistance.[33] **Acute uncomplicated cystitis** in women can be effectively and inexpensively treated, before the infecting organism is known, with a three-day course of oral trimethoprim/sulfamethoxazole. In areas where the prevalence of *E. coli* resistant to trimethoprim/sulfamethoxazole exceeds 15% to 20%, or in women with risk factors for resistance, a 3-day course of a fluoroquinolone such as ciprofloxacin or levofloxacin or a 7-day course of nitrofurantoin could be substituted.[34] A single dose of fosfomycin is another alternative.[35] Based on results of susceptibility testing, nitrofurantoin, amoxicillin or a cephalosporin can be used to treat UTIs in pregnant women[36], but nitrofurantoin should not be given near term or during labor or delivery because it can cause hemolytic anemia in the newborn.

Acute uncomplicated pyelonephritis can often be managed with a 7-10 day course of ciprofloxacin or levofloxacin.[37]

Complicated UTIs that recur after treatment, occur in patients with indwelling urinary catheters, or are acquired in hospitals or nursing homes, are more likely to be due to antibiotic-resistant gram-negative bacilli, *S. aureus* or enterococci. A fluoroquinolone, oral amoxicillin/clavulanate or an oral third-generation cephalosporin such as cefpodoxime, cefdinir or ceftibuten can be useful in treating such infections in outpatients. In hospitalized patients with complicated UTIs, treatment with a third-generation cephalosporin, a fluoroquinolone, ticarcillin/clavulanate, piperacillin/tazobactam, imipenem, doripenem or meropenem is recommended.

PROSTATITIS — Acute bacterial prostatitis may be due to enteric gram-negative bacteria, especially *E. coli* and *Klebsiella* spp., or to *P. aeruginosa* or *Enterococcus* spp.,[38] but a bacterial pathogen is often not identified. Occasionally, a sexually transmitted organism such as *N. gonorrhoeae*, *Chlamydia trachomatis* or *Ureaplasma urealyticum* is responsible. Chronic bacterial prostatitis, although often idiopathic, may be caused by the same bacteria as acute prostatitis, or by *S. aureus* or coagulase-negative staphylococci.[39]

An oral fluoroquinolone with activity against *P. aeruginosa* (ciprofloxacin or levofloxacin) is a reasonable choice for initial treatment of acute bacterial prostatitis in a patient who does not require hospitalization. Trimethoprim/sulfamethoxazole could be used as an alternative. Fluoroquinolones are no longer recommended for treatment of *N. gonorrhoeae*; if gonorrhea is suspected, IV ceftriaxone is recommended.[40]

For more severe prostatitis, an IV fluoroquinolone or third-generation cephalosporin may be used. Prostatic abscesses may require drainage in addition to antimicrobial treatment. Chronic bacterial prostatitis is generally treated with a long (4-12 week) course of an oral fluoroquinolone or trimethoprim/sulfamethoxazole.

INTRA-ABDOMINAL INFECTIONS

Most intra-abdominal infections, such as **cholangitis** and **diverticulitis**, are due to enteric gram-negative organisms, most commonly *E. coli,* but also *Klebsiella* or *Proteus* spp. Enterococci and anaerobes, particularly *Bacteroides fragilis*, are also common. Changes in bowel flora, such as occur in hospitalized patients treated with antibiotics, lead to an increased risk of infections due to *Pseudomonas* and *Candida* spp. Many intra-abdominal infections, particularly abscesses, are polymicrobial.

Empiric therapy should cover both aerobic and anaerobic enteric gram-negative organisms. For community-acquired infection of mild to moderate severity, monotherapy with piperacillin/tazobactam, ertapenem, imipenem or meropenem would be a reasonable first choice.[41] Cefotetan is an alternative. A fluoroquinolone such as moxifloxacin, or tigecycline alone[9] can be used in patients allergic to beta-lactams. In severely ill patients and those with prolonged hospitalization, treatment should include coverage for *Pseudomonas.* Reasonable choices would include an antipseudomonal penicillin (piperacillin/tazobactam) or a carbapenem (imipenem, meropenem or doripenem). Ceftazidime, cefepime, aztreonam or ciprofloxacin, each plus metronidazole for *B. fragilis* coverage, could also be given.

Clostridium difficile is the most common identifiable cause of antibiotic-associated diarrhea. In recent years, a more toxic epidemic strain has emerged, causing an increase in the incidence and severity of *C. difficile* **infection** (CDI).[42] Oral metronidazole can be used to treat mild or moderate CDI. Patients with severe disease and those with delayed response to metronidazole should be treated with oral vancomycin. First recurrences of CDI can be treated with either metronidazole or vancomycin, but for multiple recurrences, longer courses of oral vancomycin with slow tapering or pulsed doses should be used.[43,44]

SEPSIS SYNDROME

For treatment of sepsis syndromes, the choice of drugs should be based on the probable source of infection, the causative organism and the immune status of the patient. The choice should also reflect local patterns of bacterial resistance.[45]

A third- or fourth-generation cephalosporin (cefotaxime, ceftizoxime, ceftriaxone, ceftazidime or cefepime), piperacillin/tazobactam, ticarcillin/clavulanate, imipenem, meropenem, doripenem or aztreonam can be used to treat sepsis caused by most strains of gram-negative bacilli. Among the cephalosporins, ceftazidime has less activity against gram-positive cocci and cephalosporins other than ceftazidime and cefepime have limited activity against *P. aeruginosa*. Piperacillin/tazobactam, imipenem, doripenem and meropenem are active against most strains of *P. aeruginosa* and are active against anaerobes. Aztreonam is active against many strains of *P. aeruginosa,* but has no activity against gram-positive bacteria or anaerobes.

For initial treatment of life-threatening sepsis in adults, a third- or fourth-generation cephalosporin (cefotaxime, ceftriaxone, ceftazidime or cefepime), piperacillin/tazobactam, imipenem, doripenem or meropenem, each plus vancomycin, is recommended. Some experts would add an aminoglycoside or a fluoroquinolone for a brief period (2-3 days).[46,47]

When **bacterial endocarditis** is suspected and therapy must be started before the pathogen is identified, a combination of ceftriaxone and vancomycin can be used. Many Medical Letter consultants would also add low-dose gentamicin to cover the 5% of cases caused by *Enterococcus*.

Recombinant human activated protein C *(Xigris)* is occasionally used in combination with standard therapy for treatment of severe sepsis. Its use should be limited to adult patients with severe sepsis and evidence of dysfunction in more than one organ, and with no bleeding risk.[48]

FEVER AND NEUTROPENIA — Selection of antibacterials in patients with febrile neutropenia is usually made with little information about a causative organism.[49] Gram-positive bacteria account for the majority of microbiologically confirmed infections in patients with neutropenia (especially in patients with central venous catheters), but enteric gram negative organisms and *Pseudomonas* spp. also occur, and the origins of infection (e.g. neutropenic enteritis) are frequently polymicrobial.[50,51]

For empiric treatment of fever in patients with neutropenia, ceftazidime, piperacillin/tazobactam, imipenem, doripenem, meropenem or cefepime would be a reasonable first choice, with or without an aminoglycoside. Addition of vancomycin may be necessary for treatment of neutropenic patients who remain febrile despite antibiotics or who may have bacteremia caused by methicillin-resistant staphylococci or penicillin-resistant viridans streptococci. When the response to antibacterials is poor, the possibility of fungemia, especially with *Candida* spp., should be considered.

Studies in low-risk hospitalized adults show that when neutropenia is expected to last less than 10 days, oral ciprofloxacin with amoxicillin/

clavulanate is as effective as intravenous ceftazidime or ceftriaxone plus amikacin.[52]

MULTIPLE-ANTIBIOTIC-RESISTANT ENTEROCOCCI — Many *Enterococcus* spp., particularly *E. faecium,* are now resistant to penicillin and ampicillin, to gentamicin or streptomycin or both, and to vancomycin. Some of these strains are susceptible *in vitro* to chloramphenicol, doxycycline or, rarely, to fluoroquinolones, but clinical results with these drugs have been variable. Linezolid, daptomycin and tigecycline are active against many gram-positive organisms, including both *E. faecium* and *E. faecalis*; resistance to these drugs has been relatively rare. Quinupristin/dalfopristin, which is not commonly used because of its toxicity and drug interactions, is active against most strains of vancomycin-resistant *E. faecium,* but not *E. faecalis*.[53] Polymicrobial surgical infections that include antibiotic-resistant enterococci may respond to antibiotics aimed at the other organisms. When antibiotic-resistant enterococci cause endocarditis, surgical replacement of the infected valve may be required. UTIs caused by resistant enterococci may respond nevertheless to ampicillin or amoxicillin, which reach very high concentrations in urine; nitrofurantoin or fosfomycin can also be used.

TABLES BEGIN ON PAGE 56.

1. AK May. Skin and soft tissue infections. Surg Clin North Am 2009; 89:403.
2. RM Klevens et al. Invasive methicillin-resistant *Staphylococcus aureus* infections in the United States. JAMA 2007; 298:1763.
3. J Edelsberg et al. Trends in US hospital admissions for skin and soft tissue infections. Emerg Infect Dis 2009; 15:1516.
4. JS Gerber et al. Trends in the incidence of methicillin-resistant *Staphylococcus aureus* infection in children's hospitals in the United States. Clin Infect Dis 2009; 49:65.
5. SD Kobayashi and FR DeLeo. An update on community-associated MRSA virulence. Curr Opin Pharmacol 2009; 9:545.
6. DA Anaya and EP Dellinger. Necrotizing soft-tissue infection: diagnosis and management. Clin Infect Dis 2007; 44:705.

7. RS Daum. Skin and soft tissue infections caused by methicillin-resistant *Staphylococcus aureus*. N Engl J Med 2007; 357:380.
8. LG Miller et al. Clinical and epidemiologic characteristics cannot distinguish community-associated methicillin-resistant *Staphylococcus aureus* infection from methicillin-susceptible *S. aureus* infection: a prospective investigation. Clin Infect Dis 2007; 44:471.
9. Tigecycline *(Tygacil)*. Med Lett Drugs Ther 2005; 47:73.
10. RC Moellering Jr. Current treatment options for community-acquired methicillin-resistant *Staphylococcus aureus* infection. Clin Infect Dis 2008; 46:1032.
11. DL Stevens et al. Practice guidelines for the diagnosis and management of skin and soft-tissue infections. Clin Infect Dis 2005; 41:1373.
12. BA Lipsky et al. Diagnosis and treatment of diabetic foot infections. Clin Infect Dis 2004; 39;885.
13. I García-De La Torre and A Nava-Zavala. Gonococcal and nongonococcal arthritis. Rheum Dis Clin North Am 2009; 35:63.
14. JR Samuel and FK Gould. Prosthetic joint infections: single versus combination therapy. J Antimicrob Chemother 2010; 65:18.
15. I Byren et al. Pharmacotherapy of diabetic foot osteomyelitis. Expert Opin Pharmacother 2009; 10:3033.
16. MT Fitch and D van de Beek. Emergency diagnosis and treatment of adult meningitis. Lancet Infect Dis 2007; 7:191.
17. KS Kim. Acute bacterial meningitis in infants and children. Lancet Infect Dis 2010; 10:32.
18. D van de Beek et al. Nosocomial bacterial meningitis. N Engl J Med 2010; 362:146.
19. F Allerberger and M Wagner. Listeriosis: a resurgent foodborne infection. Clin Microbiol Infect 2010; 16:16.
20. Vancomycin dosing and monitoring. Med Lett Drugs Ther 2009; 51: 25.
21. D van de Beek et al. Corticosteroids for acute bacterial meningitis (Review). Cochrane Database Syst Rev 2007; 1:CD004405.
22. Committee on Infectious Diseases in LK Pickering eds, 2009 Red Book: Report of the Committee on Infectious Diseases 28th ed, Evanston III: American Academy of Pediatrics 2009, page 528.
23. I Brook. Acute and chronic bacterial sinusitis. Infect Dis Clin North Am 2007; 21:427.
24. A Zalmanovici and J Yaphe. Intranasal steroids for acute sinusitis. Cochrane Database Syst Rev 2009; 4:CD005149.
25. S Sethi and TF Murphy. Infection in the pathogenesis and course of chronic obstructive pulmonary disease. N Engl J Med 2008; 359:2355.
26. ML Alcaide and AL Bisno. Pharyngitis and epiglottitis. Infect Dis Clin North Am 2007; 21:449.
27. AL Myers et al. Genetic commonality of macrolide-resistant group A beta hemolytic streptococcus pharyngeal strains. Ann Clin Microbiol Antimicrob 2009; 8:33.
28. J Aspa et al. Pneumococcal antimicrobial resistance: therapeutic strategy and management in community-acquired pneumonia. Expert Opin Pharmacother 2008; 9:229.

29. LA Mandell et al. Infectious Diseases Society of America/American Thoracic Society consensus guidelines on the management of community-acquired pneumonia in adults. Clin Infect Dis 2007; 44 Suppl 2: S27.
30. SG Jenkins et al. Trends in antibacterial resistance among Streptococcus pneumoniae isolated in the USA: update from PROTEKT US Years 1-4. Ann Clin Microbiol Antimicrob 2008; 7:1.
31. AN Kieninger and PA Lipsett. Hospital-acquired pneumonia: pathophysiology, diagnosis, and treatment. Surg Clin North Am 2009; 89:439.
32. DRP Guay. Contemporary management of uncomplicated urinary tract infections. Drugs 2008; 68:1169.
33. TM Hooton et al. Acute uncomplicated cystitis in an era of increasing antibiotic resistance: a proposed approach to empirical therapy. Clin Infect Dis 2004; 39:75.
34. K Gupta et al. Increasing antimicrobial resistance and the management of uncomplicated community-acquired urinary tract infections. Ann Intern Med 2001; 135:41.
35. BJ Knottnerus et al. Fosfomycin tromethamine as second agent for the treatment of acute, uncomplicated urinary tract infections in adult female patients in The Netherlands? J Antimicrob Chemother 2008; 62:356.
36. AM Macejko and AJ Schaeffer. Asymptomatic bacteriuria and symptomatic urinary tract infections during pregnancy. Urol Clin North Am 2007; 34:35.
37. FM Wagenlehner et al. An update on uncomplicated urinary tract infections in women. Curr Opin Urol 2009; 19:368.
38. BM Benway and TD Moon. Bacterial prostatitis. Urol Clin North Am 2008; 35:23.
39. AB Murphy et al. Chronic prostatitis: management strategies. Drugs 2009; 69:71.
40. Centers for Disease Control and Prevention (CDC). Update to CDC's sexually transmitted diseases treatment guidelines, 2006: fluoroquinolones no longer recommended for treatment of gonococcal infections. MMWR Morbid Mortal Wkly Rep 2007; 56:332.
41. JS Solomkin et al. Diagnosis and management of complicated intra-abdominal infection in adults and children: guidelines by the Surgical Infection Society and the Infectious Diseases Society of America. Clin Infect Dis 2010; 50:133.
42. LV McFarland. Renewed interest in a difficult disease: *Clostridium difficile* infections—epidemiology and current treatment strategies. Curr Opin Gastroenterol 2009; 25:24.
43. S Johnson. Recurrent *Clostridium difficile* infection: a review of risk factors, treatments, and outcomes. J Infect 2009; 58:403.
44. SH Cohen et al. Clinical practice guidelines for *Clostridium difficile* infection in adults: 2010 update by the society for healthcare epidemiology of America (SHEA) and the infectious diseases society of America (IDSA). Infect Control Hosp Epidemiol 2010; 31:431.
45. A Kumar. Optimizing antimicrobial therapy in sepsis and septic shock. Crit Care Clin 2009; 25:733.
46. L Leibovici et al. Aminoglycoside drugs in clinical practice: an evidence-based approach. J Antimicrob Chemother 2009; 63:246.
47. ST Micek et al. Empiric combination antibiotic therapy is associated with improved outcome against sepsis due to Gram-negative bacteria: a retrospective analysis. Antimicrob Agents Chemother 2010; 54:1742.

48. S Toussaint and H Gerlach. Activated protein C for sepsis. N Engl J Med 2009; 361:2646.
49. C Viscoli et al. Infections in patients with febrile neutropenia: epidemiology, microbiology, and risk stratification. Clin Infect Dis 2005; 40:S240.
50. C Cordonnier et al. Epidemiology and risk factors for Gram-positive coccal infections in neutropenia: toward a more targeted antibiotic strategy. Clin Infect Dis 2003; 36:149.
51. WT Hughes et al. 2002 guidelines for the use of antimicrobial agents in neutropenic patients with cancer. Clin Infect Dis 2002; 34:730.
52. KG Moores. Safe and effective outpatient treatment of adults with chemotherapy-induced neutropenic fever. Am J Health Syst Pharm 2007; 64:717.
53. JL Wang and PR Hsueh. Therapeutic options for infections due to vancomycin-resistant enterococci. Expert Opin Pharmacother 2009; 10:785.

CHOICE OF ANTIBACTERIAL DRUGS

Drug of First Choice	Alternative Drugs

GRAM-POSITIVE COCCI
Enterococcus spp.[1]

    endocarditis or other severe infection: penicillin G or ampicillin + gentamicin or streptomycin[2]

                  vancomycin + gentamicin or streptomycin[2]; linezolid[3]; daptomycin; quinupristin/dalfopristin[5]; telavancin; tigecycline

    uncomplicated urinary tract infection: ampicillin or amoxicillin

                  nitrofurantoin; a fluoroquinolone[6]; fosfomycin

---

* Resistance may be a problem; susceptibility tests should be used to guide therapy.
1. Disk susceptibility testing may not provide adequate information; β-lactamase assays, "E" tests and dilution tests for susceptibility should be used in serious infections.
2. Aminoglycoside resistance is increasingly common among enterococci; treatment options include ampicillin 2 g IV q4h, continuous infusion of ampicillin, a combination of ampicillin plus a fluoroquinolone, or a combination of ampicillin, imipenem and vancomycin.
3. Reversible bone marrow suppression has occurred, especially with therapy for more than two weeks. Linezolid is an MAO inhibitor and can interact with serotonergic and adrenergic drugs and with tyramine-containing foods (JJ Taylor et al, Clin Infect Dis 2006; 43:180).
4. Daptomycin should not be used to treat pneumonia.
5. Quinupristin/dalfopristin is not active against *Enterococcus faecalis*.
6. Among the fluoroquinolones, levofloxacin, gemifloxacin and moxifloxacin have excellent *in vitro* activity against most *S. pneumoniae*, including penicillin- and cephalosporin-resistant strains. Levofloxacin, gemifloxacin and moxifloxacin also have good activity against many strains of *S. aureus*, but resistance has become frequent among methicillin-resistant strains. Gemifloxacin is associated with a high rate of rash; other fluoroquinolones are preferred. Ciprofloxacin has the greatest activity against *Pseudomonas aeruginosa*. For urinary tract infections, norfloxacin can be used. For tuberculosis, levofloxacin, ofloxacin, ciprofloxacin or moxifloxacin could be used (Treat Guidel Med Lett 2010; 8:43). Ciprofloxacin, ofloxacin, levofloxacin and moxifloxacin are available for IV use. None of these agents is recommended for children or pregnant women.

Continued on next page.

CHOICE OF ANTIBACTERIAL DRUGS (continued)

Drug of First Choice	Alternative Drugs

GRAM-POSITIVE COCCI (continued)

Staphylococcus aureus or epidermidis
 methicillin-susceptible
     a penicillinase-resistant   a cephalosporin[8,9]; vancomycin;
       penicillin[7]   imipenem or meropenem;
                                       clindamycin; linezolid[3]; dapto-
                                         mycin[4]; a fluoroquinolone[6];
                                         telavancin

---

* Resistance may be a problem; susceptibility tests should be used to guide therapy.

7. For oral use against staphylococci, dicloxacillin is preferred; for severe infections, a parenteral formulation (nafcillin or oxacillin) should be used. Ampicillin, amoxicillin, carbenicillin, ticarcillin and piperacillin are not effective against penicillinase-producing staphylococci. The combinations of clavulanate with amoxicillin or ticarcillin, sulbactam with ampicillin, and tazobactam with piperacillin may be active against these organisms.

8. Cephalosporins have been used as alternatives to penicillins in patients allergic to penicillins, but such patients may also have allergic reactions to cephalosporins.

9. For parenteral treatment of staphylococcal or non-enterococcal streptococcal infections, a first-generation cephalosporin such as cefazolin can be used. For oral therapy, cephalexin can be used. The second-generation cephalosporins cefamandole, cefprozil, cefuroxime, cefotetan and cefoxitin are more active than the first-generation drugs against gram-negative bacteria. Cefamandole is no longer available. Cefuroxime is active against ampicillin-resistant strains of *H. influenzae*. Cefoxitin is the most active of the cephalosporins against *B. fragilis*. The third-generation cephalosporins cefotaxime, cefoperazone, ceftizoxime, ceftriaxone and ceftazidime and the fourth-generation cefepime have greater activity than the second-generation drugs against enteric gram-negative bacilli. Ceftazidime has poor activity against many gram-positive cocci and anaerobes, and ceftizoxime has poor activity against penicillin-resistant *S. pneumoniae*. Cefepime has *in vitro* activity against gram-positive cocci similar to that of cefotaxime and ceftriaxone and somewhat greater activity against enteric gram-negative bacilli. The activity of cefepime against *P. aeruginosa* is similar to that of ceftazidime.Cefixime, cefpodoxime, cefdinir, ceftibuten and cefditoren are oral cephalosporins with more activity than second-generation cephalosporins against facultative gram-negative bacilli; they have no useful activity against anaerobes or *P. aeruginosa*, and cefixime and ceftibuten have no useful activity against staphylococci. With the exception of cefoperazone (which can cause bleeding), ceftazidime and cefepime, the activity of all currently available cephalosporins against *P. aeruginosa* is poor or inconsistent.

Continued on next page.

CHOICE OF ANTIBACTERIAL DRUGS (continued)

Drug of First Choice	**Alternative Drugs**

GRAM-POSITIVE COCCI (continued)

*Staphylococcus aureus or epidermidis (continued)
methicillin-resistant[10]

vancomycin ± gentamicin ± rifampin[11]	linezolid[3]; daptomycin[4]; tigecycline[12]; a fluoroquinolone[6]; trimethoprim/sulfamethoxazole; quinupristin/dalfopristin; doxycycline[12]; telavancin

Streptococcus pyogenes (group A[13]) and groups C and G

penicillin G or V[14]	clindamycin; erythromycin; a cephalosporin[8,9]; vancomycin; clarithromycin[15]; azithromycin; linezolid[3]; daptomycin[4]; telavancin

Streptococcus, group B

penicillin G or ampicillin	a cephalosporin[8,9]; vancomycin; daptomycin[4]; erythromycin; telavancin

* **Resistance may be a problem; susceptibility tests should be used to guide therapy.**

10. Many strains of coagulase-positive and coagulase-negative staphylococci are resistant to penicillinase-resistant penicillins; these strains are also resistant to cephalosporins and carbapenems and are often resistant to fluoroquinolones, trimethoprim/sulfamethoxazole and clindamycin. Community-acquired MRSA often is susceptible to clindamycin and trimethoprim/sulfamethoxazole.
11. Rifampin is recommended if prosthetic valve or hardware is present.
12. Tetracyclines and tigecycline, a derivative of minocycline, are generally not recommended for pregnant women or children less than 8 years old.
13. For serious soft-tissue infection due to group A streptococci, clindamycin may be more effective than penicillin. Group A streptococci may, however, be resistant to clindamycin; therefore, some Medical Letter consultants suggest using both clindamycin and penicillin, with or without IV immune globulin, to treat serious soft-tissue infections. Surgical debridement is usually needed for necrotizing soft tissue infections due to group A streptococci. Group A streptococci may also be resistant to erythromycin, azithromycin and clarithromycin.
14. Penicillin V (or amoxicillin) is preferred for oral treatment of infections caused by non-penicillinase-producing streptococci. For initial therapy of severe infections, penicillin G, administered parenterally, is the first choice. For somewhat longer action in less severe infections due to group A streptococci, pneumococci or *Treponema pallidum*, procaine penicillin G, an IM formulation, can be given once or twice daily, but is seldom used now. Benzathine penicillin G, a slowly absorbed preparation, is usually given in a single monthly injection for prophylaxis of rheumatic fever, once for treatment of group A streptococcal pharyngitis and once or more for treatment of syphilis.
15. Not recommended for use in pregnancy.

Continued on next page.

CHOICE OF ANTIBACTERIAL DRUGS (continued)

Drug of First Choice	Alternative Drugs
GRAM-POSITIVE COCCI (continued)	
Streptococcus, viridans group[1]	
penicillin G ± gentamicin	a cephalosporin[8,9]; vancomycin; telavancin
Streptococcus bovis	
penicillin G	a cephalosporin[8,9]; vancomycin; telavancin
Streptococcus, anaerobic or *Peptostreptococcus*	
penicillin G	clindamycin; a cephalosporin[8,9]; vancomycin; telavancin
Streptococcus pneumoniae[16] (pneumococcus)	
penicillin-susceptible (MIC ≤2 mcg/mL)	
penicillin G or V[14]; amoxicillin	a cephalosporin[8,9]; erythromycin; azithromycin; clarithromycin[15]; levofloxacin, gemifloxacin or moxifloxacin[6]; meropenem, imipenem, doripenem or ertapenem; trimethoprim/ sulfamethoxazole; clinda- mycin; a tetracycline[12]; van- comycin; telavancin
penicillin-intermediate resistance (MIC 4 mcg/mL)	
penicillin G IV (12 million units/day for adults); ceftria- xone or cefotaxime	levofloxacin, gemifloxacin or moxifloxacin[6]; vancomycin; clindamycin; telavancin

* Resistance may be a problem; susceptibility tests should be used to guide therapy.
16. Some strains of *S. pneumoniae* are resistant to erythromycin, clindamycin, trimethoprim/sul- famethoxazole, clarithromycin, azithromycin and chloramphenicol, and resistance to the newer flu- oroquinolones is rare but increasing. Nearly all strains tested so far are susceptible to linezolid and quinupristin/dalfopristin *in vitro*.

Continued on next page.

CHOICE OF ANTIBACTERIAL DRUGS (continued)

Drug of First Choice	Alternative Drugs
GRAM-POSITIVE COCCI (continued)	
Streptococcus pneumoniae[16] (pneumococcus) (continued) penicillin-high-level resistance (MIC $\geq$8 mcg/mL)	
meningitis: vancomycin + ceftriaxone or cefotaxime, $\pm$ rifampin	
other infections: vancomycin + ceftriaxone or cefotaxime; levofloxacin, gemifloxacin or moxifloxacin[6]	linezolid[3]; quinupristin/dalfopristin; telavancin
GRAM-NEGATIVE COCCI	
Moraxella (Branhamella) catarrhalis	
cefuroxime[8]; a fluoroquinolone[6]	trimethoprim/sulfamethoxazole; amoxicillin/clavulanate; erythromycin; clarithromycin[15]; azithromycin; doxycycline[12]; cefotaxime[8]; ceftizoxime[8]; ceftriaxone[8]; cefpodoxime[8]
Neisseria gonorrhoeae (gonococcus)[17]	
ceftriaxone[8]	cefixime[8]; cefotaxime[8]; penicillin G[18]

* **Resistance may be a problem; susceptibility tests should be used to guide therapy.**
17. Patients with gonorrhea should be treated presumptively for co-infection with *C. trachomatis* with azithromycin or doxycycline. Fluoroquinolones are no longer recommended for treatment (Centers for Disease Control and Prevention (CDC). MMWR Morbid Mortal Wkly Rep 2007; 56:332).
18. Not recommended unless the isolate is known to be susceptible.

Continued on next page.

CHOICE OF ANTIBACTERIAL DRUGS (continued)

Drug of First Choice	Alternative Drugs
GRAM-NEGATIVE COCCI (continued)	
Neisseria meningitidis[19] (meningococcus)	
penicillin G	cefotaxime[8]; ceftizoxime[8]; ceftriaxone[8]; chloramphenicol[18]; a sulfonamide[21]; a fluoroquinolone[6]
GRAM-POSITIVE BACILLI	
*Bacillus anthracis [22] (anthrax)	
ciprofloxacin[6]; a tetracycline[12]	penicillin G; amoxicillin; erythromycin; imipenem; clindamycin; levofloxacin[6]
Bacillus cereus, subtilis	
vancomycin	imipenem or meropenem; clindamycin
Clostridium perfringens [23]	
penicillin G; clindamycin	metronidazole; imipenem, meropenem, doripenem or ertapenem; chloramphenicol[20]
Clostridium tetani [24]	
metronidazole	penicillin G; doxycycline[12]

* Resistance may be a problem; susceptibility tests should be used to guide therapy.
19. Rare strains of *N. meningitidis* are resistant or relatively resistant to penicillin. A fluoroquinolone or rifampin is recommended for prophylaxis after close contact with infected patients.
20. Because of the possibility of serious adverse effects, this drug should be used only for severe infections when less hazardous drugs are ineffective.
21. Sulfonamide-resistant strains are frequent in the US; sulfonamides should be used only when susceptibility is established by susceptibility tests.
22. For post-exposure prophylaxis, ciprofloxacin for 4 weeks if given with vaccination, and 60 days if not given with vaccination, might prevent disease; if the strain is susceptible, doxycycline is an alternative (JG Bartlett et al, Clin Infect Dis 2002; 35:851).
23. Debridement is primary. Large doses of penicillin G are required. Hyperbaric oxygen therapy may be a useful adjunct to surgical debridement in management of the spreading, necrotizing type of infection.
24. For prophylaxis, a tetanus toxoid booster and, for some patients, tetanus immune globulin (human) are required.

Continued on next page.

Drugs for Bacterial Infections

CHOICE OF ANTIBACTERIAL DRUGS (continued)

Drug of First Choice	Alternative Drugs
GRAM-POSITIVE BACILLI (continued)	
Clostridium difficile [25]	
metronidazole (oral)	vancomycin (oral)
Corynebacterium diphtheriae[26]	
erythromycin	penicillin G
Corynebacterium, jeikeium	
vancomycin	penicillin G + gentamicin; erythromycin
*Erysipelothrix rhusiopathiae	
penicillin G	erythromycin; a cephalosporin[8,9]; a fluoroquinolone[6]
Listeria monocytogenes	
ampicillin ± gentamicin	trimethoprim/sulfamethoxazole
ENTERIC GRAM-NEGATIVE BACILLI	
*Campylobacter fetus	
a third-generation cephalosporin[9]; gentamicin	ampicillin; imipenem or meropenem
*Campylobacter jejuni	
erythromycin or azithromycin	a fluoroquinolone[6]; a tetracycline[12]; gentamicin

* Resistance may be a problem; susceptibility tests should be used to guide therapy.
25. In order to decrease the emergence of vancomycin-resistant enterococci in hospitals and to reduce costs, most clinicians now recommend use of metronidazole first in treatment of patients with mild to moderate *C. difficile* infection (CDI), with oral vancomycin used only for seriously ill patients or those who do not respond to metronidazole. First recurrences of CDI can be treated with either metronidazole or vancomycin, but for multiple recurrences, oral vancomycin should be used.
26. Antitoxin is primary; antimicrobials are used only to halt further toxin production and to prevent the carrier state.

Continued on next page.

CHOICE OF ANTIBACTERIAL DRUGS (continued)

Drug of First Choice	**Alternative Drugs**
ENTERIC GRAM-NEGATIVE BACILLI (continued)	
Citrobacter freundi	
imipenem or meropenem[27]	a fluoroquinolone[6]; ertapenem; doripenem; amikacin; tigecycline[12]; doxycycline[12]; trimethoprim/sulfamethoxazole; cefotaxime[8,27], ceftizoxime[8,27], ceftriaxone[8,27], cefepime[8,27], or ceftazidime[8,27]
Enterobacter spp.	
imipenem or meropenem[27]; cefepime[8,27]	gentamicin, tobramycin or amikacin; trimethoprim-sulfamethoxazole; ciprofloxacin[6]; ticarcillin/clavulanate[28] or piperacillin/tazobactam[28]; aztreonam[27]; cefotaxime, ceftizoxime, ceftriaxone, or ceftazidime[8,27]; tigecycline[12]

* Resistance may be a problem; susceptibility tests should be used to guide therapy.
27. In severely ill patients, many Medical Letter consultants would add gentamicin, tobramycin or amikacin.
28. In severely ill patients, many Medical Letter consultants would add gentamicin, tobramycin or amikacin (but see footnote 42).

Continued on next page.

Drugs for Bacterial Infections

CHOICE OF ANTIBACTERIAL DRUGS (continued)

Drug of First Choice	Alternative Drugs

ENTERIC GRAM-NEGATIVE BACILLI (continued)

*Escherichia coli [30]

cefotaxime, ceftriaxone, ceftazidime or cefepime[8,27]	ampicillin ± gentamicin, tobramycin or amikacin; gentamicin, tobramycin or amikacin; amoxicillin/clavulanate; ticarcillin/clavulanate[28]; piperacillin/tazobactam[28]; ampicillin/sulbactam[27]; trimethoprim/sulfamethoxazole; imipenem, meropenem, doripenem or ertapenem[27,29]; aztreonam[27]; a fluoroquinolone[6]; another cephalosporin[8,9]; tigecycline[12]

*Klebsiella pneumoniae [30]

cefotaxime, ceftriaxone or cefepime[8,25]	imipenem, meropenem, doripenem or ertapenem[27,29]; gentamicin, tobramycin or amikacin; amoxicillin/clavulanate; ticarcillin/clavulanate[28]; piperacillin/tazobactam[28]; ampicillin/sulbactam[27]; trimethoprim/sulfamethoxazole; aztreonam[27]; a fluoroquinolone[6]; another cephalosporin[8,9]; tigecycline[12]

29. A carbapenem is the drug of choice when extended-spectrum beta-lactamases (ESBLs) are present.
30. For an acute, uncomplicated urinary tract infection, before the infecting organism is known, the drug of first choice is trimethoprim/sulfamethoxazole. Antibacterial treatment of gastroenteritis due to *E. coli* O157:H7 may increase toxin release and risk of hemolytic uremic syndrome and is not recommended (Centers for Disease Control and Prevention (CDC). Morbid Mortal Wkly Rep, MMWR 2006; 55:1045).

Continued on next page.

CHOICE OF ANTIBACTERIAL DRUGS (continued)

Drug of First Choice	Alternative Drugs

ENTERIC GRAM-NEGATIVE BACILLI (continued)

Proteus mirabilis[30]

ampicillin[31]	a cephalosporin[8,9,27]; ticarcillin/clavulanate or piperacillin/tazobactam[28]; gentamicin, tobramycin or amikacin; trimethoprim/sulfamethoxazole; imipenem, meropenem, doripenem or ertapenem[27]; aztreonam[27]; a fluoroquinolone[6]; chloramphenicol[20]

Proteus, indole-positive (including *Providencia rettgeri, Morganella morganii,* and *Proteus vulgaris*)

cefotaxime, ceftriaxone, cefepime or ceftazidime[8,27]	imipenem, meropenem, doripenem or ertapenem[27]; gentamicin, tobramycin or amikacin; amoxicillin/clavulanate; ticarcillin/clavulanate[28]; piperacillin/tazobactam[28]; ampicillin/sulbactam[27]; aztreonam[27]; trimethoprim-sulfamethoxazole; a fluoroquinolone[6]

* Resistance may be a problem; susceptibility tests should be used to guide therapy.
31. Large doses (6 grams or more daily) are usually necessary for systemic infections. In severely ill patients, some Medical Letter consultants would add gentamicin, tobramycin or amikacin.

Continued on next page.

CHOICE OF ANTIBACTERIAL DRUGS (continued)

Drug of First Choice	Alternative Drugs
ENTERIC GRAM-NEGATIVE BACILLI (continued)	
Providencia stuartii	
cefotaxime, ceftriaxone, cefepime or ceftazidime[8,27]	imipenem, meropenem, doripenem or ertapenem[27]; ticarcillin/clavulanate [28]; piperacillin/tazobactam[28]; gentamicin, tobramycin or amikacin; aztreonam[27]; trimethoprim/sulfamethoxazole; a fluoroquinolone[6]
Salmonella typhi (typhoid fever)[32]	
a fluoroquinolone[6] or ceftriaxone[8]	chloramphenicol[20]; trimethoprim/sulfamethoxazole; ampicillin; amoxicillin; azithromycin[33]
Other Salmonella spp. [34]	
cefotaxime[8] or ceftriaxone[8] or a fluoroquinolone[6]	ampicillin or amoxicillin; trimethoprim/sulfamethoxazole; chloramphenicol[20]
Serratia spp.	
imipenem or meropenem[27]	gentamicin or amikacin; cefotaxime, ceftizoxime, ceftriaxone, cefepime or ceftazidime[8,27]; aztreonam[27]; trimethoprim/sulfamethoxazole; a fluoroquinolone[6]
Shigella spp.	
a fluoroquinolone[6]	azithromycin; trimethoprim/sulfamethoxazole; ampicillin; ceftriaxone[8]

* **Resistance may be a problem; susceptibility tests should be used to guide therapy.**
32. A fluoroquinolone or amoxicillin is the drug of choice for *S. typhi* carriers (CM Parry et al, N Engl J Med 2002; 347:1770).
33. RW Frenck Jr, et al, Clin Infect Dis 2000; 31:1134.
34. Most cases of *Salmonella* gastroenteritis subside spontaneously without antimicrobial therapy. Immunosuppressed patients, young children and the elderly may benefit the most from antibacterials.

Continued on next page.

CHOICE OF ANTIBACTERIAL DRUGS (continued)

Drug of First Choice	Alternative Drugs
ENTERIC GRAM-NEGATIVE BACILLI (continued)	
Yersinia enterocolitica	
trimethoprim/sulfamethoxazole	a fluoroquinolone[6]; gentamicin, tobramycin or amikacin; cefotaxime[8]
OTHER GRAM-NEGATIVE BACILLI	
Acinetobacter	
imipenem or meropenem[27]	an aminoglycoside; ciprofloxacin[6]; trimethoprim/sulfamethoxazole; ticarcillin/clavulanate[28] or piperacillin/tazobactam[28]; ceftazidime[27]; tigecycline[12] doxycycline[12]; sulbactam[35]; colistin[20]
Aeromonas	
trimethoprim/sulfamethoxazole	gentamicin or tobramycin; imipenem; a fluoroquinolone[6]
Bacteroides	
metronidazole	imipenem, meropenem or ertapenem; amoxicillin/clavulanate, ticarcillin/clavulanate, piperacillin/tazobactam or ampicillin/sulbactam; chloramphenicol[20]
Bartonella henselae or *quintana* (bacillary angiomatosis, trench fever)	
erythromycin	azithromycin; doxycycline[12]
Bartonella henselae [36] (cat scratch bacillus)	
azithromycin	erythromycin; ciprofloxacin[6]; trimethoprim/sulfamethoxazole; gentamicin; rifampin

* Resistance may be a problem; susceptibility tests should be used to guide therapy.
35. Sulbactam may be useful to treat multi-drug resistant *Acinetobacter*. It is only available in combination with ampicillin as *Unasyn*. Medical Letter consultants recommend 3 g IV q4h.
36. Role of antibiotics is not clear (DA Conrad, Curr Opin Pediatr 2001; 13:56).

Continued on next page.

CHOICE OF ANTIBACTERIAL DRUGS (continued)

Drug of First Choice	Alternative Drugs
OTHER GRAM-NEGATIVE BACILLI (continued)	
Bordetella pertussis (whooping cough)	
azithromycin; erythromycin; clarithromycin[15]	trimethoprim/sulfamethoxazole
Brucella spp.	
a tetracycline[12] + rifampin	a tetracycline[12] + streptomycin or gentamicin; chloramphenicol[20] ± streptomycin; trimethoprim/sulfamethoxazole ± gentamicin; ciprofloxacin[6] + rifampin
Burkholderia cepacia	
trimethoprim/sulfamethoxazole	ceftazidime[8]; chloramphenicol[20]; imipenem
Burkholderia (Pseudomonas) mallei (glanders)	
streptomycin + a tetracycline[12]	streptomycin + chloramphenicol[20]; imipenem
Burkholderia (Pseudomonas) pseudomallei (melioidosis)	
imipenem; ceftazidime[8]	meropenem; chloramphenicol[20] + doxycycline[12] + trimethoprim/sulfamethoxazole; amoxicillin/clavulanate
Calymmatobacterium granulomatis (granuloma inguinale)	
trimethoprim/sulfamethoxazole	doxycycline[12] or ciprofloxacin[6] ± gentamicin
Capnocytophaga canimorsus [37]	
penicillin G	cefotaxime, ceftizoxime or ceftriaxone[8]; imipenem or eropenem; vancomycin; a fluoroquinolone[6]; clindamycin

* Resistance may be a problem; susceptibility tests should be used to guide therapy.
37. C Pers et al, Clin Infect Dis 1996; 23:71.

Continued on next page.

CHOICE OF ANTIBACTERIAL DRUGS (continued)

Drug of First Choice	Alternative Drugs

OTHER GRAM-NEGATIVE BACILLI (continued)

Eikenella corrodens
    ampicillin — erythromycin; azithromycin; clarithromycin[15]; doxycycline[12]; amoxicillin/clavulanate; ampicillin/sulbactam; ceftriaxone[8]

Francisella tularensis (tularemia)[38]
    gentamicin (or streptomycin) + a tetracycline[12] — ciprofloxacin[6]; chloramphenicol[20]

Fusobacterium
    penicillin G; metronidazole — clindamycin; cefoxitin[8]; chloramphenicol[20]

Gardnerella vaginalis (bacterial vaginosis)
    oral metronidazole[39] — topical clindamycin or metronidazole; oral clindamycin

Haemophilus ducreyi (chancroid)
    azithromycin or ceftriaxone — ciprofloxacin[6] or erythromycin

Haemophilus influenzae
    meningitis, epiglottitis, arthritis and other serious infections:
    cefotaxime or ceftriaxone[8] — cefuroxime[8] (not for meningitis); chloramphenicol[20]; meropenem

    upper respiratory infections and bronchitis:
    trimethoprim/sulfamethoxazole — cefuroxime[8]; amoxicillin/clavulanate; cefuroxime axetil[8]; cefpodoxime[8]; cefaclor[8]; cefotaxime[8]; ceftizoxime[8]; ceftriaxone[8]; cefixime[8]; doxycycline[12]; clarithromycin[15]; azithromycin; a fluoroquinolone[6]; ampicillin or amoxicillin

---

* **Resistance may be a problem; susceptibility tests should be used to guide therapy.**
38. For post-exposure prophylaxis, doxycycline or ciprofloxacin begun during the incubation period and continued for 14 days might prevent disease (Med Lett Drugs Ther 2001; 43:87).
39. Metronidazole is effective for bacterial vaginosis even though it is not usually active *in vitro* against *Gardnerella*.

Continued on next page.

CHOICE OF ANTIBACTERIAL DRUGS (continued)

Drug of First Choice	Alternative Drugs
OTHER GRAM-NEGATIVE BACILLI (continued)	
*Helicobacter pylori [40]	
proton pump inhibitor[41] + clarithromycin[15] + either amoxicillin or metronidazole	bismuth subsalicylate + metronidazole + tetracycline HCl[12] + either a proton pump inhibitor[41] or H$_2$-blocker[41]
Legionella species	
azithromycin or a fluoroquinolone[6] ± rifampin	doxycycline[12] ± rifampin; trimethoprim/sulfamethoxazole; erythromycin
Leptotrichia buccalis	
penicillin G	doxycycline[12]; clindamycin; erythromycin
Pasteurella multocida	
penicillin G	doxycycline[12]; a second- or third-generation cephalosporin[8,9]; amoxicillin/clavulanate; ampicillin/sulbactam
*Pseudomonas aeruginosa	
urinary tract infection:	
ciprofloxacin[6]	levofloxacin[6]; piperacillin/tazobactam; ceftazidime[8]; cefepime[8]; imipenem, meropenem or doripenem; aztreonam; tobramycin, gentamicin or amikacin

* **Resistance may be a problem; susceptibility tests should be used to guide therapy.**

40. Eradication of *H. pylori* with various antibacterial combinations, given concurrently with a proton pump inhibitor or H$_2$-blocker, has led to rapid healing of active peptic ulcers and low recurrence rates.

41. Proton pump inhibitors available in the US are omeprazole (*Prilosec*, and others), lansoprazole (*Prevacid*), pantoprazole (*Protonix*), esomeprazole (*Nexium*) and rabeprazole (*Aciphex*). Available H$_2$-blockers include cimetidine (*Tagamet*, and others), famotidine (*Pepcid*, and others), nizatidine (*Axid*, and others) and ranitidine (*Zantac*, and others).

Continued on next page.

CHOICE OF ANTIBACTERIAL DRUGS (continued)

Drug of First Choice	Alternative Drugs

OTHER GRAM-NEGATIVE BACILLI (continued)

Pseudomonas aeruginosa (continued)
    other infections:

piperacillin/tazobactam or ticarcillin/clavulanate, **plus/minus** tobramycin, gentamicin or amikacin[42]	ceftazidime[8]; ciprofloxacin[6]; imipenem, meropenem or doripenem; aztreonam; cefepime[8] **plus/minus** tobramycin, gentamicin or amikacin

Spirillum minus (rat bite fever)

penicillin G	doxycycline[12]; streptomycin[20]

Stenotrophomonas maltophilia

trimethoprim/sulfamethoxazole	ticarcillin/clavulanate[28]; minocycline[12]; a fluoroquinolone[6]; tigecycline[12]

Streptobacillus moniliformis (rat bite fever; Haverhill fever)

penicillin G	doxycycline[12]; streptomycin[20]

Vibrio cholerae (cholera)[43]

a tetracycline[12]	a fluoroquinolone[6]; trimethoprim/sulfamethoxazole; azithromycin

Vibrio vulnificus

a tetracycline[12]	cefotaxime[8]; ciprofloxacin[15]

Yersinia pestis (plague)

streptomycin ± a tetracycline[12]	chloramphenicol[20]; gentamicin; trimethoprim/sulfamethoxazole; ciprofloxacin[15]

* **Resistance may be a problem; susceptibility tests should be used to guide therapy.**
42. Neither gentamicin, tobramycin, netilmicin or amikacin should be mixed in the same bottle with carbenicillin, ticarcillin, mezlocillin or piperacillin for IV administration. When used in high doses or in patients with renal impairment, these penicillins may inactivate the aminoglycosides.
43. Antibiotic therapy is an adjunct to and not a substitute for prompt fluid and electrolyte replacement. Reduced susceptibility of *Vibrio cholerea* against tetracyclines and fluoroquinolones has been reported.

Continued on next page.

CHOICE OF ANTIBACTERIAL DRUGS (continued)

Drug of First Choice	Alternative Drugs
MYCOBACTERIA	
Mycobacterium tuberculosis[44]	
isoniazid + rifampin + pyrazinamide ± ethambutol or streptomycin[20]	a fluoroquinolone[6]; cycloserine[20]; capreomycin[20] or kanamycin[20] or amikacin[20]; ethionamide[20]; paraaminosalicylic acid[20]
Mycobacterium kansasii[44]	
isoniazid + rifampin ± ethambutol or streptomycin[20]	clarithromycin[15] or azithromycin; ethionamide[20]; cycloserine[20]
Mycobacterium avium complex[44]	
treatment: azithromycin or clarithromycin[15], plus ethambutol ± rifabutin	ciprofloxacin[6]; amikacin[20]
prophylaxis: clarithromycin[15] or azithromycin ± rifabutin	
Mycobacterium fortuitum/chelonae[44] complex	
amikacin + clarithromycin[15]	cefoxitin[8]; rifampin; a sulfonamide; doxycycline[12]; ethambutol; linezolid[3]
Mycobacterium marinum (balnei)[45]	
minocycline[12]	trimethoprim/sulfamethoxazole; rifampin; clarithromycin[15]; doxycycline[12]
Mycobacterium leprae (leprosy)[44]	
dapsone + rifampin ± clofazimine	minocycline[12]; ofloxacin[6]; clarithromycin[15]

* **Resistance may be a problem; susceptibility tests should be used to guide therapy.**
44. Multidrug regimens are necessary for successful treatment. Drugs listed as alternatives are substitutions for primary regimens and are meant to be used in combination. For additional treatment recommendations for tuberculosis, see Treat Guidel Med Lett 2009; 7:75.
45. Most infections are self-limited without drug treatment.

Continued on next page.

CHOICE OF ANTIBACTERIAL DRUGS (continued)

Drug of First Choice	**Alternative Drugs**
ACTINOMYCETES	
Actinomyces israelii (actinomycosis)	
penicillin G	doxycycline[14]; erythromycin; clindamycin
Nocardia	
trimethoprim/sulfamethoxazole	sulfisoxazole; amikacin[20]; a tetracycline[12]; ceftriaxone; imipenem or meropenem; cycloserine[20]; linezolid[3]
Rhodococcus equi	
vancomycin ± a fluoroquinolone[6], rifampin, imipenem or meropenem; amikacin	erythromycin
Tropheryma whippelii[46] (Whipple's disease)	
trimethoprim/sulfamethoxazole	penicillin G; a tetracycline[12]; ceftriaxone
CHLAMYDIAE	
Chlamydia trachomatis	
trachoma: azithromycin	doxycycline[12]; a sulfonamide (topical plus oral)
inclusion conjunctivitis:	
erythromycin (oral or IV)	a sulfonamide
pneumonia: erythromycin	a sulfonamide
urethritis, cervicitis:	
azithromycin or doxycycline[12]	erythromycin; ofloxacin[6]; amoxicillin
lymphogranuloma venereum:	
a tetracycline[12]	erythromycin
Chlamydophila (formerly *Chlamydia*) *pneumoniae*	
erythromycin; a tetracycline[12]; clarithromycin[15] or azithromycin	a fluoroquinolone[6]

* Resistance may be a problem; susceptibility tests should be used to guide therapy.
46. F Fenollar et al, N Engl J Med 2007; 356:55.

Continued on next page.

CHOICE OF ANTIBACTERIAL DRUGS (continued)

Drug of First Choice	Alternative Drugs
CHLAMYDIAE (continued)	
Chlamydophila (formerly *Chlamydia*) *psittaci* (psittacosis; ornithosis)	
a tetracycline[12]	chloramphenicol[20]
EHRLICHIA	
Anaplasma phagocytophilum (formerly *Ehrlichia phagocytophila*)	
doxycycline[12]	rifampin
Ehrlichia chaffeensis	
doxycycline[12]	chloramphenicol[20]
Ehrlichia ewingii	
doxycycline[12]	
MYCOPLASMA	
Mycoplasma pneumoniae	
erythromycin; a tetracycline[12]; clarithromycin[15] or azithromycin	a fluoroquinolone[6]
Ureaplasma urealyticum	
azithromycin	erythromycin; a tetracycline[12]; clarithromycin[15]; ofloxacin[6]
RICKETTSIOSES	
Rickettsia rickettsii (Rocky Mountain spotted fever)	
doxycycline[12]	a fluoroquinolone[6]; chloramphenicol[20]
Rickettsia typhi (endemic typhus-murine)	
doxycycline[12]	a fluoroquinolone[6]; chloramphenicol[20]
Rickettsia prowazekii (epidemic typhus-louseborne)	
doxycycline[12]	a fluoroquinolone[6]; chloramphenicol[20]
Orientia tsutsugamushi (scrub typhus)	
doxycycline[12]	a fluoroquinolone[6]; chloramphenicol[20]

* Resistance may be a problem; susceptibility tests should be used to guide therapy.

Continued on next page.

CHOICE OF ANTIBACTERIAL DRUGS (continued)

Drug of First Choice	Alternative Drugs
RICKETTSIOSES (continued)	
Coxiella burnetii (Q fever)	
doxycycline[12]	a fluoroquinolone[6]; chloramphenicol[20]
SPIROCHETES	
Borrelia burgdorferi (Lyme disease)[47]	
doxycycline[12]; amoxicillin; cefuroxime axetil[8]	ceftriaxone[8]; cefotaxime[8]; penicillin G; azithromycin; clarithromycin[15]
Borrelia recurrentis (relapsing fever)	
a tetracycline[12]	penicillin G; erythromycin
Leptospira	
penicillin G	doxycycline[12]; ceftriaxone[8,48]
Treponema pallidum (syphilis)	
penicillin G[14]	doxycycline[12]; ceftriaxone[8]
Treponema pertenue (yaws)	
penicillin G	doxycycline[12]

* Resistance may be a problem; susceptibility tests should be used to guide therapy.

47. For treatment of erythema migrans, uncomplicated facial nerve palsy, mild cardiac disease and arthritis, oral therapy is satisfactory; for other neurologic or more serious cardiac disease, parenteral therapy with ceftriaxone, cefotaxime or penicillin G is recommended. For recurrent arthritis after an oral regimen, another course of oral therapy or a parenteral drug may be given (Med Lett Drugs Ther 2005; 47:41).
48. JM Vinetz, Clin Infect Dis 2003; 36:1514; T Panaphot et al, Clin Infect Dis 2003; 36:1507.

DOSAGE OF ORAL ANTIBACTERIAL DRUGS

Drug	Formulations
AZITHROMYCIN – generic	250, 500, 600 mg tabs[2,3]
Zithromax	
ZMax	2 g ER susp
CEPHALOSPORINS	
Cefaclor – generic	250, 500 mg caps[2]
Ceclor	125, 187, 250, 375 mg chewable tabs
Raniclor	
extended-release – generic	375, 500 mg ER tabs
Cefadroxil – generic	500 mg caps; 1 g tabs[2]
Duricef	
Cefdinir – generic	300 mg caps[2]
Omnicef	
Cefditoren – *Spectracef*	200, 400 mg tabs
Cefpodoxime – generic	100, 200 mg tabs[2]
Vantin	
Cefprozil – generic	250, 500 mg tabs[2]
Cefzil	
Ceftibuten – *Cedax*	400 mg caps[2]
Cefuroxime axetil – generic	125, 250, 500 mg tabs[2]
Ceftin	
Cephalexin – generic	250, 500 mg tabs[2]; 250, 500 mg caps
Keflex	250, 500 mg caps[2]
CLARITHROMYCIN – generic	250, 500 mg tabs[2]
Biaxin	
extended-release – generic	500 mg ER tabs
Biaxin XL	
CLINDAMYCIN – generic	75, 150, 300 mg caps[2,3]
Cleocin	

1. Doses may vary with site of infection, infecting organism and patient renal function.
2. Suspension formulation also available.

Usual Adult Dosage[1]	Usual Pediatric Dosage[1]
500 mg day 1, then 250 mg days 2-5	5-12 mg/kg q24h
2 g single dose	
500 mg q8h	6.6-13.3 mg/kg q8h
500 mg q12h	
1 gram daily	15 mg/kg q12h
300 mg q12h	7 mg/kg q12h or 14 mg/kg q24h
400 mg q12h	
200 mg q12h	10 mg/kg q24h or 5 mg/kg q12h
500 mg q12h	15 mg/kg q12h
400 mg daily	9 mg/kg q24h
500 mg bid	10-15 mg/kg q12h
500 mg q6h	6.25-25 mg/kg q6h
500 mg q12h	7.5 mg/kg q12h
1000 mg q24h	
300 mg q6h	2-8 mg/kg q6-8h

3. Injectable formulation also available.

Continued on next page.

DOSAGE OF ORAL ANTIBACTERIAL DRUGS (continued)

Drug	Formulations
ERYTHROMYCIN	
base, delayed-release capsules	250 mg caps
generic	
ERYC	
base, enteric-coated tablets	
Ery-tab	250, 333, 500 mg tabs
FLUOROQUINOLONES	
Ciprofloxacin – generic	100, 250, 500, 750 mg tabs[2,3]
Cipro	
extended release – generic	500, 1000 ER tabs
Cipro XR	
Gemifloxacin – *Factive*	320 mg tabs
Levofloxacin – *Levaquin*	250, 500, 750 mg tabs[2,3]
Moxifloxacin – *Avelox*	400 mg tabs[3]
Norfloxacin – *Noroxin*	400 mg tabs
Ofloxacin – generic	200, 300, 400 mg tabs
FOSFOMYCIN – *Monurol*	3 g powder
LINEZOLID – *Zyvox*	600 mg tabs[2,3]
KETOLIDE	
Telithromycin – *Ketek*	300, 400 mg tabs
METRONIDAZOLE	
generic	250, 500 mg tabs, 375 mg caps[3]
Flagyl	
generic	750 mg ER tabs
Flagyl ER	
NITROFURANTOIN	
macrocrystals – generic	25, 50, 100 mg caps
Macrodantin	
monohydrate-macrocrystals–	100 mg caps
generic	
Macrobid	

4. Pediatric dose for post-exposure prophylaxis for anthrax is 10-15 mg/kg bid.

Usual Adult Dosage[1]	Usual Pediatric Dosage[1]
500 mg q6h	7.5-12.5 mg/kg q6h
500 mg q6h	7.5-12.5 mg/kg q6h
500 mg q12h	see footnote 4
1000 mg q24h	
320 mg daily	
500 mg daily	
400 mg daily	
400 mg bid	
400 mg q12h	
3 grams once	
600 mg q12h	10 mg/kg q8h[5]
800 mg daily	
500 mg tid	30 mg/kg/d divided q6h
750 mg once/day	
100 mg q6h	1.25-1.75 mg/kg q6h
100 mg q12h	

5. For children ≤11 years of age. Usual dose for children ≥12 years old is 600 mg q12h.

Continued on next page.

DOSAGE OF ORAL ANTIBACTERIAL DRUGS (continued)

Drug	Formulations
PENICILLINS	
Penicillin V[6] – generic	250, 500 mg tabs[2]
Amoxicillin – generic	250, 500 mg caps; 500, 875 mg tabs;
Amoxil	125, 200, 250, 400 mg chewable tabs[2]
Amoxicillin/clavulanate[7]	250/125, 500/125, 875/125 tabs;
Augmentin	200/28.5, 400/57mg chewable tabs[2]
Augmentin XR [8]	1000/62.5 mg ER tabs
Ampicillin – generic	250, 500 mg caps[2]
Principen	
Dicloxacillin – generic	125, 250, 500 mg caps[2]
TETRACYCLINES	
Doxycycline	50, 100 mg caps[2]
generic (capsules)	
Vibramycin	
generic (tablets)	100 mg tabs
Vibra-tabs	
Minocycline – generic	50, 75, 100 mg caps[3]
Minocin	
extended release – generic	45, 90, 135 mg ER tabs
Solodyn	45, 65, 90, 115, 135 mg ER tabs
Tetracycline HCl – generic	250, 500 mg caps,
Sumycin	tabs[2]

6. One mg is equal to 1600 units.
7. Dosage based on amoxicillin content. For doses of 500 or 875 mg, 500-mg or 875-mg tablets should be used, because multiple smaller tablets would contain too much clavulanate. 125 mg/5 mL oral suspension contains 31.25 mg clavulanate; 250-mg/5 mL oral suspension contains 62.5 mg clavulanate.

Usual Adult Dosage[1]	Usual Pediatric Dosage[1]
500 mg q6h	6.25-12.5 mg/kg q6h
500 mg q8h	6.6-13.3 mg/kg q8h or 15 mg/kg q12h
875 mg q12h	6.6-13.3 mg/kg q8h or 15 mg/kg q12h
2000 mg q12h	
500 mg q6h	12.5-25 mg/kg q6h
500 mg q6h	3.125-12.5 mg/kg q6h
100 mg bid	2.2 mg/kg q12-24h[9]
200 mg once, then 100 mg bid	
1 mg/kg daily	
500 mg q6h	6.25-12.5 mg/kg q6h[9]

8. Dosage based on amoxicillin content.
9. Not recommended for children <8 years old.

Continued on next page.

DOSAGE OF ORAL ANTIBACTERIAL DRUGS (continued)

Drug	Formulations
TRIMETHOPRIM/SULFAMETHOXAZOLE	
generic	400/80 mg tabs[2,3]
Bactrim	
Septra	
double strength (DS) –	800/160 mg tabs
generic	
Bactrim DS	
Septra DS	
VANCOMYCIN[2,10]	
Vancocin	125, 250 mg caps

10. Some pharmacies use the intravenous formulation for oral administration, which costs less.

Usual Adult Dosage[1]	Usual Pediatric Dosage[1]
1 tablet q6h	4-5 mg/kg (TMP) q6h
1 DS tablet q12h	
125 mg q6h	40 mg/kg/d divided q6-8h

Ceftaroline Fosamil *(Teflaro)* — A New IV Cephalosporin
Originally published in The Medical Letter – January 2011; 53:5

The FDA has approved ceftaroline fosamil *(Teflaro* – Forest), an intra-venous (IV) cephalosporin, for treatment of acute bacterial skin and skin structure infections, including those caused by methicillin-resistant *Staphylococcus aureus* (MRSA), and for treatment of community-acquired bacterial pneumonia in adults. It is the first beta-lactam antibi-otic approved for treatment of MRSA.

MECHANISM OF ACTION — Like other beta-lactams, ceftaroline binds to penicillin-binding proteins (PBPs), inhibiting cell wall synthe-sis. Unlike other currently available beta-lactams, it has a high affinity *in vitro* for PBP2a, a unique PBP encoded by the *mecA* gene in MRSA.[1]

STANDARD TREATMENT[2] **— Skin and Skin-Structure Infection – Uncomplicated** skin and skin-structure infections in immunocompe-tent patients are commonly due to *S. aureus*, *Streptococcus pyogenes* (group A streptococci) or *Streptococcus agalactiae* (group B strepto-cocci). Patients hospitalized for such infections have generally been treated with an IV beta-lactam such as nafcillin or cefazolin. In the past few years, however, MRSA has become the predominant cause of sup-purative skin infection in many parts of the US. When MRSA is isolated or suspected (e.g., the patient was recently treated with antibiotics, is known to be colonized, has a history of recent previous hospitalization, or is in a geographic area of high prevalence) in a hospitalized patient, vancomycin, linezolid or daptomycin has been added to or substituted for the beta-lactam.

Complicated skin and skin-structure infections, such as those that occur in patients with burns, diabetes mellitus, infected pressure ulcers and trau-matic or surgical wound infections, may also be caused by gram-negative bacilli, such as *Escherichia coli* and *Pseudomonas aeruginosa*, or can be

SOME TRADE NAMES

Ampicillin/sulbactam – *Unasyn**	Daptomycin – *Cubicin*
Azithromycin – *Zithromax**	Imipenem/cilastatin – *Primaxin*
Aztreonam – *Azactam**	Levofloxacin – *Levaquin*
Cefazolin*	Linezolid – *Zyvox*
Cefepime – *Maxipime**	Meropenem – *Merrem**
Cefotaxime – *Claforan**	Moxifloxacin – *Avelox*
Ceftaroline – *Teflaro*	Nafcillin*
Ceftazidime – *Fortaz, Tazicef**	Piperacillin/tazobactam – *Zosyn**
Ceftriaxone – *Rocephin**	Ticarcillin/clavulanate – *Timentin*
Clarithromycin – *Biaxin**	Vancomycin – *Vancocin**

*Available generically

polymicrobial. For such infections in hospitalized patients, ampicillin/sulbactam, piperacillin/tazobactam, ticarcillin/clavulanate, imipenem or meropenem have generally been given, together with vancomycin, linezolid or daptomycin until MRSA is ruled out.

Community-Acquired Pneumonia – The pathogen responsible for community-acquired bacterial pneumonia (CAP) is often not confirmed, but *Streptococcus pneumoniae* and the "atypicals" *Mycoplasma pneumoniae*, *Chlamydophila pneumoniae* (formerly *Chlamydia pneumoniae*) and *Legionella* spp. are frequent pathogens. Other causes include *Haemophilus influenzae*, *S. aureus* and occasionally other gram-negative bacilli and anaerobic mouth organisms. In CAP requiring hospitalization, either an IV beta-lactam such as ceftriaxone or cefotaxime plus a macrolide such as azithromycin, or monotherapy with a fluoroquinolone with good activity against *S. pneumoniae* (levofloxacin or moxifloxacin alone), has been recommended pending culture results.

ANTIBACTERIAL SPECTRUM — Overall, the antibacterial spectrum of ceftaroline is most similar to that of ceftriaxone, but with better gram-positive activity. Ceftaroline is active *in vitro* against both methicillin-susceptible and methicillin-resistant *S. aureus* (MSSA and MRSA) and against various streptococci, including penicillin-susceptible, penicillin-resistant, and cephalosporin-resistant isolates of *S. pneumoniae*. It is also active *in vitro* against vancomycin-intermediate *S. aureus* (VISA) and hetero-vancomycin-intermediate *S. aureus* (h-VISA).[3] Like other cephalosporins, ceftaroline does not have clinically significant activity against *Enterococcus*.

Among gram-negative organisms, ceftaroline is highly active *in vitro* against *E. coli, Klebsiella pneumoniae, Citrobacter freundii* and *Enterobacter cloacae* that do not produce extended-spectrum beta-lactamases (ESBL). It is somewhat less active than ceftriaxone, ceftazidime or cefepime against *Proteus mirabilis*, *Morganella morganii*, *Serratia marcescens* and *Providencia* spp. It is not active against *Acinetobacter* spp., *P. aeruginosa* or ceftazidime-resistant *Enterobacteriaceae* spp. (including amp C overproducers and ESBL-producing strains).[4]

Ceftaroline is generally active *in vitro* against gram-positive anaerobes and some gram-negative anaerobes, but not against *Bacteroides fragilis*.[5]

CLINICAL STUDIES — Skin and Skin-Structure Infection – Two clinical trials in more than 1300 patients with complicated skin and skin structure infections compared ceftaroline 600 mg IV every 12 hours to vancomycin plus aztreonam (1 g of each every 12 hours) for 5-14 days. Patients with diabetic foot ulcers, decubitus ulcers, extensive burns, or known or suspected *Pseudomonas* infection were excluded from the trials. Clinical cure rates in the clinically evaluable population were similar (91.6% with ceftaroline vs. 92.7% with vancomycin plus aztreonam) in the pooled results. Among 330 patients with MRSA infection, clinical cure rates were 93.4% with ceftaroline vs. 94.3% with vancomycin plus aztreonam.[6]

Community-Acquired Pneumonia – Two clinical trials compared ceftaroline 600 mg IV every 12 hours to ceftriaxone 1 g every 24 hours for

PHARMACOLOGY

Drug class	Cephalosporin antibiotic
Formulations available	400-mg, 600-mg vials (refrigerated)
Route	Intravenous
Dosage	600 mg every 12 hours
Renal dosage adjustment	Based on creatinine clearance: 31-50 mL/min: 400 mg every 12 hours 15-30 mL/min: 300 mg every 12 hours <15 mL/min (ESRD): 200 mg every 12 hours
Administration	Over 1 hour; each dose must be diluted in 250 mL before infusion
Plasma concentrations	Cmax: 21.3 mcg/mL AUC: 56.3 mcg/h/mL
Metabolism	Ceftaroline fosamil prodrug converted to ceftaroline in plasma by phosphatases with subsequent hydrolysis to inactive metabolite
Excretion	Primarily renal; ~50% as unchanged ceftaroline
Elimination half-life	~2.6 hours

5-7 days for treatment of community-acquired pneumonia in a total of about 1200 hospitalized patients. Both trials excluded patients with known or suspected infection with MRSA or an atypical pathogen. In the clinically evaluable population, ceftaroline was non-inferior to ceftriaxone in the rate of clinical cure (84.3% vs. 77.7%) in the combined analysis.[7]

ADVERSE EFFECTS — The most common adverse reactions associated with ceftaroline use in clinical trials were diarrhea (5%), nausea (4%), and rash (3%). Direct Coombs' test seroconversion from negative to positive occurred in about 10% of patients, but clinically significant drug-induced hemolysis was rare. *Clostridium difficile*-associated diarrhea was reported in 2 patients during clinical trials. Ceftaroline is classified as category B (no evidence of risk) for use in pregnancy.

COST — A single 600-mg vial of *Teflaro* costs $41.00, according to the manufacturer.

CONCLUSION — Ceftaroline *(Teflaro)* is the first beta-lactam antibiotic with activity against MRSA. It has been effective for treatment of skin and skin structure infections, including those caused by MRSA, but some patients with complicated infections were excluded from clinical trials. Whether it is effective for treatment of other MRSA infections, including pneumonia, remains to be established.

1. A Villegas-Estrada et al. Co-opting the cell wall in fighting methicillin-resistant Staphylococcus aureus: potent inhibition of PBP 2a by two anti-MRSA beta-lactam antibiotics. J Am Chem Soc 2008; 130:9212.
2. Drugs for bacterial infections. Treat Guidel Med Lett 2010; 8:43.
3. L Saravolatz et al. In vitro activity of ceftaroline against community-associated methicillin-resistant, vancomycin-intermediate, vancomycin-resistant, and daptomycin-nonsusceptible Staphylococcus aureus isolates. Antimicrob Agents Chemother 2010; 54:3027.
4. Y Ge et al. In vitro profiling of ceftaroline against a collection of recent bacterial clinical isolates from across the United States. Antimicrob Agents Chemother 2008; 52:3398.
5. DM Citron et al. In vitro activity of ceftaroline against 623 diverse strains of anaerobic bacteria. Antimicrob Agents Chemother 2010; 54:1627.
6. GR Corey et al. Integrated analysis of CANVAS 1 and 2: phase 3, multicenter, randomized, double-blind studies to evaluate the safety and efficacy of ceftaroline versus vancomycin plus aztreonam in complicated skin and skin-structure infection. Clin Infect Dis 2010; 51:641.
7. TM File Jr, et al. Integrated analysis of FOCUS 1 and FOCUS 2: randomized, doubledblinded, multicenter phase 3 trials of the efficacy and safety of ceftaroline fosamil versus ceftriaxone in patients with community-acquired pneumonia. Clin Infect Dis 2010; 51:1395.

Treatment of *Clostridium Difficile* Infection
Originally published in The Medical Letter – February 2011; 53:14

Clostridium difficile infection (CDI) is the most common infectious cause of healthcare-associated diarrhea in adults. The incidence and severity of CDI have increased in recent years with the emergence of an epidemic virulent strain (NAP1/BI/027).[1,2] Common risk factors include admission to a healthcare facility, increasing age and severity of underlying illness, gastric acid suppression and exposure to antimicrobials, particularly clindamycin, ampicillin, cephalosporins or fluoroquinolones.[3,4] Patients who develop CDI while receiving a precipitating antibiotic should have the antibiotic discontinued, if possible, or switched to another appropriate antimicrobial with a lower risk of CDI.[5]

INITIAL EPISODE — Antidiarrheal drugs do not decrease the severity or duration of CDI. All patients with CDI should be treated with an appropriate antimicrobial; oral metronidazole and oral vancomycin have been the drugs of choice for many years. Oral administration of vancomycin results in very high concentrations in the intestinal lumen and little or no systemic absorption. Metronidazole can be given intravenously to patients who cannot take oral drugs.

Oral metronidazole 500 mg 3 times daily for 10-14 days is recommended for patients with **mild to moderate** CDI. Patients whose symptoms progress or fail to improve after 5-7 days (some Medical Letter consultants say 3-5 days) should be switched to oral vancomycin.

Patients with **severe** CDI should be treated with oral vancomycin 125 mg 4 times daily for 10-14 days.[6] Infectious disease experts recommend that patients with an increase in serum creatinine 1.5 times baseline or a white blood cell count of $\geq$15,000 cells/mm^3 should be considered as having severe disease. Other factors associated with severe disease include age >65 years old, hypoalbuminemia, immunocompromised state and the severity of the underlying illness.

DRUGS FOR CDI

Drug	Usual Dosage	Cost[1]
Metronidazole[2] – generic	500 mg PO 3x/d	$12.99
Flagyl (Pfizer)		180.00
Vancomycin – Vancocin HCl (Viropharma)	125 mg PO 4x/d	1101.11[3]

1. Cost of 10 days' treatment at drugstore.com; accessed February 14, 2011.
2. Not approved by the FDA for this indication. IV metronidazole can be used in patients who are unable to take oral drugs.
3. Oral vancomycin is not available generically. Vancomycin for intravenous use can be prepared for oral use at a much lower cost.

Although controlled trials are lacking, most Medical Letter consultants treat patients with **fulminant** CDI (refractory hypotension, ileus, and/or toxic megacolon) with both intravenous (IV) metronidazole 500 mg every 6-8 hours and oral vancomycin 125-500 mg every 6 hours.[4] IV administration of vancomycin is not effective for treatment of CDI. Vancomycin can be administered by retention enema if complete ileus is present, but colonic perforation is a concern. In patients with fulminant CDI that does not respond promptly to metronidazole and vancomycin, colectomy can be life saving.

RECURRENCE — Most CDI recurrences develop within the first 60 days after cessation of therapy, with the greatest risk in the first two weeks. The recurrence rate after an initial episode of CDI is typically 20-25%, regardless of whether the initial treatment was metronidazole or oral vancomycin. Patients who develop one recurrent episode have up to a 35% chance of having another recurrence, and patients with at least 3 CDI episodes have up to a 65% chance of additional recurrences.[5]

First recurrences of CDI should be treated like the first episode (metronidazole for mild to moderate CDI and oral vancomycin for severe CDI).

Subsequent recurrences are often treated with 10-14 days of oral vancomycin followed by a prolonged tapered or pulsed regimen of oral vancomycin (e.g., one week each of 125 mg 4 times daily, 3 times daily, twice daily, once daily, every other day, and then every 3 days for 2 weeks) to allow for *C. difficile* spore germination and restoration of normal gut flora.[5] Prolonged courses of metronidazole are not recommended because they can cause potentially severe peripheral neuropathy and because the drug is generally not detectable in stool once diarrhea resolves.

OTHER OPTIONS — Fidaxomicin is an investigational antibiotic more active *in vitro* than vancomycin against *C. difficile*. A double-blind study in 629 patients with CDI compared 10 days treatment with fidaxomicin 200 mg twice daily to vancomycin 125 mg 4 times daily. The treatments were similarly effective (88.2% vs. 85.8% rate of clinical cure). Among patients with non-NAP1 strains, there were fewer recurrences in the fidoxamicin group (15.4% vs. 25.3%).[7] Fidaxomicin is currently under review by the FDA.

Fecal flora restoration by administration of stool through a nasogastric tube, colonoscopy or enema has had reported efficacy of about 90% in preventing recurrent CDI, but randomized trials are lacking.[8,9,10]

A few case series have suggested that **rifaximin** *(Xifaxan)*, a non-absorbed rifamycin approved for treatment of traveler's diarrhea, might be helpful in preventing recurrences of CDI.[11,12] Use of rifaximin can lead to rapid development and spread of resistance to rifamycins.

Nitazoxanide *(Alinia)* is approved for treatment of diarrhea due to *Giardia* or *Cryptosporidium*. Two small randomized trials demonstrated response rates in treatment of CDI equivalent to those of metronidazole or oral vancomycin.[13,14]

Some case reports have described success with use of **IV immunoglobulin (IVIG)** as adjunctive therapy for both fulminant CDI and multiple recurrences of CDI. The presumed mechanism of action is passive immunity against *C. difficile* toxins.[15]

Monoclonal antibodies against *C. difficile* toxins as an adjunct to metronidazole or oral vancomycin significantly reduced CDI recurrence (7.1% vs. 25% with placebo) in a double-blind, randomized trial in 200 patients.[16] These antibodies had no effect on the severity or duration of the initial infection, and they are not available commercially.

A few case reports have described successful use of the IV antimicrobial **tigecycline** *(Tygacil)* as adjunctive therapy for severe CDI.[17,18]

Probiotics have been used to treat or prevent recurrences of CDI, but data on their safety and efficacy are insufficient to recommend such use.[19]

CONCLUSION — Oral metronidazole should be used for initial treatment or first recurrences of mild to moderate *Clostridium difficile* infection (CDI). Oral vancomycin is the drug of choice for severe CDI. For patients with multiple recurrences of CDI, a prolonged pulsed or tapered dose of oral vancomycin can be used.

1. VG Loo et al. A predominantly clonal multi-institutional outbreak of Clostridium difficile-associated diarrhea with high morbidity and mortality. N Engl J Med 2005; 353:2442.
2. LC McDonald et al. An epidemic, toxin gene-variant strain of Clostridium difficile. N Engl J Med 2005; 353:2433.
3. ER Dubberke et al. Clostridium difficile-associated disease in a setting of endemicity: identification of novel risk factors. Clin Infect Dis 2007; 45:1543.
4. SH Cohen et al. Clinical practice guidelines for Clostridium difficile infection in adults: 2010 update by the Society for Healthcare Epidemiology of America (SHEA) and the Infectious Diseases Society of America (IDSA). Infect Control Hosp Epidemiol 2010; 31:431.
5. DN Gerding et al. Treatment of Clostridium difficile infection. Clin Infect Dis 2008; 46 Suppl1:S32.
6. FA Zar et al. A comparison of vancomycin and metronidazole for the treatment of Clostridium difficile-associated diarrhea, stratified by disease severity. Clin Infect Dis 2007; 45:302.

7. TJ Louie et al. Fidaxomicin versus vancomycin for Clostridium difficile infection. N Engl J Med 2011; 364:422.

8. JS Bakken. Fecal bacteriotherapy for recurrent Clostridium difficile infection. Anaerobe 2009; 15:285.

9. SS Yoon and LJ Brandt. Treatment of refractory/recurrent C. difficile-associated disease by donated stool transplanted via colonoscopy. A case series of 12 patients. J Clin Gastroenterol 2010; 44:562.

10. F Rohlke et al. Fecal flora reconstitution for recurrent Clostridium difficile infection: results and methodology. J Clin Gastroenterol; 2010; 44:567.

11. S Johnson et al. Rifaximin redux: treatment of recurrent Clostridium difficile infections with rifaximin immediately post-vancomycin treatment. Anaerobe 2009; 15:290.

12. KW Garey et al. Rifaximin in treatment of recurrent Clostridium difficile-associated diarrhea: an uncontrolled pilot study. J Clin Gastroenterol 2009; 43:91.

13. DM Musher et al. Nitazoxanide for the treatment of Clostridium difficile colitis. Clin Infect Dis 2006; 43:421.

14. DM Musher et al. Nitazoxanide versus vancomycin in Clostridium difficile infection: a randomized, double-blind study. Clin Infect Dis 2009; 48:e41.

15. J O'Horo and N Safdar. The role of immunoglobulin for the treatment of Clostridium difficile infection: a systematic review. Int J Infect Dis 2009; 13:663.

16. I Lowy et al. Treatment with monoclonal antibodies against Clostridium difficile toxins. N Engl J Med 2010; 362:197.

17. CL Lu et al. Severe and refractory Clostridium difficile infection successfully treated with tigecycline and metronidazole. Int J Antimicrob Agents 2010; 35:311.

18. BL Herpers et al. Intravenous tigecycline as adjunctive or alternative therapy for severe refractory Clostridium difficile infection. Clin Infect Dis 2009; 48:1732.

19. LV McFarland. Meta-analysis of probiotics for the prevention of antibiotic associated diarrhea and the treatment of Clostridium difficile disease. Am J Gastroenterol 2006; 101:812.

Drugs for MRSA with Reduced Susceptibility to Vancomycin
Originally published in The Medical Letter – May 2009; 51:36

The recent *Medical Letter* article on vancomycin dosing and monitoring[1] briefly mentioned use of an alternative antibiotic for treatment of methicillin-resistant *Staphylococcus aureus* (MRSA) with reduced susceptibility to vancomycin. Some readers have asked for more information on this subject.

REDUCED SUSCEPTIBILITY TO VANCOMYCIN — Microbiology laboratories generally report isolates of MRSA as "susceptible" to vancomycin when the minimum inhibitory concentration (MIC) is ≤ 2 mg/L. Recent guidelines suggest considering an alternative antibiotic when the MIC is ≥ 2 mg/L.[2]

ALTERNATIVES TO VANCOMYCIN — For complicated skin or soft tissue infections caused by MRSA with reduced susceptibility to vancomycin, either **daptomycin** *(Cubicin)* or **linezolid** *(Zyvox)* would be a reasonable choice. Linezolid, which is available for both oral and IV use, is bacteriostatic and may not be effective for treatment of endocarditis; it is not recommended for use in catheter-associated bacteremias. Linezolid can cause bone marrow suppression, particularly if it is used for more than 10 days.

When bacteremia is present, especially when it is due to right-sided endocarditis, daptomycin, which is given IV, would be a better choice, unless the patient has concomitant pneumonia (daptomycin is inactivated by surfactant). Daptomycin is rapidly bactericidal, but some *S. aureus* strains with decreased susceptibility to vancomycin have decreased susceptibility to daptomycin as well.

Other drugs that may be effective against some strains of MRSA include **quinupristin-dalfopristin** *(Synercid)*, which causes thrombophlebitis and has substantial potential for adverse drug interactions, and **tigecycline** *(Tygacil)*, which achieves only low serum concentrations and is bacteriostatic. Another alternative is **trimethoprim-sulfamethoxazole**

(*Bactrim, Septra,* and others), but experience with its use in serious MRSA infections is limited.

1. Vancomycin dosing and monitoring. Med Lett Drugs Ther 2009; 51:25.
2. M Rybak et al. Therapeutic monitoring of vancomycin in adult patients: a consensus review of the American Society of Health-System Pharmacists, the Infectious Diseases Society of America, and the Society of Infectious Diseases Pharmacists. Am J Health-Syst Pharm 2009; 66:82.

Vancomycin Dosing and Monitoring
Originally published in The Medical Letter – April 2009; 51:25

Consensus recommendations for dosing and therapeutic monitoring of intravenous (IV) vancomycin (*Vancocin*, and others) were recently published.[1] IV vancomycin has been used for decades as an alternative to penicillins for treatment of serious infections due to gram-positive cocci. In recent years, the widest use of the drug has been for treatment of serious methicillin-resistant *Staphylococcus aureus* (MRSA) infections.[2]

TOXICITY — Earlier formulations of vancomycin, which contained many impurities, were associated with infusion reactions, nephrotoxicity and ototoxicity. Current formulations, however, appear to be generally free of these toxicities, at least when the standard dose is used and the patient has normal renal function and is not taking a nephrotoxic drug (such as an aminoglycoside) concurrently. The most common adverse effects, such as fever, chills and phlebitis, are unrelated to serum drug concentrations. Red man syndrome can occur if the drug is infused too quickly.

SERUM CONCENTRATIONS — **Trough serum concentrations** measured at steady state just before a dose appear to be the best predictors of vancomycin efficacy and, possibly, toxicity. Trough serum concentrations should be >10 mg/L to minimize development of resistance. Higher trough concentrations of 15-20 mg/L have been recommended to improve penetration and clinical outcome in complicated infections, such as endocarditis and hospital-acquired pneumonia, caused by *S. aureus*.

The levels of vancomycin in the blood that would produce **nephrotoxicity** are not clear, and the safety of trough concentrations of 15-20 mg/L maintained over time is not clear either. **Ototoxicity** is uncommon with current formulations of vancomycin, and there is no evidence of any correlation with serum concentrations of the drug.

Peak serum concentrations do not appear to be a predictor of vancomycin efficacy or toxicity.

DOSING — The traditional dose of IV vancomycin has been 1 g or 15 mg/kg every 12 hours. This dose may be inadequate to achieve target trough concentrations in many patients with normal renal function, so a dose of 15-20 mg/kg (based on actual, not ideal or adjusted, body weight) every 8-12 hours is now recommended. In seriously ill patients, a loading dose of 25-30 mg/kg could be considered to rapidly achieve target serum concentrations. When the vancomycin minimum inhibitory concentration (MIC) for the infecting organism is ≥2 mg/L, the new recommendations suggest considering use of an alternative antibiotic. One such alternative would be linezolid *(Zyvox).*[3]

MONITORING RECOMMENDATIONS — Measuring steady-state trough serum concentrations of vancomycin may be helpful to make sure patients are receiving adequate doses of the drug. It might also be helpful in preventing nephrotoxicity in patients receiving higher doses and longer courses of the drug, in those with diminished or changing renal function, and in those receiving nephrotoxic drugs concurrently, but the new recommendations do not specify at which serum levels vancomycin dosage should be altered to prevent nephrotoxicity, or how to alter them. Monitoring for ototoxicity is not generally recommended but might be considered in older patients and those taking other ototoxic drugs.[4] Measuring peak serum concentrations of vancomycin is not recommended.

1. M Rybak et al. Therapeutic monitoring of vancomycin in adult patients: a consensus review of the American Society of Health-System Pharmacists, the Infectious Diseases Society of America, and the Society of Infectious Diseases Pharmacists. Am J Health-Syst Pharm 2009; 66:82.
2. Treatment of community-associated MRSA infections. Med Lett Drugs Ther 2006; 48:13.
3. Choice of antibacterial drugs. Treat Guidel Med Lett 2007; 5:33.
4. A Forouzesh et al. Vancomycin ototoxicity: a reevaluation in an era of increasing doses. Antimicrob Agents Chemother 2009; 53:483.

DRUGS FOR
Tuberculosis

Original publication date – October 2009

Even though the incidence continues to decline in the United States,[1] tuberculosis (TB) is still a common cause of death worldwide, and the prevalence of drug-resistant TB poses severe challenges to its treatment and control.[2,3] Guidelines with detailed management recommendations are available from the Centers for Disease Control and Prevention (CDC), American Thoracic Society and Infectious Diseases Society of America (IDSA).[4]

DIRECTLY OBSERVED THERAPY

Poor adherence to TB therapy is the most common cause of treatment failure and can lead to drug resistance. Medical Letter consultants recommend that most patients, including those with disease due to drug-susceptible strains, take drugs for active TB under direct observation. Compared to self-administered regimens, directly observed therapy (DOT) has been shown to decrease drug resistance, relapse rates and mortality, and improve cure rates.[5,6] DOT services are available through most local and state health departments. DOT is particularly important for treatment of patients with drug-resistant infections and for those receiving intermittent regimens because these are more susceptible to failure. Patients with latent infection who are at high risk for developing active TB should also be considered for DOT.

LATENT INFECTION

Patients with latent TB infection at high risk for developing active disease include those co-infected with HIV or receiving immunosuppressive therapy, young children, close contacts of patients with recent pulmonary TB, previously untreated patients with radiographic evidence of prior TB, and those who have developed a positive tuberculin test within the previous 2 years.[7,8]

The risk of serious disease, including miliary TB and tuberculous meningitis, is highest among infants, the elderly, and patients with HIV infection or other causes of severe immunosuppression.

Immunomodulating Drugs – Recent reports indicate a high risk for development of active TB disease in patients with latent TB infection who are treated with a TNF-alpha inhibitor such as infliximab *(Remicade)*, etanercept *(Enbrel)*, adalimumab *(Humira)*, certolizumab *(Cimzia)* or golimumab *(Simponi)*. These reports include cases of extrapulmonary and disseminated disease and death. Infliximab appears to be associated with a significantly higher risk than etanercept, and with a shorter time to onset of active disease.[9,10]

Patients preparing to undergo a solid organ transplant should be evaluated for risk of TB, including 2-step TB skin testing.[11] Treatment for latent TB infection should be considered for patients with a positive test once active TB is ruled out by a chest radiograph.[12] Treatment should start before transplantation and, if not completed, continue afterward.

Diagnosis – Culture is the gold standard, but the tuberculin skin test (purified protein derivative, PPD) has been in clinical use for over a century. Recently, interferon-gamma release assays (IGRAs) that measure host cell-mediated immune response to *Mycobacterium tuberculosis* have become available for diagnosis of TB infection. Unlike PPD skin testing, IGRA results are not affected by prior immunization with Bacille Calmette-Guerin (BCG) or exposure to most nontuberculous mycobacteria.

Currently, there are three FDA-approved IGRAs – the QuantiFERON-TB Gold (QFT-G), QFT-IT and T-Spot TB assay. All detect the immune response to two *M. tuberculosis* antigens that are not present in BCG vaccines and most nontuberculous mycobacteria (exceptions are *M. kansasii*, *M. marinum* and *M. szulgai*); QFT-IT includes a third TB specific antigen. The assays have not been studied in high-risk groups such as children, healthcare workers or immunocompromised patients. They appear to have high specificity, but variable sensitivity when compared to each other (the T-spot appears to be the most sensitive) and to the TB skin test. They may be most useful in BCG-vaccinated patients and in those unlikely to return for reading of a skin test.[13-15]

Treatment – Isoniazid (INH) is the standard treatment for latent TB infection presumed to be due to drug-susceptible strains. It should be given for 9 months, daily or intermittently.[4]

An alternative regimen for treatment of latent TB, particularly for patients intolerant to isoniazid or found to be tuberculin-positive after exposure to patients with organisms resistant to isoniazid, is daily **rifampin** alone for 4 months (6 months in children).[16,17] This shorter regimen has improved adherence and may have fewer adverse effects.[18] One clinical trial found 3-4 months of isoniazid plus rifampin to be safe and possibly superior to 9 months of isoniazid alone.[19]

Drug-Resistant Latent TB Infection – There are no data-based recommendations for treatment of latent TB infection in high-risk patients with known exposure to multidrug-resistant TB (MDRTB), defined as isolates with resistance at least to isoniazid and rifampin. Regimens with two drugs to which the organism is susceptible (e.g., pyrazinamide

FIRST LINE DRUGS FOR TUBERCULOSIS

Drug/formulation	Adult dosage	
	Daily[1]	Intermittent[2]
Isoniazid (INH)[3] 100, 300 mg tabs, 50 mg/5mL syrup, 100 mg/mL inj	5 mg/kg (max 300 mg) PO, IM or IV	15 mg/kg (max 900 mg) 2-3x/wk
Rifampin *(Rifadin, Rimactane)* 150, 300 mg caps, 600 mg inj powder	10 mg/kg (max 600 mg) PO or IV	10 mg/kg (max 600 mg) 2-3x/wk
Rifabutin[4] *(Mycobutin)* 150 mg caps	5 mg/kg (max 300 mg) PO	5 mg/kg (max 300 mg) 2-3x/wk
Rifapentine *(Priftin)* 150 mg tabs	—	10 mg/kg/wk continuation phase (max 600 mg) PO
Pyrazinamide 500 mg tabs	20-25 mg/kg PO (max 2 g)	30-50 mg/kg 2x/wk (max 4 g); 3x/wk (max 3 g)
Ethambutol[5] *(Myambutol)* 100, 400 mg tabs	15-25 mg/kg PO (max 1.6 g)	20-50 mg/kg 2x/wk (max 4 g); 3x/wk (max 2.4 g)

1. Or 5x/wk DOT.
2. Intermittent therapy is usually begun after a few weeks or months of treatment with a daily regimen.
3. Pyridoxine 25-50 mg should be given to prevent neuropathy in malnourished or pregnant patients and those with HIV infection, alcoholism or diabetes.
4. For use with amprenavir, fosamprenavir, nelfinavir or indinavir, the rifabutin dose is 150 mg/day or 300 mg 3 times a week. For use with atazanavir, ritonavir alone or ritonavir combined with other protease inhibitors, and lopinavir/ritonavir *(Kaletra)*, the rifabutin dose is further decreased to 150 mg every other day or 3 times weekly. For use with efavirenz, the rifabutin dose is increased to 450 mg/day or 600 mg 2-3 times weekly. Not recommended with saquinavir alone or delavirdine.

Pediatric dosage		Main adverse effects
Daily	**Intermittent²**	**Main adverse effects**
10-15 mg/kg (max 300 mg)	20-30 mg/kg (max 900 mg) 2x/wk	Hepatic toxicity, rash, peripheral neuropathy
10-20 mg/kg (max 600 mg)	10-20 mg/kg (max 600 mg) 2x/wk	Hepatic toxicity, rash, flu-like syndrome, pruritus, drug interactions
No data available	No data available	Hepatic toxicity, flu-like syndrome, uveitis, neutropenia, drug interactions
Not approved	Not approved	Similar to rifampin
15-30 mg/kg (max 2 g)	50 mg/kg (max 2 g) 2x/wk	Arthralgias, hepatic toxicity, pruritus, rash, hyperuricemia, GI upset
15-20 mg/kg (max 1 g)	50 mg/kg (max 2.5 g) 2x/wk	Decreased red-green color discrimination, decreased visual acuity, optic neuritis

5. Usually not recommended for children when visual acuity cannot be monitored. Some clinicians use 25 mg/kg/day during first one or two months or longer if organism is isoniazid-resistant. Decrease dosage if renal function is diminished.

plus either ethambutol or a fluoroquinolone for 9-12 months) have been used, but are poorly tolerated, can be hepatotoxic and are of uncertain efficacy.[20,21]

Extensively drug-resistant TB (XDRTB), defined as isolates with resistance not only to isoniazid and rifampin but also to any fluoroquinolone and at least one of 3 other second-line drugs (capreomycin, kanamycin or amikacin), is an increasing problem worldwide; there are no data-based recommendations for treatment of latent TB following exposure to XDRTB.[22,23]

Whatever treatment is chosen, these patients should be observed for up to 2 years following exposure.

ACTIVE DISEASE

All initial isolates of *M. tuberculosis* should be tested for antimicrobial susceptibility, but results generally do not become available for at least 2-4 weeks.[24] Standard treatment of active TB includes a **2-month initial phase** and a **continuation phase of either 4 or 7 months**, depending on the presence or absence of cavitary disease at the time of diagnosis and the results of sputum cultures taken at 2 months (see table on next page). Patients should be monitored monthly for adverse reactions, adherence and response to treatment.

Initial Therapy – Until susceptibility results are available, empiric initial treatment should include 4 drugs: isoniazid, rifampin, pyrazinamide and ethambutol. When susceptibility to isoniazid, rifampin and pyrazinamide has been documented, ethambutol can be omitted.[26] Patients who cannot take pyrazinamide, such as those with severe liver disease or gout, should take isoniazid, rifampin and ethambutol.

Immunomodulators are usually stopped in patients who develop active TB. The timing of restarting the biologic agent while still on TB treat-

DURATION OF CONTINUATION THERAPY[1]

Cavity on Chest X-ray	Drugs	Sputum culture taken at 2 mos	Duration (months)[2]
No	INH/RIF	Negative	4
	or INH/RPT[3]		4
No	INH/RIF	Positive[4]	4 or 7
	or INH/RPT[3]		7
Yes	INH/RIF	Negative	4 or 7
Yes	INH/RIF	Positive	7

INH = Isoniazid; RIF = rifampin; RPT = rifapentine
1. For treatment of drug-susceptible disease after two months of initial therapy.
2. Always 7 months for patients who could not take pyrazinamide as part of the initial regimen.
3. RPT is a treatment option only for non-pregnant, HIV-negative adults without cavitary or extrapulmonary disease who are smear-negative at 2 months.
4. If the culture is positive and the patient is taking INH/RPT, some Medical Letter consultants would switch to INH/RIF.

ment is controversial; some clinicians wait until the disease improves before restarting.

Continuation Therapy – Two factors that increase the risk of treatment failure and relapse are cavitary disease at presentation and a positive sputum culture taken at 2 months. For patients with drug-susceptible infection and one or no risk factors, the continuation phase of treatment should include isoniazid and rifampin for 4 months. For patients with both risk factors, those with initial resistance to pyrazinamide or those unable to take it as part of the initial regimen, the continuation phase should be extended to 7 months.

For HIV-negative patients without cavitary disease who have negative sputum smears after 2 months of therapy, rifapentine (a long-acting rifamycin), given once weekly for 4 months by DOT, is an option.[25]

SOME SECOND-LINE DRUGS

Drug	Daily adult dosage
Streptomycin[1]	15 mg/kg IM or IV (max 1 g)
Capreomycin (Capastat)	15 mg/kg IM or IV (max 1 g)
Kanamycin (Kantrex, and others)	15 mg/kg IM or IV (max 1 g)
Amikacin (Amikin)	15 mg/kg IM or IV (max 1 g)
Cycloserine[2] (Seromycin)	10-15 mg/kg (max 500 mg bid) PO
Ethionamide (Trecator-SC)	15-20 mg/kg in 2 doses (max 500 mg bid) PO
Levofloxacin (Levaquin)	500-1000 mg PO or IV
Moxifloxacin (Avelox)	400 mg PO or IV
Aminosalicylic acid (PAS; Paser)	8-12 g in 2-3 doses PO

1. Streptomycin is generally given 5-7 times per week (15 mg/kg, or a maximum of 1 g per dose) for an initial 2 to 12 week period, and then (if needed) 2 to 3 times per week (20 to 30 mg/kg, or a maximum of 1.5 g per dose). For patients >59 years old, dosage is reduced to 10 mg/kg (max 750 mg). Dosage should be decreased if renal function is diminished.
2. Some authorities recommend pyridoxine 50 mg for every 250 mg of cycloserine to decrease the incidence of adverse neurological effects.

Rifapentine should not be used if the patient has extrapulmonary TB or co-infection with HIV, is younger than 12 years of age or pregnant, or if drug susceptibility is unknown.

If sputum cultures remain positive after 4 months of treatment, nonadherence to treatment or infection with drug-resistant TB should be considered. Treatment duration should be prolonged in such patients.

TB osteomyelitis is usually treated for 6-9 months. Tuberculous meningitis is usually treated for a total of 9-12 months. Addition of a corticos-

Daily pediatric dosage	Main adverse effects
20-40 mg/kg	Vestibular and auditory toxicity, renal damage
15-30 mg/kg	Auditory and vestibular toxicity, renal damage, electrolyte disturbances
15-30 mg/kg	Auditory toxicity, renal damage
15-30 mg/kg	Auditory toxicity, renal damage
10-15 mg/kg	Psychiatric symptoms, seizures
15-20 mg/kg	GI and hepatic toxicity, hypothyroidism
See footnote 3	GI toxicity, CNS effects, rash, dysglycemia
See footnote 3	GI toxicity, CNS effects, rash, dysglycemia
200-300 mg/kg, in 2-4 doses (max 10 g)	GI disturbance

3. According to the American Academy of Pediatrics, although fluoroquinolones are generally contraindicated in children <18 years old, their use may be justified in special circumstances. Medical Letter consultants would use these drugs to treat children with MDRTB.

teroid for 1-2 months should be considered for tuberculous pericarditis or meningitis.[26]

Culture-Negative TB – Patients with evidence of pulmonary disease, 3 negative sputum cultures for *M. tuberculosis* before treatment, and clinical improvement on treatment have "culture-negative TB". In these patients, some experts shorten the continuation phase with isoniazid and rifampin to 2 months. Others believe that these patients should be treated for 6 months or longer.

Drug Intolerance – Adverse effects from first line anti-TB drugs are common.[4,25] Pyrazinamide is probably the most hepatotoxic of the first-line drugs.[27] In patients with asymptomatic hepatic toxicity, sequential rechallenge with isoniazid and rifampin often permits their use for the duration of treatment.[28]

For patients who cannot tolerate rifamycins, alternative regimens include 9-12 months of isoniazid, ethambutol and pyrazinamide, with or without a fluoroquinolone (levofloxacin or moxifloxacin). These two fluoro-quinolones are well tolerated in patients with drug-induced hepatic dysfunction [29] and are commonly used in combination with ethambutol and injectable drugs.[28] Levofloxacin appears to be safe for long-term use in patients with drug-resistant TB. Moxifloxacin may be more active than levofloxacin against *M. tuberculosis*, but clinical data are limited.

Isoniazid plus ethambutol for 18 months has also been used for patients intolerant of rifamycins. Rifabutin has been substituted for rifampin in standard regimens for some patients who could not take rifampin because of intolerance or unacceptable drug interactions (such as HIV co-infected patients on a protease inhibitor or patients with solid organ transplants).[12]

Intermittent Treatment – Intermittent 4-drug regimens (isoniazid, pyraz-inamide, rifampin, ethambutol) with **2 or 3 doses per week** are effective for treatment of active TB. All intermittent regimens should be given by DOT. Intermittent therapy is most commonly used in the continuation phase, after 2 months of daily (or 5x/wk) therapy during the initiation phase. It should never be used for treatment of drug-resistant TB.

A **once-weekly** continuation-therapy regimen of isoniazid plus rifapen-tine (instead of rifampin), started after 2 months of standard initial therapy, is also effective for drug-susceptible TB in selected patients.[4,25] This regimen has, however, been associated with development of rifamycin resistance in HIV-infected patients and should not be used in such patients.[30,31]

Twice-weekly intermittent regimens have also been associated with rifamycin resistance in HIV co-infected patients with low CD4 counts; such patients should receive daily or 3x/wk therapy. **Thrice-weekly** continuation regimens may also be preferable for other immunocompromised patients and for patients with cavitary disease.[32]

Fixed-Dose Combinations – A combination formulation of rifampin, isoniazid and pyrazinamide *(Rifater)* is approved by the FDA for the initial 2 months of daily anti-tuberculosis therapy. A combination of rifampin and isoniazid (*Rifamate*, and others) has been available in the US since 1975. Fixed-dose combinations may be particularly useful for patients self-administering their therapy.[33]

DRUG-RESISTANT TB DISEASE

Resistance to Isoniazid – Patients with TB resistant to isoniazid can be treated with rifampin, pyrazinamide and ethambutol for 6-9 months. If the organism is susceptible, streptomycin is an alternative to ethambutol. Patients who cannot tolerate pyrazinamide can take rifampin and ethambutol for 12 months. A fluoroquinolone or an injectable drug (capreomycin, amikacin, kanamycin or streptomycin) is sometimes added, especially if the patient cannot tolerate pyrazinamide or if there is extensive disease, but does not change treatment duration. Isoniazid may be beneficial in patients with TB resistant only to low concentrations of the drug.

Multidrug Resistance – Recommendations for treatment of MDRTB and XDRTB are based on limited data. MDRTB and XDRTB should be treated daily with ≥4 drugs to which the organism is susceptible.

When MDRTB is likely, or in patients with a history of treatment for TB, some experienced clinicians start with combinations of 5-7 drugs before laboratory susceptibility data become available. Typically, empiric therapy for suspected MDRTB includes isoniazid, rifampin, ethambutol, pyrazinamide, an aminoglycoside (streptomycin, kanamycin or amikacin) or capreomycin, a fluoroquinolone, and either cycloserine, ethionamide or aminosalicylic acid (PAS).[3,34,35] The regimen should include all active first-line drugs (e.g., pyrazinamide, ethambutol), plus a fluoroquinolone and one injectable drug.

For XDRTB, treatment options are even more limited and usually all drugs to which the organism is suscept-ible are used. Linezolid at a dose of 300-1200 mg daily, in combination with other anti-TB agents, appears to have some efficacy, but clinical trial data are lacking, adverse effects, particularly peripheral neuropathy, are common with prolonged use of high doses, and the drug is expensive.[36] Nevertheless, comprehensive management of XDRTB has resulted in outcomes not dissimilar to those with MDRTB, at least in HIV-negative patients.[37]

Monthly bacteriologic results (smear and culture) should be monitored and treatment continued for 18-24 months, or 12-18 months after the culture becomes negative. The parenteral drug should be continued for 6 months after culture conversion. Surgical resection has improved outcome in some patients and should be considered if cultures fail to become negative after 3-4 months of appropriate treatment.[38]

HIV-INFECTED PATIENTS

Testing for HIV infection is recommended for all patients with TB. Persons with HIV, once infected with *M. tuberculosis*, are at markedly increased risk of developing active TB disease. HIV-infected patients with a history of prior untreated or inadequately treated TB disease should be re-evaluated for active disease regardless of age or results of tests for latent TB infection. If active TB disease is ruled out, patients should receive treatment for latent TB infection. HIV-infected persons who have had recent close contact with a patient with active TB disease should receive empiric treatment for latent infection regardless of age, results of tests for TB infection, or history of previous treatment.

To minimize the emergence of drug-resistant TB, co-infected patients in the continuation phase of TB treatment should take medication once daily or, with DOT, three times weekly.[39] Twice-weekly regimens have been associated with acquisition of rifamycin resistance in patients with CD4 cell counts <100 cells/mm^3.[40] Once-weekly isoniazid/rifapentine is not recommended for TB treatment in HIV-infected patients because it has been associated with development of rifamycin resistance.[31]

Patients Not on HAART – Starting highly active antiretroviral therapy (HAART) during anti-TB therapy improves survival and virologic outcome.[41-43] Using fixed-dose combinations in the HAART regimen along with fixed-dose anti-TB drugs may facilitate adherence. The optimal regimen and timing for initiating HAART are unknown.

A rifamycin-based anti-TB regimen should be used if at all possible. Both efavirenz *(Sustiva)* and nevirapine *(Viramune)* can be used at standard doses with rifampin.[44] Efavirenz-based HAART may have a lower risk of hepatic toxicity when used with rifampin than nevirapine-based regimens.

Patients on HAART – Rifamycins induce hepatic CYP450 enzymes, especially CYP3A4, and can accelerate metabolism of protease inhibitors and some non-nucleoside reverse transcriptase inhibitors (NNRTIs), decreasing their serum concentrations, possibly to ineffective levels. The degree to which each drug induces CYP3A4 differs: rifampin is the most potent and rifabutin the least. In addition, rifabutin is a substrate of CYP3A4; protease inhibitors decrease its metabolism, increasing serum concentrations and possibly toxicity.

Standard 4-drug treatment regimens including rifampin can be given to HIV-infected patients with active TB who are simultaneously receiving HAART if the HAART regimen consists of efavirenz or nevirapine and two nucleoside reverse transcriptase inhibitors (NRTIs).[45]

Two alternative TB/HAART regimens are based on **rifabutin**, which appears to be as effective as rifampin against TB and has less effect on protease inhibitor concentrations. The first substitutes low-dose rifabutin (150 mg once/day or 300 mg 3x/week) for rifampin in the standard TB regimen (i.e., isoniazid, rifabutin, pyrazinamide and ethambutol) and uses higher-than-usual doses of indinavir *(Crixivan)* or nelfinavir *(Viracept)*, or standard doses of amprenavir *(Agenerase)* or fosamprenavir *(Lexiva)*, as the HIV protease inhibitor. The second decreases the rifabutin dose further to 150 mg every other day or 3 times weekly and uses a HAART regimen that includes standard doses of atazanavir *(Reyataz)*, ritonavir/lopinavir *(Kaletra)* or ritonavir alone or combined with other protease inhibitors. Saquinavir *(Invirase)* alone should not be used. Higher rifabutin doses (450 mg daily or 600 mg 2-3 times per week) are needed if the HAART regimen contains efavirenz.

Newer Antiretroviral Agents – The dose of maraviroc *(Selzentry)* must be increased to 600 mg twice daily when given with rifampin; when coadministered with rifabutin, no change in the doses of either drug is needed. Current recommendations state that the dose of raltegravir *(Isentress)* does not need to be adjusted for coadministration with either rifampin or rifabutin. Etravirine *(Intelence)* and rifampin should not be used together. Standard doses of etravirine may be safe to use with rifabutin. No data are available on the use of these drugs in patients with active TB.

TB IN PREGNANCY

Active TB disease during pregnancy requires treatment. The treatment of **latent TB infection** during pregnancy is more problematic because of the risk of hepatotoxicity and the scarcity of data on the risk of teratogenicity. In general, it is recommended that treatment for latent TB be delayed until 2 or 3 months after delivery. However, for women who are HIV-positive or have been recently infected with TB, initiation of therapy should not be delayed.

Treatment of **active TB disease** should be initiated in pregnancy when there is a moderate to high suspicion of disease because the risk to the fetus is much greater than the risk of adverse drug effects. The initial regimen should include isoniazid, rifampin and ethambutol. Each of these drugs crosses the placenta, but none are teratogenic. Pyrazinamide has not been extensively studied in pregnancy, but some Medical Letter consultants would use it in addition to isoniazid, rifampin and ethambutol.[46] If pyrazinamide is not used, treatment should be extended for a total of at least 9 months. Pyrazinamide is always recommended as part of the initial regimen in pregnant women who are HIV co-infected or when drug resistance is suspected.

Limited data are available on the treatment of MDRTB in pregnancy. Regimens using various combinations of amikacin, ethionamide, PAS, cycloserine, capreomycin and fluoroquinolones have been successful without causing fetal adverse effects, even though these drugs are generally not considered safe in pregnancy.[47,48]

ADVERSE EFFECTS

Isoniazid – Serum aminotransferase activity increases in 10-20% of patients taking isoniazid, especially in the early weeks of treatment, but often returns to normal even when the drug is continued. Severe liver damage due to isoniazid is less common than previously thought. It is more likely to occur in patients more than 35 years old. Clinical monitoring should occur monthly; monitoring of serum transaminases is not routinely recommended except for patients with pre-existing liver disease and those at increased risk for isoniazid hepatotoxicity, such as patients who drink alcohol regularly. Medical Letter consultants recommend stopping isoniazid when serum aminotransferase activity reaches five times the upper limit of normal or if the patient has symptoms of hepatitis. In patients with active TB disease it can usually be restarted later.[28,49] Rechallenge with isoniazid is not recommended for patients with latent TB infection.

Peripheral neuropathy occurs rarely and can usually be prevented by sup-plementation with pyridoxine (vitamin B6, 25-50 mg/day), which is rec-ommended for patients with chronic alcohol use, diabetes, chronic renal failure or HIV infection, and for those who are pregnant, breastfeeding or malnourished. Some Medical Letter consultants routinely use pyridoxine for all patients taking isoniazid. Pyridoxine does not need to be given to a nursing infant unless the baby is also being given isoniazid.

Rifamycins – Rifampin is potentially hepatotoxic. GI disturbances, morbilliform rash and thrombocytopenic purpura can occur. Whenever possible, rifampin should be continued despite minor adverse reactions such as pruritus and gastrointestinal upset. When taken erratically, the drug can cause a febrile "flu-like" syndrome and, very rarely, shortness of breath, hemolytic anemia, shock and acute renal failure. Patients should be warned that rifampin may turn urine, tears and other body fluids reddish-orange and can permanently stain contact lenses and lens implants.

Rifampin is an inducer of CYP isozymes 3A4, 2C9, 2C19, 2D6, 2B6 and 2C8. It can increase the metabolism and decrease the effect of many other drugs, including hormonal contraceptives, sulfonylureas, corticosteroids, warfarin, quinidine, methadone, delavirdine, etravirine, clarithromycin, ketoconazole, itraconazole and fluconazole, as well as protease inhibitors, the CCR5-antagonist maraviroc, and most statins (e.g., ator-vastatin, simvastatin).[50]

Rifabutin and **rifapentine** have adverse effects similar to those of rifampin. At higher doses, rifabutin can also cause uveitis, skin hyper-pigmentation and neutropenia, but is less likely than rifampin to interact with other drugs.

Other Drugs – Pyrazinamide can cause gastrointestinal disturbances, hepatotoxicity, arthralgias and hyperuricemia, and can block the hypouricemic action of allopurinol (*Zyloprim*, and others). It is the most common cause of hepatotoxicity and of drug rash among the first-line agents; some patients are able to continue the drug despite the rash. **Ethambutol** can cause optic neuritis, but only very rarely when using a dosage of 15 mg/kg daily. Testing of visual acuity and color perception should be performed at the start of therapy, and monthly thereafter. The decision to use ethambutol in children too young to have visual acuity monitored must take into consideration the risk/benefit for each particular patient.[51]

Streptomycin causes ototoxicity (usually vestibular disturbance) and, less frequently, renal toxicity. **Amikacin** and **kanamycin** can cause tinnitus and high-frequency hearing loss. These drugs and **capreomycin** can also cause renal and vestibular toxicity. Capreomycin in particular can cause severe electrolyte disturbances. **Cycloserine** can cause psychiatric symptoms and seizures. **Ethionamide** has been associated with gastrointestinal, hepatic and thyroid toxicity. A delayed-release granular formulation of **aminosalicylic acid** (PAS) has better gastrointestinal tolerability than older formulations. **Fluoroquinolones** are usually well-tolerated, but can cause gastrointestinal and CNS disturbances, and dysglycemia can occur, particularly in the elderly and in patients with diabetes. Fluoroquinolones are associated with an increased risk of tendon rupture. This risk is further increased in patients over 60 years of age, in patients taking corticosteroid drugs and in those with kidney, heart or lung transplants.

CONCLUSION

All initial isolates of *M. tuberculosis* should be tested for antimicrobial susceptibility. Initial therapy for most patients with active TB should include at least isoniazid, rifampin, pyrazinamide and ethambutol until susceptibility is known. Directly observed therapy (DOT) by a healthcare worker should be offered to all patients with active TB to minimize treatment failure, relapse and the emergence of drug resistance. It is especially important for patients on intermittent regimens. Confirmed multidrug-resistant tuberculosis and extensively drug-resistant tuberculosis

Drugs for Tuberculosis

(MDRTB and XDRTB) should be treated with DOT in collaboration with a clinician familiar with management of these conditions. Regimens for MDR and XDR TB must include at least 4 drugs to which the organism is susceptible; the duration of therapy usually should be 18-24 months.

(MDRTB and XDRTB) should be treated with DOT in collaboration with a clinician familiar with management of these conditions. Regimens for MDR and XDR TB must include at least 4 drugs to which the organism is susceptible; the duration of therapy usually should be 18-24 months.

1. CDC. Reported Tuberculosis in the United States, 2007. Atlanta, GA: U.S. Department of Health and Human Services, CDC, September 2008.
2. G Maartens and RJ Wilkinson. Tuberculosis. Lancet 2007; 370:2030.
3. A Wright et al. Epidemiology of antituberculosis drug resistance 2002-07: an updated analysis of the Global Project on Anti-Tuberculosis Drug Resistance Surveillance. Lancet 2009; 373:1861. Epub 2009 Apr 15.
4. American Thoracic Society; CDC; Infectious Diseases Society of America. Treatment of tuberculosis. MMWR Recomm Rep 2003; 52 (RR-11):1.
5. TR Frieden and SS Munsiff. The DOTS strategy for controlling the global tuberculosis epidemic. Clin Chest Med 2005; 26:197.
6. K DeRiemer et al. Does DOTS work in populations with drug-resistant tuberculosis? Lancet 2005; 365:1239.
7. CR Horsburgh Jr. Priorities for the treatment of latent tuberculosis infection in the United States. N Engl J Med 2004; 350:2060.
8. KP Cain et al. Tuberculosis among foreign-born persons in the United States: achieving tuberculosis elimination. Am J Respir Crit Care Med 2007; 175:75.
9. RS Wallis. Tumour necrosis factor antagonists: structure, function, and tuberculosis risks. Lancet Infect Dis. 2008; 8:601.
10. JJ Gomez-Reino et al. Risk of tuberculosis in patients treated with tumor necrosis factor antagonists due to incomplete prevention of reactivation of latent infection. Arthritis Rheum. 2007; 57:756.
11. Centers for Disease Control and Prevention (CDC). Guidelines for the investigation of contacts of persons with infectious tuberculosis. MMWR Recomm Rep 2005; 54 (RR-15):1.
12. JM Aguado et al. Tuberculosis in solid-organ transplant recipients: consensus statement of the group for the study of infection in transplant recipients (GESITRA) of the Spanish Society of Infectious Diseases and Clinical Microbiology. Clin Infect Dis 2009; 48:1276.
13. Centers for Disease Control and Prevention (CDC). Guidelines for using the QuantiFERON®-TB Gold test for detecting Mycobacterium tuberculosis infection, United States. MMWR Recomm Rep 2005;54 (RR-15):49.
14. M Pai et al. Systematic review: T-cell-based assays for the diagnosis of latent tuberculosis infection: an update. Ann Intern Med 2008; 149:177.
15. M Bocchino et al. IFN-gamma release assays in tuberculosis management in selected high-risk populations. Expert Rev Mol Diagn 2009; 9:165.
16. KR Page et al. Improved adherence and less toxicity with rifampin vs isoniazid for treatment of latent tuberculosis: a retrospective study. Arch Intern Med 2006; 166:1863.
17. A Lardizabal et al. Enhancement of treatment completion for latent tuberculosis infection with 4 months of rifampin. Chest 2006; 130:1712.

18. J Landry and D Menzies. Preventive chemotherapy. Where has it got us? Where to go next? Int J Tuberc Lung Dis. 2008; 12:1352.
19. NP Spyridis et al.The effectiveness of a 9-month regimen of isoniazid alone versus 3- and 4-month regimens of isoniazid plus rifampin for treatment of latent tuberculosis infection in children: results of an 11-year randomized study. Clin Infect Dis 2007; 45:715. Epub 2007 Aug 6.
20. T Papastavros et al. Adverse events associated with pyrazinamide and levofloxacin in the treatment of latent multidrug-resistant tuberculosis. CMAJ 2002; 167:131.
21. R Ridzon et al. Asymptomatic hepatitis in persons who received alternative preventive therapy with pyrazinamide and ofloxacin. Clin Infect Dis 1997; 24:1264.
22. Centers for Disease Control and Prevention (CDC). Revised definition of extensively drug-resistant tuberculosis. MMWR Morb Mortal Wkly Rep 2006; 55:1176.
23. NR Gandhi et al. Extensively drug-resistant tuberculosis as a cause of death in patients co-infected with tuberculosis and HIV in a rural area of South Africa. Lancet 2006; 368:1575.
24. GL Woods. The mycobacteriology laboratory and new diagnostic techniques. Infect Dis Clin North Am 2002; 16:127.
25. H Blumberg et al. Update on the treatment of tuberculosis and latent tuberculosis infection. JAMA 2005; 293:2776.
26. GE Thwaites et al. Dexamethasone for the treatment of tuberculous meningitis in adolescents and adults. N Engl J Med 2004; 351:1741.
27. D Yee et al. Incidence of serious side effects from first-line antituberculosis drugs among patients treated for active tuberculosis. Am J Respir Crit Care Med 2003; 167:1472.
28. JJ Saukkonen et al. for the ATS (American Thoracic Society) Hepatotoxicity of Antituberculosis Therapy Subcommittee. An official ATS statement: hepatotoxicity of antituberculosis therapy. Am J Resp Crit Care Med 2006; 174:935.
29. CC Ho et al. Safety of fluoroquinolone use in patients with hepatotoxicity induced by anti-tuberculosis regimens. Clin Infect Dis 2009; 48:1526.
30. FM Gordin. Rifapentine for the treatment of tuberculosis: is it all it can be? Am J Respir Crit Care Med 2004; 169:1176.
31. A Vernon et al. Acquired rifamycin monoresistance in patients with HIV-related tuberculosis treated with once-weekly rifapentine and isoniazid. Tuberculosis Trials Consortium. Lancet 1999; 353:1843.
32. KC Chang et al. Dosing schedules of 6-month regimens and relapse for pulmonary tuberculosis. Am J Resp Crit Care Med 2006; 174:1153. Epub 2006 Aug 14.
33. B Blomberg and B Fourie. Fixed-dose combination drugs for tuberculosis: application in standardised treatment regimens. Drugs 2003; 63:535.
34. JA Caminero. Treatment of multidrug-resistant tuberculosis: evidence and controversies. Int J Tuberc Lung Dis 2006; 10:829.
35. JS Mukherjee et al. Programmes and principles in treatment of multidrug-resistant tuberculosis. Lancet 2004; 363:474.
36. WJ Koh et al. Daily 300 mg dose of linezolid for the treatment of intractable multidrug-resistant and extensively drug-resistant tuberculosis. J Antimicrob Chemother 2009; 64:388.

37. CD Mitnick et al. Comprehensive treatment of extensively drug-resistant tuberculosis. N Engl J Med 2008; 359:563.

38. ED Chan et al. Treatment and outcome analysis of 205 patients with multi-drug resistant tuberculosis. Am J Respir Crit Care Med 2004; 169:1103.

39. Centers for Disease Control and Prevention (CDC). Acquired rifamycin resistance in persons with advanced HIV disease being treated for active tuberculosis with intermittent rifamycin-based regimens. MMWR Morb Mortal Wkly Rep 2002; 51:214.

40. RE Nettles et al. Risk factors for relapse and acquired rifamycin resistance after directly observed tuberculosis treatment: a comparison by HIV serostatus and rifamycin use. Clin Infect Dis 2004; 38:731.

41. A Boulle et al. Outcomes of nevirapine- and efavirenz-based antiretroviral therapy when coadministered with rifampicin-based antitubercular therapy. JAMA 2008; 300:530.

42. AD Harries et al. Providing HIV care for co-infected tuberculosis patients: a perspective from sub-Saharan Africa. Int J Tuberc Lung Dis 2009; 13:6.

43. M Velasco et al. Effect of simultaneous use of highly active antiretroviral therapy on survival of HIV-infected patients with tuberculosis. J Acquir Immune Defic Syndr 2009; 50:148.

44. www.aidsinfo.nih.gov. Accessed September 8, 2009.

45. Centers for Disease Control and Prevention (CDC). Managing drug interactions in the treatment of HIV-related tuberculosis. Available at http://www.cdc.gov/tb/publications/guidelines/TB_HIV_Drugs/PDF/tbhiv.pdf. Accessed September 1, 2009.

46. G Bothamley. Drug treatment for tuberculosis during pregnancy: safety considerations. Drug Saf 2001; 24:553.

47. E Palacios et al. Drug-resistant tuberculosis and pregnancy: treatment outcome of 38 cases in Lima, Peru. Clin Infect Dis 2009; 48:1413.

48. KD Lessnau and S Qarah. Multidrug-resistant tuberculosis in pregnancy: case report and review of the literature. Chest 2003; 123:953.

49. SS Munsiff et al. Clinical Policies and Protocols (TB manual), Bureau of Tuberculosis Control, 4th Edition. March 2008, New York City Department of Health and Mental Hygiene, New York, NY. Available at http://www.nyc.gov/html/doh/downloads/pdf/tb/tb-protocol.pdf. Accessed September 1, 2009.

50. Medical Letter Adverse Drug Interactions Program.

51. World Health Organization. Ethambutol efficacy and toxicity: literature review and recommendations for daily and intermittent dosage in children. Available at http://whqlibdoc.who.int/hq/2006/who_htm_ tb_2006.365_eng.pdf. Accessed September 1, 2009.

ANTIMICROBIAL PROPHYLAXIS FOR Surgery

Original publication date – June 2009

Antimicrobial prophylaxis can decrease the incidence of infection, particularly surgical site infection, after certain procedures. Recommendations for prevention of surgical site infection are listed in the table that begins on page 122. Antimicrobial prophylaxis for dental procedures to prevent endocarditis is discussed in The Medical Letter 2007; 49:99.

CHOICE OF A PROPHYLACTIC AGENT

An effective prophylactic regimen should be directed against the most likely infecting organisms, but need not eradicate every potential pathogen. For most procedures, the first-generation cephalosporin **cefazolin** (*Ancef*, and others), which is active against many staphylococci and streptococci, remains effective. For procedures that might involve exposure to bowel anaerobes, including *Bacteroides fragilis*, the second-generation cephalosporins **cefoxitin** (*Mefoxin*, and others) and **cefotetan** are more active than cefazolin against these organisms. **Cefazolin** plus **metronidazole** (*Flagyl*, and others), or **ampicillin/sulbactam** (*Unasyn*, and others) alone, are reasonable alternatives.[1] **Cefuroxime** (*Zinacef*, and others) is a second-generation cephalosporin with little activity against *B. fragilis*, but it can be used instead of cefazolin in non-cardiac thoracic or orthopedic operations. In institutions where surgical site infections are frequently due to methicillin-resistant *Staphylococcus* *aureus* (MRSA) or methicillin-resistant coagulase-negative staphylococci, **vancomycin** (*Vancocin*, and others) can be used for prophylaxis, but it may not be more effective than cefazolin in these settings and such use could lead to emergence of vancomycin-resistant organisms.[2]

Screening for MRSA – Pre-operative identification of patients colonized with MRSA and subsequent decolonization using intranasal mupirocin (*Bactroban*, and others) remains controversial.[3,4] Intranasal mupirocin has been shown to decrease the rate of post-operative infections with MRSA in some patients who were colonized before surgery.[5,6] The Society of Thoracic Surgeons recommends decolonization with mupirocin prior to cardiac surgery for all patients without documented negative testing (via nasopharyngeal swab and culture or PCR) for MRSA.[7]

Decontamination with an oral formulation of chlorhexidine gluconate (*Peridex*, and others) has also been tried with some success.[8,9] However, other studies using chlorhexidine bathing have not found any impact on surgical site infection.[10,11]

TIMING AND NUMBER OF DOSES

It has been common practice to give antibiotics at the time of anesthesia induction, which results in adequate serum and tissue levels. For procedures lasting less than 4 hours, Medical Letter consultants recommend a single intravenous dose of an antimicrobial started within 60 minutes before the initial skin incision. If vancomycin or a fluoroquinolone is used, the infusion should begin 60-120 minutes before the incision to minimize the risk of antibiotic-associated reactions around the time of anesthesia induction and to ensure adequate tissue levels of the drug at the time of the initial incision.

Additional Doses – Published studies of antimicrobial prophylaxis often use one or two doses postoperatively in addition to one dose just before surgery; most Medical Letter consultants believe that postoperative doses are usually unnecessary and can increase the risk of antimicrobial resistance.

INDICATIONS

Cardiac Surgery – Preoperative antibiotics can decrease the incidence of infection after cardiac surgery, and intraoperative redosing has been associated with a decreased risk of postoperative infection in procedures lasting >400 minutes.[12] Single-dose prophylaxis or 24-hour prophylaxis may be as effective as 48-hour prophylaxis.[13] There is no evidence of benefit beyond 48 hours.

Antimicrobial prophylaxis for prevention of **device-related infections** has not been rigorously studied, but is generally used before placement of electrophysiologic devices, ventricular assist devices, ventriculoatrial shunts and arterial patches.[14] Studies of antimicrobial prophylaxis for implantation of **permanent pacemakers** and **cardioverter-defibrillators** have shown a significant reduction in the incidence of wound infection, inflammation and skin erosion.[15,16]

Gastrointestinal Surgery – Antimicrobial prophylaxis is recommended for **esophageal** surgery in the presence of obstruction, which increases the risk of infection. After **gastroduodenal** surgery, the risk of infection is high when gastric acidity and gastrointestinal motility are diminished by obstruction, hemorrhage, gastric ulcer or malignancy, or by therapy with an H_2-blocker or proton pump inhibitor, and is also high in patients with morbid obesity.[17] One dose of cefazolin before surgery can decrease the incidence of postoperative infection in these circumstances. Prophylaxis is not indicated for routine gastroesophageal endoscopy, but most clinicians use it before placement of a percutaneous gastrostomy.[18-20]

Preoperative antibiotics are used routinely for **bariatric surgery**, including adjustable gastric banding, vertical banded gastroplasty, Roux-en-y

ANTIMICROBIAL PROPHYLAXIS FOR SURGERY

Nature of Operation	Common Pathogens
CARDIAC	
	Staphylococcus aureus, S. epidermidis
GASTROINTESTINAL	
Esophageal, gastroduodenal	Enteric gram-negative bacilli, gram-positive cocci
Biliary tract	Enteric gram-negative bacilli, enterococci, clostridia
Colorectal	Enteric gram-negative bacilli, anaerobes, enterococci
Appendectomy, non-perforated[8]	Same as for colorectal

1. Parenteral prophylactic antimicrobials can be given as a single IV dose begun 60 minutes or less before the operation. For prolonged operations (>4 hours), or those with major blood loss, additional intraoperative doses should be given at intervals 1-2 times the half-life of the drug (ampicillin/sulbactam q2-4 hours, cefazolin q2-5 hours, cefuroxime q3-4 hours, cefoxitin q2-3 hours, clindamycin q3-6 hours, vancomycin q6-12 hours, and metronidazole q6-8 hours [DW Bratzler et al. Clin Infect Dis 2004; 38:1706]) for the duration of the procedure in patients with normal renal function. If vancomycin or a fluoroquinolone is used, the infusion should be started 60-120 minutes before the initial incision in order to minimize the possibility of an infusion reaction close to the time of induction of anesthesia and to have adequate tissue levels at the time of incision.
2. Some consultants recommend an additional dose when patients are removed from bypass during open-heart surgery.
3. Vancomycin can be used in hospitals in which methicillin-resistant *S. aureus* and *S. epidermidis* are a frequent cause of postoperative wound infection, patients previously colonized with MRSA, or for those who are allergic to penicillins or cephalosporins. Rapid IV administration may cause hypotension, which could be especially dangerous during induction of anesthesia. Even when the drug is

Recommended Antimicrobials	Adult Dosage Before Surgery[1]
cefazolin	1-2 g IV[2]
OR vancomycin[3]	1 g IV
High risk[4] only: cefazolin[5]	1-2 g IV
High risk[6] only: cefazolin[5]	1-2 g IV
Oral: neomycin + erythromycin base[7]	
OR + metronidazole[7]	
Parenteral: cefoxitin[5] or cefotetan[5]	1-2 g IV
OR cefazolin	1-2 g IV
+ metronidazole	0.5 g IV
OR ampicillin/sulbactam[5]	3 g IV
cefoxitin[5] or cefotetan[5]	1-2 g IV
OR cefazolin	1-2 g IV
+ metronidazole	0.5 g IV
OR ampicillin/sulbactam[5]	3 g IV

given over 60 minutes, hypotension may occur; treatment with diphenhydramine (*Benadryl*, and others) and further slowing of the infusion rate may be helpful. Some experts would give 15 mg/kg of vancomycin to patients weighing more than 75 kg, up to a maximum of 1.5 g, with a slower infusion rate (90 minutes for 1.5 g). For operations in which enteric gram-negative bacilli are common pathogens, many Medical Letter consultants would add another drug such as an aminoglycoside (gentamicin, tobramycin or amikacin).

4. Morbid obesity, esophageal obstruction, decreased gastric acidity or gastrointestinal motility.
5. For patients allergic to penicillins and cephalosporins, clindamycin with either gentamicin, ciprofloxacin, levofloxacin or aztreonam is a reasonable alternative. Fluoroquinolones should not be used for prophylaxis in cesarean section.
6. Age >70 years, acute cholecystitis, non-functioning gall bladder, obstructive jaundice or common duct stones.
7. 1 g of neomycin plus 1 g of erythromycin at 1 PM, 2 PM and 11 PM or 2 g of neomycin plus 2 g of metronidazole at 7 PM and 11 PM the day before an 8 AM operation.
8. For a ruptured viscus, therapy is often continued for about five days.

Continued on next page.

ANTIMICROBIAL PROPHYLAXIS FOR SURGERY (continued)

Nature of Operation	Common Pathogens
GENITOURINARY	
Cystoscopy alone	Enteric gram-negative bacilli, enterococci
Cystoscopy with manipulation or Upper tract instrumentation[10]	Enteric gram-negative bacilli, enterococci
Open or laparoscopic surgery[11]	Enteric gram-negative bacilli, enterococci
GYNECOLOGIC AND OBSTETRIC	
Vaginal, abdominal or laparoscopic hysterectomy	Enteric gram-negative bacilli, anaerobes, Gp B strep, enterococci
Cesarean section	same as for hysterectomy
Abortion	same as for hysterectomy
HEAD AND NECK SURGERY	
Incisions through oral or pharyngeal mucosa	Anaerobes, enteric gram-negative bacilli, S. aureus
NEUROSURGERY	
	S. aureus, S. epidermidis

9. Urine culture positive or unavailable, preoperative catheter, transrectal prostatic biopsy, placement of prosthetic material.
10. Shockwave lithotripsy, ureteroscopy.
11. Including percutaneous renal surgery, procedures with entry into the urinary tract, and those involving implantation of a prosthesis. If manipulation of bowel is involved prophylaxis is given according to colorectal guidelines.

	Recommended Antimicrobials	Adult Dosage Before Surgery[1]
	High risk[9] only:	
	ciprofloxacin	500 mg PO or 400 mg IV
OR	trimethoprim-sulfamethoxazole	1 DS tablet
	ciprofloxacin	500 mg PO or 400 mg IV
OR	trimethoprim-sulfamethoxazole	1 DS tablet
	cefazolin[5]	1-2 g IV
	cefoxitin[5], cefotetan[5] or cefazolin[5]	1-2 g IV
OR	ampicillin/sulbactam[5]	3 g IV
	cefazolin[5]	1-2 g IV
	doxycycline	300 mg PO[12]
	clindamycin	600-900 mg IV
OR	cefazolin	1-2 g IV
	+ metronidazole	0.5 g IV
	cefazolin	1-2 g IV
OR	vancomycin[3]	1 g IV

12. Divided into 100 mg one hour before the abortion and 200 mg one half hour after.

Continued on next page.

Nature of Operation	Common Pathogens
OPHTHALMIC	S. epidermidis, S. aureus, streptococci, enteric gram-negative bacilli, Pseudomonas spp.
ORTHOPEDIC	S. aureus, S. epidermidis
THORACIC (NON-CARDIAC)	S. aureus, S. epidermidis, streptococci, enteric gram-negative bacilli
VASCULAR Arterial surgery involving a prosthesis, the abdominal aorta, or a groin incision	S. aureus, S. epidermidis, enteric gram-negative bacilli
Lower extremity amputation for ischemia	S. aureus, S. epidermidis, enteric gram-negative bacilli, clostridia

13. If a tourniquet is to be used in the procedure, the entire dose of antibiotic must be infused prior to its inflation.

bypass and biliopancreatic diversion, but no controlled trials supporting such use are available.

Antimicrobial prophylaxis is recommended before **biliary tract** surgery for patients with a high risk of infection, such as those more than 70 years old and those with acute cholecystitis, a non-functioning gallbladder, obstructive jaundice or common duct stones. Similar guidelines apply to antibiotic prophylaxis of endoscopic retrograde cholan-

Recommended Antimicrobials	Adult Dosage Before Surgery[1]
gentamicin, tobramycin, ciprofloxacin, gatifloxacin, levofloxacin, moxifloxacin, ofloxacin or neomycin-gramicidin-polymyxin B	multiple drops topically over 2 to 24 hours
OR cefazolin	100 mg subconjunctivally
cefazolin[13]	1-2 g IV
or cefuroxime[13]	1.5 g IV
OR vancomycin[3,13]	1 g IV
cefazolin or	1-2 g IV
cefuroxime	1.5 g IV
OR vancomycin[3]	1 g IV
cefazolin	1-2 g IV
OR vancomycin[3]	1 g IV
cefazolin	1-2 g IV
OR vancomycin[3]	1 g IV

giopancreatography (ERCP).[21,22] Prophylactic antibiotics are generally not necessary for low-risk patients undergoing elective laparoscopic cholecystectomy.[23,24]

Preoperative antibiotics can decrease the incidence of infection after **colorectal** surgery; for elective operations, an oral regimen of neomycin (not available in Canada) plus either erythromycin or metronidazole appears to be as effective as parenteral drugs. Many surgeons in the US use a combination of oral and parenteral agents; whether such combinations are more effective than just one or the other is unclear. Several meta-analyses indicate that mechanical bowel preparation (similar to a colonoscopy prep) before elective colorectal surgery is not helpful in preventing infection.[25-28]

Preoperative antimicrobials can decrease the incidence of infection after surgery for acute appendicitis.[29,30] If perforation has occurred, antibiotics are often used therapeutically rather than prophylactically and are continued for 5-7 days. In studies of penetrating abdominal and intestinal injuries, however, a short course (12-24 hours) was as effective as 5 days of therapy.[31-33]

Genitourinary Surgery – Medical Letter consultants do not recommend antimicrobial prophylaxis before cystoscopy without manipulation (dilation, biopsy, fulguration, resection or ureteral instrumentation) in patients with sterile urine. When cystoscopy with manipulation is planned, the urine culture is positive or unavailable, or an indwelling urinary catheter is present, patients should either be treated to sterilize the urine before surgery or receive a single preoperative dose of an agent active against the likely microorganisms.

Antimicrobial prophylaxis decreases the incidence of postoperative bacteriuria and septicemia in patients with sterile preoperative urine undergoing **transurethral prostatectomy** and **transrectal prostatic biopsies**.[34-36] Prophylaxis is also used for ureteroscopy, shock wave lithotripsy, percutaneous renal surgery, open laparoscopic procedures, and when a **urologic prosthesis** (penile implant, artificial sphincter, synthetic pubovaginal sling, bone anchors for pelvic floor reconstruction) will be placed.[37]

Gynecology and Obstetrics – Antimicrobial prophylaxis decreases the incidence of infection after vaginal or abdominal **hysterectomy**.[38] Prophylaxis is also used for laparoscopic hysterectomies. Antimicrobials can prevent infection after elective and non-elective **cesarean section;** dosing prior to skin incision appears to be more effective than dosing after clamping.[39-41] Antimicrobial prophylaxis can also prevent infection after **elective abortion**.[42]

Head and Neck Surgery – Prophylaxis with antimicrobials has decreased the incidence of surgical site infection after oncologic head and neck operations that involve an incision through the oral or pharyngeal mucosa.[43] One study, however, found no benefit from antimicrobial prophylaxis in patients undergoing open reduction or internal fixation of mandibular fractures.[44]

Neurosurgery – An antistaphylococcal antibiotic can decrease the incidence of infection after **craniotomy**.[45,46] In **spinal surgery**, the infection rate after conventional lumbar discectomy is low, but the serious consequences of a surgical site infection have led many surgeons to use perioperative antibiotics. One meta-analysis concluded that antibiotic prophylaxis prevents infection even in low-risk spinal surgery.[47] Infection rates are higher after prolonged spinal surgery or spinal procedures involving fusion or insertion of foreign material, and prophylactic antibiotics are generally used.[48] Some studies of antimicrobial prophylaxis for implantation of permanent **cerebrospinal fluid shunts** have shown lower infection rates with use of prophylactic antibiotics; the benefits of antimicrobial prophylaxis for ventriculostomy placement remains uncertain.[49]

Ophthalmic Surgery – Data are limited on the effectiveness of antimicrobial prophylaxis for ophthalmic surgery, but most ophthalmologists use antimicrobial eye drops for prophylaxis, and some also give a subconjunctival injection of an antimicrobial or add antimicrobial drops to the intraocular irrigation solution.[50] There is no consensus supporting a particular choice, route or duration of antimicrobial prophylaxis.[51] Preoperative povidone-iodine applied to the skin and conjunctiva has been associated with a lower incidence of culture-proven endophthalmitis.[52] There is no evidence that prophylactic antibiotics are needed for procedures that do not invade the globe.

Orthopedic Surgery – Prophylactic antistaphylococcal drugs administered preoperatively can decrease the incidence of both early and delayed infection following joint replacement and after surgical repair of **closed fractures**.[53,54] They also decrease the rate of infection when hip and other closed fractures are treated with internal fixation by nails, plates, screws or wires, and in compound or open fractures. Whether single-dose or 24-hour prophylactic use of antibiotics is superior is unclear.[55,56] A retrospective review of patients undergoing diagnostic and operative **arthroscopic surgery** concluded that antibiotic prophylaxis is not indicated, but that view is controversial.[57,58]

Thoracic (Non-Cardiac) Surgery – Antibiotic prophylaxis is used routinely in thoracic surgery, but supporting data remain sparse. In one study, a single preoperative dose of cefazolin before **pulmonary resection** led to a decrease in the incidence of surgical site infection, but not of pneumonia or empyema.[59] A retrospective review of 312 patients who underwent major lung resection found that 24% developed post-operative pneumonia despite antibacterial prophylaxis; the study did not evaluate surgical site infections.[60] Other trials have found that multiple doses of a cephalosporin can prevent infection after **closed-tube thoracostomy** for chest trauma with hemo- or pneumothorax.[61] Insertion of chest tubes for other indications, such as spontaneous pneumothorax, does not require antimicrobial prophylaxis.

Vascular Surgery – Preoperative administration of a cephalosporin decreases the incidence of postoperative surgical site infection after arterial reconstructive surgery on the abdominal aorta, vascular operations on the leg that include a groin incision, and amputation of the lower extremity for ischemia.[62,63] Many experts also recommend prophylaxis for implantation of any vascular prosthetic material, such as grafts for vascular access in hemodialysis. Prophylaxis is not indicated for carotid endarterectomy or brachial artery repair without prosthetic material.

Other Procedures – Antimicrobial prophylaxis is generally not indicated for cardiac catheterization, varicose vein surgery, most dermatologic[64] and plastic surgery, arterial puncture, thoracentesis, paracentesis, repair of simple lacerations, outpatient treatment of burns, dental extractions or root canal therapy because the incidence of surgical site infections is low.

The need for prophylaxis in breast surgery, herniorrhaphy and other "clean" surgical procedures has been controversial. Medical Letter consultants generally do not recommend surgical prophylaxis for these procedures because of the low rate of infection and the potential adverse effects of prophylaxis in such a large number of patients; some recommend prophylaxis for procedures involving placement of prosthetic material (e.g., synthetic mesh, saline implants, tissue expanders).

1. DW Bratzler and DR Hunt. The surgical infection prevention and surgical care improvement projects: national initiatives to improve outcomes for patients having surgery. Clin Infect Dis 2006; 43:322.
2. G Zanetti and R Platt. Antibiotic prophylaxis for cardiac surgery: does the past predict the future? Clin Infect Dis 2004; 38:1364.
3. M Trautmann et al. Intranasal mupirocin prophylaxis in elective surgery. A review of published studies. Chemotherapy 2008; 54:9.
4. M van Rijen et al. Mupirocin ointment for preventing Staphylococcus aureus infections in nasal carriers. Cochrane Database Syst Rev 2008; (4): CD006216.
5. NK Shrestha et al. Safety of targeted perioperative mupirocin treatment for preventing infections after cardiac surgery. Ann Thorac Surg 2006; 81:2183.
6. MM van Rijen and JA Kluytmans. New approaches to prevention of staphylococcal infection in surgery. Curr Opin Infect Dis 2008; 21:380.
7. R Engelman et al. The Society of Thoracic Surgeons practice guidelines series: antibiotic prophylaxis in cardiac surgery, part II: antibiotic choice. Ann Thorac Surg 2007; 83:1569.
8. P Segers et al. Prevention of nosocomial infection in cardiac surgery by decontamination of the nasopharynx and oropharynx with chlorhexidine gluconate: a randomized controlled trial. JAMA 2006; 296:2460.
9. SL Richer and BL Wenig. The efficacy of preoperative screening and the treatment of methicillin-resistant Staphylococcus aureus in an otolaryngology surgical practice. Otolaryngol Head Neck Surg 2009; 140:29.

10. DF Veiga et al. Randomized controlled trial of the effectiveness of chlorhexidine showers before elective plastic surgical procedures. Infect Control Hosp Epidemiol 2009; 30:77.

11. J Webster and S Osborne. Preoperative bathing or showering with skin antiseptics to prevent surgical site infection. Cochrane Database Syst Rev 2007; (2): CD004985.

12. G Zanetti et al. Intraoperative redosing of cefazolin and risk for surgical site infection in cardiac surgery. Emerg Infect Dis 2001; 7:828.

13. FH Edwards et al. The Society of Thoracic Surgeons practice guidelines series: antibiotic prophylaxis in cardiac surgery, part I: duration. Ann Thorac Surg 2006; 81:397.

14. LM Baddour et al. Nonvalvular cardiovascular device-related infections. Circulation 2003; 108:2015.

15. JC deOliveira et al. Efficacy of antibiotic prophylaxis before the implantation of pacemakers and cardioverter-defibrillators. Circ Arrhythmia Electrophysiol 2009; 2:29.

16. MR Sohail et al. Risk factors analysis of permanent pacemaker infection. Clin Infect Dis 2007; 45:166.

17. AJ Chong and EP Dellinger. Infectious complications of surgery in morbidly obese patients. Curr Treat Options Infect Dis 2003; 5:387.

18. S Banerjee et al. Antibiotic prophylaxis for GI endoscopy. Gastrointest Endosc 2008; 67:791.

19. NS Jafri et al. Meta-analysis: antibiotic prophylaxis to prevent peristomal infection following percutaneous endoscopic gastrostomy. Aliment Pharmacol Ther 2007; 94:647.

20. S Mahadeva et al. Antibiotic prophylaxis tailored to local organisms reduces percutaneous gastrostomy site infection. Int J Clin Prac 2009; 29:1086.

21. JS Mallery et al. Complications of ERCP. Gastrointest Endosc 2003; 57:633.

22. PB Cotton et al. Infection after ERCP, and antibiotic prophylaxis: a sequential quality-improvement approach over 11 years. Gastrointest Endosc 2008; 67:471.

23. H Zhou and Z Hu. Meta-analysis: Antibiotic prophylaxis in elective laparoscopic cholecystectomy. Aliment Pharmacol Ther 2009, Feb 19 Epub.

24. A Choudhary et al. Role of prophylactic antibiotics in laparoscopic cholecystectomy: a meta-analysis. J Gastrointest Surg 2008; 12:1847.

25. K Slim et al. Updated systematic review and meta-analysis of randomized clincal trials on the role of mechanical bowel preparation before colorectal surgery. Ann Surg 2009; 249:203.

26. G Gravante et al. Mechanical bowel preparation for colorectal surgery: a meta-analysis on abdominal and systemic complications on almost 5,000 patients. Int J Colorectal Dis 2008; 23:1145.

27. CE Pineda et al. Mechanical bowel preparation in intestinal surgery: a meta-analysis and review of the literature. J Gastrointest Surg 2008; 12:2037.

28. KK Guenaga et al. Mechanical bowel preparation for elective colorectal surgery. Cochrane Database Syst Rev 2009; (1):CD001544.

29. BR Andersen et al. Antibiotics versus placebo for prevention of postoperative infection after appendicectomy. Cochrane Database Syst Rev 2003; 2:CD001439.

30. LM Mui et al. Optimum duration of prophylactic antibiotics in acute non-perforated appendicitis. ANZ J Surg 2005; 75:425.

31. EP Dellinger et al. Efficacy of short-course antibiotic prophylaxis after penetrating intestinal injury. A prospective randomized trial. Arch Surg 1986; 121:23.

32. A Bozorgzadeh et al. The duration of antibiotic administration in penetrating abdominal trauma. Am J Surg 1999; 177:125.

33. EE Cornwell 3rd et al. Duration of antibiotic prophylaxis in high-risk patients with penetrating abdominal trauma: a prospective randomized trial. J Gastrointest Surg 1999; 3:648.

34. A Berry and A Barratt. Prophylatic antibiotic use in transurethral prostatic resection: a meta-analysis. J Urol 2002; 167:571.

35. W Qiang et al. Antibiotic prophylaxis for transuretheral prostatic resection in men with preoperative urine containing less than 100,000 bacteria per ml: a systematic review. J Urol 2005; 173:1175.

36. M Aron et al. Antibiotic prophylaxis for transrectal needle biopsy of the prostate: a randomized controlled study. BJU Int 2000; 85:682.

37. JS Wolf et al. Best practice policy statement on urologic surgery antimicrobial prophylaxis. J Urol 2008; 179:1379.

38. WJ Ledger. Prophylactic antibiotics in obstetrics-gynecology: a current asset or a future liability? Expert Rev Anti Infect Ther 2006; 4:957.

39. AJ Kaimal et al. Effect of a change in policy regarding the timing of prophylactic antibiotics on the rate of postcesarean delivery surgical-site infections. Am J Obstet Gynecol 2008; 199:310.

40. MM Constantine et al. Timing of perioperative antibiotics for cesarean delivery: a meta-analysis. Am J Obstet Gynecol 2008; 199:301.

41. SA Sullivan et al. Administration of cefazolin prior to skin incision is superior to cefazolin at cord clamping in preventing postcesarean infectious morbidity: a randomized controlled trial. Am J Obstet Gynecol 2007; 196:455.

42. ACOG Practice Bulletin. Antimicrobial prophylaxis for gynecologic procedures. Obstet Gynecol 2009; 113:1180.

43. R Simo and G French.The use of prophylactic antibiotics in head and neck oncological surgery. Curr Opin Otolaryngol Head Neck Surg 2006; 14:55.

44. BA Miles et al. The efficacy of postoperative antibiotic regimens in the open treatment of mandibular fractures: a prospective randomized trial. J Oral Maxillofac Surg 2006; 64:576.

45. FG Barker II. Efficacy of prophylactic antibiotics against meningitis after craniotomy: a meta analysis. Neurosurgery 2007; 60:887.

46. FG Barker II. Efficacy of prophylactic antibiotics for craniotomy: a meta-analysis. Neurosurgery 1994; 35:484.

47. FG Barker II. Efficacy of prophylactic antibiotic therapy in spinal surgery: a meta-analysis. Neurosurgery 2002; 51:391.

48. JB Dimick et al. Spine update: antimicrobial prophylaxis in spine surgery: basic principles and recent advances. Spine 2000; 25:2544.

49. B Ratilal et al. Antibiotic prophylaxis for surgical introduction of intracranial ventricular shunts: a systematic review. J Neurosurg Pediatr 2008; 1:48.

50. DV Leaming. Practice styles and preferences of ASCRS members - 2003 survey. J Cataract Refract Surg 2004; 30:892.

51. FC DeCroos and NA Afshari. Perioperative antibiotics and anti-inflammatory agents in cataract surgery. Curr Opin Ophthalmol 2008; 19:22.

52. TA Ciulla et al. Bacterial endophthalmitis prophylaxis for cataract surgery: an evidence-based update. Ophthalmology 2002; 109:13.

53. L Prokuski. Prophylactic antibiotics in orthopaedic surgery. J Am Acad Orthop Surg 2008; 16:283.

54. WJ Gillespie and G Walenkamp. Antibiotic prophylaxis for surgery for proximal femoral and other closed long bone fractures. Cochrane Database Syst Rev 2001; 1:CD000244.

55. A Trampuz and W Zimmerli. Antimicrobial agents in orthopaedic surgery: Prophylaxis and treatment. Drugs 2006; 66:1089.

56. CJ Hauser et al. Surgical Infection Society guideline: prophylactic antibiotic use in open fractures: an evidence-based guideline. Surg Infect 2006; 7:379.

57. J Bert et al. Antibiotic prophylaxis for arthroscopy of the knee: is it necessary? Arthroscopy 2007; 23:4.

58. PR Kurzweil. Antibiotic prophylaxis for arthroscopic surgery. Arthroscopy 2006; 22:452.

59. R Aznar et al. Antibiotic prophylaxis in non-cardiac thoracic surgery: cefazolin versus placebo. Eur J Cardiothorac Surg 1991; 5:515.

60. DM Radu et al. Postoperative pneumonia after major pulmonary resections: an unsolved problem in thoracic surgery. Ann Thorac Surg 2007; 84:1669.

61. RP Gonzalez and MR Holevar. Role of prophylactic antibiotics for tube thoracostomy in chest trauma. Am Surg 1998; 64:617.

62. AH Stewart et al. Prevention of infection in peripheral arterial reconstruction: a systematic review and meta-analysis. J Vasc Surg 2007; 46:148.

63. S Homer-Vanniasinkam. Surgical site and vascular infections: treatment and prophylaxis. Int J Infect Dis 2007; 11 Suppl 1:S17.

64. TI Wright et al. Antibiotic prophylaxis in dermatologic surgery: advisory statement 2008. J Am Acad Dermatol 2008; 59:464.

Why Not Ertapenem for Surgical Prophylaxis?
Originally published in The Medical Letter – September 2009; 51:72

Some readers have asked why the June 2009 issue of *Treatment Guidelines* (Antimicrobial Prophylaxis for Surgery) did not recommend use of ertapenem *(Invanz)* for prevention of infection after elective colorectal surgery. Ertapenem is a broad-spectrum carbapenem that has been approved for such use by the FDA. Medical Letter consultants do not recommend use of broad-spectrum drugs such as ertapenem, third-generation cephalosporins such as cefotaxime *(Claforan)*, ceftriaxone *(Rocephin)*, cefoperazone *(Cefobid)*, ceftazidime *(Fortaz,* and others) or ceftizoxime *(Cefizox)*, or fourth-generation cephalosporins such as cefepime *(Maxipime)* for routine surgical prophylaxis because they are expensive, some are less active than first- or second-generation cephalosporins against staphylococci, and their spectrum of activity includes organisms rarely encountered in elective surgery. These drugs should be reserved for treatment of serious infections, particularly those likely to be caused by organisms resistant to other antimicrobials.

Recommendation for Earlier Antibiotic Prophylaxis for Cesarean Delivery

Originally published in The Medical Letter – October 2010; 52:80

The American Congress of Obstetricians and Gynecologists (ACOG) has announced a new recommendation for antibiotic prophylaxis during cesarean delivery.[1] Currently most women receive a single dose of prophylactic antibiotics after the umbilical cord has been clamped to prevent antibiotics from crossing over to the newborn. The new recommendation is for women giving birth by cesarean section to routinely receive antibiotics within one hour before the start of surgery. In the case of an emergency cesarean delivery, prophylaxis should be started as soon as possible.

Recent studies have found a lower incidence of endometritis and wound infection with preoperative antibiotic administration compared to administration post-clamping.[2-4] Whether widespread adoption of this practice could increase neonatal morbidity by masking the source of sepsis or by increasing the prevalence of resistant organisms remains to be determined.

The prophylactic antibiotic for cesarean section is cefazolin 1-2 g IV. For patients allergic to penicillins and cephalosporins, clindamycin with gentamicin would be a reasonable alternative.

1. The American College of Obstetricians and Gynecologists Committee on Obstetric Practice. Committee Opinion no. 465: Antimicrobial prophylaxis for cesarean delivery: timing of administration. Obstet Gynecol 2010; 116:791.
2. MM Constantine et al. Timing of perioperative antibiotics for cesarean delivery: a meta-analysis. Am J Obstet Gynecol 2008; 199:301.
3. FM Smaill and GML Gyte. Antibiotic prophylaxis versus no prophylaxis for preventing infection after cesarean section. Cochrane Database Syst Rev 2010: CD007482.
4. SA Sullivan et al. Administration of cefazolin prior to skin incision is superior to cefazolin at cord clamping in preventing post cesarean infectious morbidity: a randomized controlled trial. Am J Obstet Gynecol 2007; 196:455.

Antifungal Drugs

Original publication date – December 2009

The drugs of choice for treatment of some fungal infections are listed in the table that begins on the next page. Some of the indications and dosages recommended here have not been approved by the FDA. More detailed guidelines are available online from the Infectious Diseases Society of America (www.idsociety.org).

AZOLES

Azole antifungal agents inhibit synthesis of ergosterol, an essential component of the fungal cell membrane.

FLUCONAZOLE — Fluconazole (*Diflucan*, and others) is active against most *Candida* species other than *C. krusei*, which is intrinsically resistant, and many strains of *C. glabrata*, which are increasingly resistant. Fluconazole has good activity against *Coccidioides* and *Cryptococcus* spp.; higher doses may be needed against *Histoplasma capsulatum*. The drug has no clinically significant activity against most molds, including *Aspergillus* spp., *Fusarium* spp. and Zygomycetes, such as *Mucor* spp.

Adverse Effects – Fluconazole is generally well tolerated. Headache, gastrointestinal distress, facial edema, rash and pruritus can occur. Stevens-Johnson syndrome, anaphylaxis, hepatic toxicity, leukopenia and hypokalemia have been reported. Some post-marketing cases of QT

137

TREATMENT OF FUNGAL INFECTIONS

Infection		Drug
ASPERGILLOSIS		Voriconazole[2]
	or	Amphotericin B
BLASTOMYCOSIS[6]		Itraconazole
	or	Amphotericin B
CANDIDIASIS		
Vaginal[9]		
Topical therapy		Butoconazole, clotrimazole,
(intravaginal creams, ointments,		miconazole, tioconazole,
tablets, ovules or suppositories)		or terconazole
Systemic therapy		Fluconazole
Recurrent [11]		Fluconazole
Urinary[12]		Fluconazole

1. Usual adult dosage. Some drugs may need dosage adjustment for renal or hepatic dysfunction or when used with interacting drugs. The optimal duration of treatment with antifungal drugs is often unclear. Depending on the disease and its severity, they may be continued for weeks or months or, particularly in immunocompromised patients, indefinitely.
2. In one controlled trial, voriconazole was more effective than amphotericin B for treatment of invasive aspergillosis (R Herbrecht et al, N Engl J Med 2002; 347:408).
3. Not FDA-approved for this indication.
4. Children may need higher maintenance doses. According to the manufacturer, serum concentrations in children with doses of 4 mg/kg are similar to those in adults given 3 mg/kg. In the European Union, where voriconazole is licensed for use in children 2-12 years old, the recommended maintenance dosages are 7 mg/kg IV b.i.d. or 200 mg PO b.i.d., without loading doses (MO Karlsson et al. Antimicrob Agents Chemother 2009; 53:9351).
5. Dosage of amphotericin B deoxycholate given once daily. Lipid-based formulations may be preferred. Usual doses of lipid-based formulations for treatment of invasive fungal infection are: amphotericin B lipid complex *(Abelcet)* 5 mg/kg/d; liposomal amphotericin B *(AmBisome)* 3-5 mg/kg/d; amphotericin B cholesteryl sulfate *(Amphotec)* 3-4 mg/kg/d. For treatment of zygomycosis, the dosage of *AmBisome* is 5 mg/kg/d. For treatment of cryptococcal meningitis in HIV patients, the dosage of *AmBisome* is 4-6 mg/kg/d.

Dosage/Duration[1]	Alternatives
6 mg/kg IV q12h x 1d, then 4 mg/kg IV q12h or 200-300 mg PO bid ≥10 wks[4]	Posaconazole 200 mg PO tid-qid[3] Itraconazole 200 mg tid x 3d, followed by 200 mg bid Caspofungin 70 mg IV x 1d, then 50 mg IV 1x/d Micafungin 150 mg IV 1x/d
1-1.5 mg/kg/d IV[5]	
200 mg PO bid x 6-12 mos 0.5-1.0 mg/kg/d IV[5]	Fluconazole 400 mg PO 1x/d[3,7,8]
1x/d x 1-7d	
150 mg PO once[10]	Itraconazole[3] 200 mg PO bid x 1d Ketoconazole[3] 200 mg PO bid x 5d
150 mg PO 1x/wk	
200 mg IV or PO 1x/d x 7-14d	Amphotericin B 0.3-0.5 mg/kg/d IV[5] x 1-7d Flucytosine 25 mg/kg PO qid x 5-7d[13]

6. Patients with severe illness or CNS involvement should receive amphotericin B.
7. In general, a loading dose of twice the daily dose is recommended on the first day of therapy.
8. For use only in patients who cannot tolerate itraconazole or amphotericin B.
9. Non-albicans species, such as *C. glabrata* and *C. krusei*, respond to boric acid 600 mg intravaginally daily x 14d or to topical flucytosine cream (JD Sobel et al, Am J Obstet Gynecol 2003; 189:1297).
10. May be repeated in 72 hours if patient remains symptomatic.
11. JD Sobel et al, N Engl J Med 2004; 351:876.
12. Asymptomatic candiduria usually does not require treatment. Patients who are symptomatic, neutropenic, have renal allografts or are undergoing urologic manipulation and infants with low birth weight should be treated.
13. Dosage must be decreased in patients with diminished renal function.

Continued on next page.

Antifungal Drugs

TREATMENT OF FUNGAL INFECTIONS (continued)

Infection		Drug
CANDIDIASIS (continued)		
Oropharyngeal or Esophageal[14-16]		Fluconazole
	or	An echinocandin Caspofungin
		Micafungin Anidulafungin
Candidemia[15]		Fluconazole
	or	An echinocandin Caspofungin[23] Anidulafungin Micafungin
	or	Amphotericin B
COCCIDIOIDOMYCOSIS[26]		
		Itraconazole[3]
	or	Fluconazole[3]
	or	Amphotericin B

14. For uncomplicated oropharyngeal thrush, clotrimazole troches (10 mg) 5x/d or nystatin suspension 500,000 units (5 mL) qid can also be used. Azole-resistant oropharyngeal or esophageal candidiasis usually responds to amphotericin B or an echinocandin.
15. *Candida albicans* is generally highly susceptible to fluconazole. *C. krusei* infections are resistant to fluconazole. *C. glabrata* infections are often resistant to low doses, but may be susceptible to high doses of fluconazole. *C. lusitaniae* may be resistant to amphotericin B.
16. HIV-infected patients with frequent or severe recurrences of oral or esophageal candidiasis may require prophylaxis. For patients with organisms that are still susceptible, the regimen of choice is fluconazole 100-200 mg PO once daily.
17. R Ally et al, Clin Infect Dis 2001; 33:1447.
18. Duration of treatment for esophageal candidiasis is 14 to 21 days after clinical improvement.
19. For patients with oropharyngeal disease, itraconazole oral solution 200 mg (20 mL) given once daily without food is more effective than itraconazole capsules.

Dosage/Duration[1]	Alternatives
200 mg IV or PO once, then 100-200 mg 1x/d x 2-3 wks[18,20]	Voriconazole[17] 200 mg PO bid x 1-3 wks[4,18] Itraconazole[19] 200 mg PO x 1d, then 100 mg/d[20] x 1-3 wks[18] Posaconazole 100 mg bid x 1d then 100 mg 1x/d x 1-3 wks[18,21]
70 mg IV x 1d, then 50 mg IV 1x/d x 1-3 wks[18] 150 mg IV 1x/d x 1-3 wks[18] 100 mg IV x 1d, then 50 mg 1x/d x 1-3 wks[18]	Amphotericin B 0.3-0.5 mg/kg/d IV x 1-3 wks[5,18]
400 mg IV 1x/d, then PO[7,22]	Voriconazole 6 mg/kg IV q12h x 1d then 3-4 mg/kg IV bid or 200 mg PO bid[4,22]
70 mg IV x 1d, then 50 mg IV 1x/d[22] 200 mg IV x 1d, then 100 mg 1x/d[22] 100 mg IV 1x/d[22] 0.5-1 mg/kg/d IV[5,22]	
200 mg PO bid x >1 yr 400 mg PO 1x/d x >1 yr[7] 0.5-1.5 mg/kg/d IV[5] x >1 yr	

20. Use up to 400 mg/d for esophageal candidiasis.
21. For refractory oropharyngeal candidiasis, use 400 mg once/d or bid.
22. Until 2 weeks after afebrile and blood cultures negative.
23. In a large controlled trial, caspofungin was at least as effective as amphotericin B for treatment of invasive candidiasis or candidemia (J Mora-Duarte et al, N Engl J Med 2002; 347:2020).
24. Itraconazole is the drug of choice for non-meningeal coccidioidomycosis. Fluconazole is preferred for coccidioidal meningitis. Patients with meningitis who do not respond to fluconazole or itraconazole may require intrathecal amphotericin B 0.1-1.5 mg per dose at daily to weekly intervals.
25. Dosage must be decreased in patients with diminished renal function. When given with amphotericin B, some Medical Letter consultants recommend beginning flucytosine at 75 mg/kg/day divided q6h, until the degree of amphotericin nephrotoxicity becomes clear or flucytosine blood levels can be detemined.
26. For patients with HIV infection.

Continued on next page.

Antifungal Drugs

TREATMENT OF FUNGAL INFECTIONS (continued)

Infection		Drug
CRYPTOCOCCOSIS		
		Amphotericin B
	±	Flucytosine
	then	Fluconazole
Chronic suppression [26]		Fluconazole
FUSARIOSIS		
		Amphotericin B
	or	Voriconazole
HISTOPLASMOSIS		
		Amphotericin B[27]
	or	Itraconazole
Chronic suppression [26]		Itraconazole[3]
PARACOCCIDIOIDOMYCOSIS[6]		
		Itraconazole[3]
	or	Amphotericin B[28]
SCEDOSPORIOSIS (asexual form of Pseudallescheriasis)		
		Voriconazole
SPOROTRICHOSIS		
Cutaneous		Itraconazole[3]
Extracutaneous [6]		Amphotericin B
	or	Itraconazole[3]
ZYGOMYCOSIS		
		Amphotericin B

27. For severe disease, before switching to itraconazole. Amphotericin B should be continued for 4-6 weeks in patients with CNS involvement. In one study, liposomal amphotericin B *(AmBisome)* was associated with greater improvement in survival compared to amphotericin B deoxycholate (PC Johnson et al, Ann Intern Med 2002; 137:105).

Dosage/Duration[1]	Alternatives
0.5-1 mg/kg/d IV[5] x 2 wks 25 mg/kg PO qid[25] 400 mg PO 1x/d x 10 wks[7] 200 mg PO 1x/d	Itraconazole[3] 200 mg PO bid Amphotericin B 0.5-1 mg/kg IV wkly[5]
1-1.5 mg/kg/d IV[5] 6 mg/kg IV q12h x 1d, then 4 mg/kg q12h or 200 mg PO bid[4]	

0.5-1.0 mg/kg/d IV[5] x 2 wks
200 mg tid x 3d then
  200 mg PO bid x
  6 wks-≥12 mos
	Fluconazole[3] 400 mg PO 1x/d[7,8]

200 mg PO 1x/d or bid	Amphotericin[3] B 0.5-1 mg/kg IV wkly[5]
100-200 mg PO 1x/d x 6-12 mos 0.4-0.5 mg/kg/d IV[5]	Ketoconazole 200-400 mg PO 1x/d

6 mg/kg IV q12h x 1d, then
  4 mg/kg IV bid, or 200 mg
  PO bid x 12 wks[4]
	Posaconazole[3] 200 mg PO tid-qid

200 mg PO 1x/d x 3-6 mos	Terbinafine[3] 500 mg PO bid Saturated solution of potassium iodide 1-5 mL PO tid Fluconazole[3,7] 400-800 mg PO 1x/d
0.7-1 mg/kg/d IV[5] x 6-12 wks 200 mg PO 1x/d x 12 mos	
1-1.5 mg/kg/d IV[5] x 6-10 wks	Posaconazole[3,29] 200 mg PO tid-qid

28. Initial treatment of severely ill patients. To be followed by itraconazole.
29. Posaconazole has been used after mucormycosis was clinically improved and oral alimentation was sufficient to enhance absorption (AM Tobon et al, Clin Infect Dis 2003; 36:1488).

prolongation and torsades de pointes have also been reported. Fluconazole is teratogenic in animals (pregnancy category C).

Drug Interactions – Fluconazole is a strong inhibitor of CYP2C9 and 2C19 *(in vitro)* and a moderate inhibitor of CYP3A4; it may increase serum concentrations of drugs metabolized by these enzymes.[1] Concomitant administration of rifampin can lower serum concentrations of fluconazole. Concurrent use of fluconazole with other drugs known to prolong the QT interval, particularly those metabolized by CYP2C9, 2C19 or 3A4, may increase the risk of QT prolongation and torsades de pointes.[1,2]

ITRACONAZOLE — Itraconazole (*Sporanox*, and others) has a broader spectrum of activity than fluconazole. It is active against a wide variety of fungi including *Cryptococcus neoformans*, *Aspergillus* spp., *Blastomyces dermatitidis*, *Coccidioides* spp., *H. capsulatum*, *Paracoccidioides brasiliensis*, *Sporothrix* spp. and dermatophytes. It is also active against most species of *Candida*. Itraconazole has no clinically significant activity against *Scedosporium* spp.*, Fusarium* spp., *Scopulariopsis* spp. or Zygomycetes.

Itraconazole is available orally in both capsules and solution; an IV formulation is no longer being produced in the US. Absorption after oral dosing is variable. The solution is more bioavailable than the capsules. The capsules should be taken with food, while the solution is absorbed best without food.

Adverse Effects – The most common adverse effects of itraconazole are nausea, vomiting and rash. Stevens-Johnson syndrome and serious hepatic toxicity can occur. The drug can cause hypokalemia, edema and hypertension. Negative inotropic effects and congestive heart failure have been reported; itraconazole should not be used in patients with a history of heart failure or ventricular dysfunction. Peripheral neuropathy, visual disturbances, hearing loss and tinnitus have also been reported. Itraconazole is teratogenic in rats (pregnancy category C).

Drug Interactions – The absorption of itraconazole from capsules is reduced by drugs that decrease gastric acidity, such as antacids, H_2-receptor blockers or proton pump inhibitors.

Itraconazole is a substrate of CYP3A4 and P-glycoprotein (P-gp); its metabolism may be affected by both inducers and inhibitors of these pathways.[1]

Itraconazole is a strong inhibitor of CYP3A4 and may significantly increase serum concentrations of drugs metabolized by this enzyme.[3] It is contraindicated for use with some drugs that are metabolized by CYP3A4, particularly those known to prolong the QT interval.[2] Itraconazole may increase the serum concentrations and negative inotropic effects of calcium channel blockers. It is also a P-gp inhibitor and can increase serum concentrations of P-gp substrates.[1]

VORICONAZOLE — Voriconazole *(Vfend)* has a spectrum of activity similar to that of itraconazole but appears to be more active against *Aspergillus* spp. and most species of *Candida,* including *C. glabrata* and *C. krusei.* Unlike itraconazole, voriconazole is active against *Fusarium* spp. and *Scedosporium* spp. It is not active against *Sporothrix* spp.or Zygomycetes; infection with these organisms has developed during treatment with voriconazole. In a randomized trial of initial treatment of invasive aspergillosis, voriconazole improved survival compared to amphotericin B and caused fewer severe adverse effects.[4]

Patients with mild to moderate hepatic insufficiency should receive a normal loading dose of voriconazole, but half the maintenance dose. Serum concentrations of voriconazole may need monitoring; they vary from patient to patient and with the formulation used (lower with capsules and higher with the solution).[5,6] Children need a higher per-kg dose than adults because they clear the drug more rapidly.[7]

Adverse Effects – Transient visual disturbances including blurred vision, photophobia and altered perception of color or image have occurred in about 20% of patients treated with voriconazole. Rash (including Stevens-Johnson syndrome), photosensitivity, increased transaminase levels, confusion and hallucinations have also occurred. In patients with creatinine clearance <50 mL/min, the oral formulation is preferred because the solubilizing agent in the IV formulation (sulfobutyl ether beta-cyclodextrin) can accumulate and cause toxicity. Anaphylactoid infusion reactions have occurred. Voriconazole is teratogenic in animals (pregnancy category D).

Drug Interactions – Voriconazole is a substrate of CYP2C19, 2C9, 3A4 and P-gp. Drugs that inhibit or induce one or more of these clearance pathways may significantly alter serum concentrations of voriconazole.[1] Patients deficient in CYP2C19 (about 3-5% of Caucasians and African-Americans and about 15% of Asians do not express it) may have 2- to 4-fold higher serum concentrations of voriconazole.

Voriconazole is an inhibitor *(in vitro)* of CYP2C9, 3A4 and, to a lesser extent, 2C19; it may significantly increase serum concentrations of drugs metabolized by these enzymes. Concurrent use of voriconazole with other drugs that prolong the QT interval, particularly those metabolized by CYP2C9, 2C19 or 3A4, may increase the risk of QT prolongation and torsades de pointes.[1,2]

POSACONAZOLE — Posaconazole *(Noxafil)*, the newest triazole,[8] has an antifungal spectrum similar to that of itraconazole, but its *in vitro* activity is about twice as great; it can be used to treat *Fusarium* spp. and *Scedosporium* spp. and has up to 4-fold greater activity against many species of *Mucor*, such as *Absidia* spp. Posaconazole is only available for oral use and must be taken with meals for optimal absorption.

Clinical Studies – A randomized, open-label clinical trial of posacona-zole for **prophylaxis** against fungal infections found that 602 adults who were neutropenic as a result of induction chemotherapy for acute myel-ogenous leukemia (AML) or myelodysplastic syndrome (MDS) had fewer invasive mycoses (including aspergillosis) and lower mortality rates when taking posaconazole (200 mg t.i.d.) compared to those taking fluconazole (400 mg once/day) or itraconazole (200 mg b.i.d.).[9] A dou-ble-blind randomized trial in 600 adults with graft-versus-host disease following allogeneic hematopoietic stem cell transplantation (HSCT) found posaconazole similar to fluconazole in preventing invasive mycoses and superior in preventing invasive aspergillosis and death.[10]

HIV-infected patients with oropharyngeal or esophageal candidiasis refractory to **treatment** with fluconazole or itraconazole have responded to posaconazole; in one study, 75% of these patients achieved cure or improvement after 28 days of treatment.[11] Posaconazole is not approved in the US for salvage therapy of invasive mycoses, but it has been used suc-cessfully for this indication in patients with invasive aspergillosis. It has also been used off-label to treat coccidioidomycosis and zygomycosis.[12-15]

Adverse Effects – Posaconazole has a safety profile comparable to that of fluconazole; dry mouth, rash, headache, diarrhea, fatigue, nausea, vomit-ing, QT prolongation and abnormal liver function have been reported, but infrequently lead to drug discontinuation. Arrhythmias, toxic epidermal necrolysis, angioedema and anaphylaxis have been rare. Posaconazole causes skeletal malformations in rats (pregnancy category C).

Drug Interactions – Posaconazole is primarily metabolized through UDP glucuronidation and is also a substrate of P-gp.[1] Any drug that inhibits or induces these clearance pathways may alter serum concentra-tions of posaconazole. Drugs that increase gastric pH, such as proton pump inhibitors, H_2-receptor blockers or antacids, may decrease the absorption of posaconazole. Posaconazole is a strong inhibitor of CYP3A4 and may increase serum concentrations of drugs that are

TREATMENT OF ONYCHOMYCOSIS AND TINEA PEDIS

Infection		Drug
ONYCHOMYCOSIS[2,3]		
		Terbinafine
	or	Itraconazole
TINEA PEDIS[6]		
		Terbinafine cream[7]
	or	Topical azoles (i.e. clotrimazole, miconazole, econazole)

1. Usual adult dosage. Some drugs may need dosage adjustment for renal or hepatic dysfunction or when used with interacting drugs.
2. Nail specimens should be obtained prior to any drug therapy to confirm the diagnosis of onychomycosis.
3. Topical treatment with ciclopirox 8% nail laquer (*Penlac*, and others) is indicated for treatment of mild-to-moderate onychomycosis caused by *T. rubium* that does not involve the lunula. Ciclopirox is less effective than systemic therapy, but has no systemic side effects or drug interactions.

metabolized by this enzyme.[3] Posaconazole is contraindicated for use with sirolimus, ergot alkaloids, and CYP3A4 substrates that also prolong the QT interval. It should be used with caution with other drugs known to prolong the QT interval.[2]

KETOCONAZOLE — Ketoconazole (*Nizoral*, and others) is seldom used now. Other azoles are preferred because they have fewer adverse effects.

Adverse Effects – Anorexia, nausea and vomiting are common with higher doses (>400 mg/day) of ketoconazole. Pruritus, rash, dizziness and photophobia may occur. Ketoconazole can decrease plasma testosterone concentrations and cause gynecomastia, decreased libido and erectile dysfunction in men and menstrual irregularities in women. High

Dosage/Duration[1]	Alternatives
250 mg PO once/d x 12 wks[4]	
200 mg PO once/d x 3 mos[4] or 200 mg PO bid 1 wk/mo x 3 mos[4]	Fluconazole[5] 150-300 mg PO once wkly x 6-12 mos[4]
twice daily application x 1-2 wks	Fluconazole[5] 150 mg PO once/wk x 1-4 wks
once or twice daily application x 4 wks	

4. Duration for toenail infection. Duration of treatment for fingernail infection: 6 weeks with terbinafine, 2 months with itraconazole and 3-6 months with fluconazole.
5. Not FDA-approved for this indication.
6. Topical treatment of "athlete's foot" is adequate for mild cases. Relapse is common and requires prolonged treatment (>4 wks).
7. Other topical non-azoles, including butenafine and naftifine may also be used, but the duration of treatment should then be increased to 2-4 weeks.

doses may inhibit adrenal steroidogenesis and decrease plasma cortisol concentrations. Hepatic toxicity, including fatal hepatic necrosis, can occur. Ketoconazole is teratogenic in animals (pregnancy category C).

Drug Interactions – Ketoconazole is a strong inhibitor of CYP3A4 and other metabolic pathways; it can significantly increase serum concentrations of many other drugs.[3] The absorption of ketoconazole is significantly reduced by drugs that increase gastric pH, such as proton pump inhibitors, H[2]-receptor blockers and antacids.

ECHINOCANDINS

Echinocandins inhibit synthesis of ß (1, 3)-D-glucan, an essential component of the fungal cell wall. Their potential for adverse effects in humans is low due to the absence in mammalian cells of enzymes involved in glucan synthesis. Caspofungin, anidulafungin and micafungin all have activity against most *Candida* species, including those resistant to azoles. Their activity against molds appears to be confined to *Aspergillus*. All 3 echinocandins are given intravenously once daily, do not require dose adjustment for renal failure, do not significantly interact with other drugs, and appear to be similar to each other in efficacy and safety.[16]

CASPOFUNGIN — Caspofungin (*Cancidas*) is FDA-approved for treatment of esophageal candidiasis, candidemia, intra-abdominal abscesses, peritonitis, and pleural space infections due to *Candida*. It is also approved for empiric treatment of presumed fungal infections in febrile, neutropenic patients and for treatment of invasive aspergillosis in patients who are refractory to or intolerant of other therapies. Data on its use for primary treatment of aspergillosis are lacking.

Adverse Effects – Although generally well tolerated, caspofungin occasionally causes rash, fever, nausea, vomiting, headache, hypokalemia and mild hepatic toxicity. Stevens-Johnson syndrome and exfoliative dermatitis have been reported. Anaphylaxis has occurred. Dosage should be reduced in patients with moderate hepatic dysfunction. Caspofungin is embryo-toxic in animals (pregnancy category C).

Drug Interactions – Rifampin, carbamazepine, dexamethasone, efavirenz, nevirapine and phenytoin may increase the clearance of caspofungin. An increase in caspofungin dosage to 70 mg daily (70 mg/m^2/day in children, max 70 mg) should be considered when it is co-administered with these drugs. Caspofungin can decrease serum concentrations of tacrolimus.

MICAFUNGIN — Micafungin (*Mycamine*) is FDA-approved for treatment of esophageal candidiasis and prevention of invasive candidiasis in autologous or allogeneic stem cell transplant recipients. It is also approved for treatment of candidemia and deeply invasive candidiasis.

Approval was based on showing noninferiority in 2 large randomized clinical trials in patients with invasive candidiasis, one comparing mica-fungin to liposomal amphotericin B and the other comparing it to caspo-fungin.[17,18] In an open-label, noncomparative trial, micafungin appeared to be efficacious in 12 patients with untreated and 24 patients with par-tially treated aspergillosis.[19]

Adverse Effects – Micafungin is well tolerated. Adverse effects have included rash, pruritus and facial swelling. Anaphylaxis has been rare. Fever, hepatic function abnormalities, hypokalemia, thrombocytopenia, renal dysfunction, headache, nausea, vomiting and diarrhea have been reported, but rarely limit therapy. Micafungin is teratogenic in animals (pregnancy category C).

ANIDULAFUNGIN — Anidulafungin (*Eraxis*)[20] is FDA-approved for treatment of esophageal candidiasis. It is also approved for treatment of candidemia and deeply invasive candidiasis based on a randomized, dou-ble-blind trial demonstrating noninferiority to fluconazole.[21]

Adverse Effects – Anidulafungin has a low incidence of adverse effects similar to those of caspofungin and micafungin. Unlike micafungin and caspofungin, hepatic failure does not appear to increase anidulafungin serum concentrations. Its safety in pregnancy has not been established (pregnancy category C).

AMPHOTERICIN B

Amphotericin B binds to ergosterol in the fungal cell membrane, leading to loss of membrane integrity and leakage of cell contents. Conventional amphotericin B and the newer lipid-based formulations have the same spectrum of activity and are active against most pathogenic fungi and some protozoa. They are not active against most strains of *Aspergillus terreus*, *Scedosporium apiospermum*, *Trichosporon* spp*., *Fusarium* spp. and *Candida lusitaniae*. Amphotericin B is the preferred treatment for deep fungal infections during pregnancy because of experience with its use and apparent safety.

Conventional Amphotericin B – Amphotericin B deoxycholate, the non-lipid formulation of amphotericin, is the least expensive but also the most toxic, particularly to the kidney. The development of better tolerated lipid-based formulations has led to a decrease in its use. Intravenous infusion of amphotericin B deoxycholate frequently causes fever and chills, and sometimes headache, nausea, vomiting, hypotension and tachypnea, usually beginning 1-3 hours after starting the infusion and lasting about 1 hour. The intensity of these infusion-related acute reactions tends to decrease after the first few doses. Pretreatment with acetaminophen or a nonsteroidal anti-inflammatory drug (NSAID) such as ibuprofen, diphenhydramine 25 mg IV and/or hydrocortisone 25 mg IV can decrease the severity of the reaction. Treatment with meperidine 25-50 mg IV can shorten the duration of rigors.

Nephrotoxicity is the major dose-limiting toxicity of amphotericin B deoxycholate; sodium loading with normal saline may prevent or ameliorate it and is generally recommended for patients who can tolerate a fluid load. The nephrotoxicity of amphotericin B may add to the nephrotoxicity of other drugs including cyclosporine, tacrolimus and aminoglycoside antibiotics such as gentamicin. Hypokalemia and hypomagnesemia are common and are usually due to a mild renal tubular acidosis. Weight loss, malaise, anemia, thrombocytopenia and mild leukopenia can occur. Cardiac toxicity and myopathy have been reported.

Lipid Formulations – The 3 lipid formulations of amphotericin B marketed in the US appear to be as effective as amphotericin B deoxycholate. Compared to conventional amphotericin B, acute infusion-related reactions are more severe with *Amphotec*, less severe with *Abelcet*, and least severe with *AmBisome*. Acute, severe pain in the chest, back or abdomen has occurred during the first infusion of liposomal amphotericin B.[22] The cause of the pain is unknown. Some patients have tolerated subsequent,

AMPHOTERICIN B FORMULATIONS

Drug	Usual Daily Dosage[1]	Cost[2]
Amphotericin B deoxycholate generic (Abbott)	1-1.5 mg/kg IV	$34.92
Amphotericin B lipid complex (ABLC) *Abelcet* (Enzon)	5 mg/kg IV	840.00
Liposomal amphotericin B (L-AmB) *AmBisome* (Astellas)	3-5 mg/kg IV	1318.80
Amphotericin B cholesteryl sulfate complex (ABCD) *Amphotec* (Three Rivers)	3-4 mg/kg IV	733.33

1. For invasive fungal infection.
2. Cost for one day's treatment of a 70-kg patient at the highest usual dosage according to AWP prices listed in *Redbook 2009*.

slower infusions of the drug when pretreated with diphenhydramine. Nephrotoxicity is less common with lipid-based products than with amphotericin B deoxycholate and, when it occurs, less severe. Liver toxicity, which is generally not associated with amphotericin B deoxycholate, has occurred rarely with the lipid formulations.

Cost comparisons with amphotericin B lipid formulations should take into account the fact that conventional amphotericin B deoxycholate may cause renal failure, which can increase the length of hospital stays, healthcare costs and mortality rates.[23]

OTHER DRUGS

FLUCYTOSINE – Potentially lethal, dose-related bone marrow toxicity and rapid development of resistance have occured with flucytosine

(*Ancobon*) monotherapy; it is mainly used in combination with amphotericin B for treatment of cryptococcal meningitis or systemic candidiasis. Keeping serum concentrations below 100 mcg/mL decreases toxicity, but delays in obtaining assay results often limit their utility. Flucytosine is only available for oral use in the US. Doses must be adjusted for renal dysfunction. It is classified as category C for use in pregnancy.

TERBINAFINE – Terbinafine (*Lamisil*, and others) is a synthetic allylamine approved by the FDA for treatment of onychomycosis of the toenail or fingernail due to dermatophytes. It acts by inhibiting squalene epoxidase and blocking ergosterol synthesis.

The most common adverse effects of oral terbinafine have been headache, gastrointestinal symptoms including diarrhea, dyspepsia and abdominal pain, and occasionally a taste disturbance that may persist for weeks after the drug is stopped. Rash, pruritus and urticaria, usually mild and transient, have occurred. Toxic epidermal necrolysis and erythema multiforme have been reported. Increased aminotransferase levels and serious hepatic injury have occurred. Liver function should be assessed before starting and periodically during treatment with terbinafine. Anaphylaxis, pancytopenia and severe neutropenia have also been reported. Terbinafine is classified as category B for use in pregnancy.

Drug Interactions – Terbinafine is an inhibitor of CYP2D6 and may increase serum concentrations of drugs metabolized by this enzyme.[1] Cimetidine may reduce the clearance of terbinafine. Enzyme inducers such as rifampin may increase terbinafine clearance.

COMBINATION THERAPY

Use of combination therapy for treatment of immunosuppressed patients with invasive aspergillosis, which has a high rate of morbidity and mortality despite current treatments, is controversial. *In vitro* studies and animal data suggest a potential benefit of combining an echinocandin with either an azole or amphotericin B, but clinical studies are lacking.

NEUTROPENIA

PROPHYLAXIS — High-risk neutropenic patients, such as those undergoing allogeneic and certain autologous stem cell transplants, and those with hematologic malignancy who are expected to have prolonged profound neutropenia, may require prophylactic treatment with antifungal drugs. Fluconazole (400 mg PO or IV once daily) has been used, but because of the high risk of invasive aspergillosis in these patients, some clinicians now use voriconazole (6 mg/kg every 12 hours x 2 doses, then 4-5 mg/kg every 12 hours) or posaconazole (200 mg t.i.d.) instead. Itraconazole solution, 200 mg twice daily, is an alternative but may not be well tolerated. In a prospective, randomized trial for prevention of invasive fungal infections in neutropenic patients with acute myelogenous leukemia or myelodysplastic syndrome undergoing chemotherapy, posaconazole was superior to fluconazole or itraconazole and improved survival.[9] Micafungin 50 mg/day has been recommended for prophylactic use in patients with neutropenia.[24]

FEVER AND NEUTROPENIA — For neutropenic patients with fever that persists despite treatment with antibacterial drugs, empiric addition of an antifungal drug is common practice.[25] Caspofungin and voriconazole appear to be as effective as liposomal amphotericin B.[26,27] Fluconazole and itraconazole have also been used for this indication.

1. Drug interactions. Med Lett Drugs Ther 2003; 45:46.
2. Arizona Center for Education and Research on Therapeutics. Drugs that prolong the QT interval and/or induce torsades de pointes ventricular arrhythmia. Available at www.azcert.org. Accessed November 18, 2009.
3. CYP3A and drug interactions. Med Lett Drugs Ther 2005; 47:54.
4. R Herbrecht et al. Voriconazole versus amphotericin B for primary therapy of invasive aspergillosis. N Engl J Med 2002; 347:408.
5. J Smith et al. Voriconazole therapeutic drug monitoring. Antimicrob Agents Chemother 2006; 50:1570.
6. A Pascaul et al. Voriconazole therapeutic drug monitoring in patients with mycoses improves efficacy and safety outcomes. Clin Infect Dis 2008; 46:201.
7. MO Karlsson et al. Population pharmacokinetic analysis of voricona-zole plasma concentration data from pediatric studies. Antimicrob Agents Chemother 2009; 53:935.

8. Posaconazole (Noxafil) for invasive fungal infections. Med Lett Drugs Ther 2006; 48:93.

9. OA Cornely et al. Posaconazole vs. fluconazole or itraconazole prophylaxis in patients with neutropenia. N Engl J Med 2007; 356:348.

10. AJ Ullmann et al. Posaconazole or fluconazole for prophylaxis in severe graft-versus-host disease. N Engl J Med 2007; 356:335.

11. DJ Skiest et al. Posaconazole for the treatment of azole-refractoryoropharyngeal and esophageal candidiasis in subjects with HIV infection. Clin Infect Dis 2007; 44:607.

12. TJ Walsh et al. Treatment of invasive aspergillosis with posaconazole in patients who are refractory to or intolerant of conventional therapy: an externally controlled trial. Clin Infect Dis 2007; 44:2.

13. A Cantanzaro et al. Safety, tolerance, and efficacy of posaconazole therapy in patients with nonmeningeal disseminated or chronic pulmonary coccidioidomycosis. Clin Infect Dis 2007; 45:562.

14. DA Stevens et al. Posaconazole therapy for chronic refractory coccidioidomycosis. Chest 2007; 132:952.

15. JA Van Burik et al. Posaconazole is effective as salvage therapy in zygomycosis: a retrospective summary of 91 cases. Clin Infect Dis 2006; 42:e61.

16. C Wagner et al. The echinocandins: comparison of their pharmacokinetics, pharmacodynamics and clinical applications. Pharmacology 2006; 78:161.

17. ER Kuse et al. Micafungin versus liposomal amphotericin B for candidaemia and invasive candidosis: a phase III randomised double-blind trial. Lancet 2007; 369:1519.

18. PG Pappas et al. Micafungin versus caspofungin for treatment of candidemia and other forms of invasive candidiasis. Clin Infect Dis 2007; 45:883.

19. DW Denning. Micafungin (FK463), alone or in combination with other systemic antifungal agents, for the treatment of acute invasive aspergillosis. J Infect 2006; 53:337.

20. Anidulafungin (Eraxis) for Candida infections. Med Lett Drugs Ther 2006; 48:43.

21. AC Reboli et al. Anidulafungin versus fluconazole for invasive candidiasis. N Engl J Med 2007; 356:2472.

22. MM Roden. Triad of acute infusion-related reactions associated with liposomal amphotericin B: analysis of clinical and epidemiological characteristics. Clin Infect Dis 2003; 36:1213.

23. AJ Ullmann et al. Prospective study of amphotericin B formulations in immunocompromised patients in 4 European countries. Clin Infect Dis 2006; 43:e29.

24. PG Pappas et al. Clinical practice guidelines for the management of candidiasis: 2009 update by the Infectious Disease Society of America. Clin Infect Dis 2009; 48:503.

25. WT Hughes et al. 2002 guidelines for the use of antimicrobial agents in neutropenic patients with cancer. Clin Infect Dis 2002; 34:730.

26. TJ Walsh et al. Caspofungin versus liposomal amphotericin B for empirical antifungal therapy in patients with persistent fever and neutropenia. N Engl J Med 2004; 351:1391.

27. TJ Walsh et al. Voriconazole compared with liposomal amphotericin B for empirical antifungal therapy in patients with neutropenia and persistent fever. N Engl J Med 2002; 346:225.

Miconazole *(Oravig)* for Oropharyngeal Candidiasis
Originally published in The Medical Letter – November 2010; 52:95

The FDA has approved a buccal tablet formulation of miconazole *(Oravig* – Strativa) for local treatment of oropharyngeal candidiasis in adults. Miconazole has been available for many years in topical formulations for treatment of superficial fungal infections and vulvovaginal candidiasis.[1]

OROPHARYNGEAL CANDIDIASIS — Clotrimazole troches or nystatin suspension are often used for initial treatment of mild to moderate oropharyngeal candidiasis. Compliance can be a problem because of the need for multiple doses, and recurrence is common. For treatment of recurrent or more severe disease, systemic fluconazole is often used, but development of resistance has been reported.[2]

PHARMACOLOGY — Miconazole is an azole antifungal with activity against many species of *Candida,* including some resistant to fluconazole.[3] Systemic absorption of miconazole from the buccal tablet was minimal. The average duration of buccal attachment in healthy volunteers was 15 hours.

CLINICAL STUDIES — In a randomized, investigator- blinded, non-inferiority study in 282 patients with oropharyngeal candidiasis who had received radiotherapy for head and neck cancer, complete or partial response occurred in 56% of patients treated with buccal miconazole 50 mg once daily for 14 days and in 49% of those using 125 mg of oral miconazole gel (not available in the US) applied 4 times daily.[4]

A non-inferiority, double-blind, double-dummy trial in patients with HIV and oropharyngeal candidiasis randomized 476 patients to 14 days' treatment with 50 mg of buccal miconazole once daily or to clotrimazole troches 10 mg 5 times/day. The rate of clinical cure in patients treated with miconazole (68%) was non-inferior to that in patients treated with clotri-

SOME DRUGS FOR OROPHARYNGEAL CANDIDIASIS

	Dosage	Cost[1]
Clotrimazole – generic	10 mg troche 5x/d	$89.99
Mycelex		122.99
Fluconazole[2] – generic	200 mg x1, then 100 mg/d PO	54.99
Diflucan		198.96
Miconazole –	50 mg buccal tablet once/d	270.00[3]
Oravig		

1. Cost of 14 days' treatment based on prices at drugstore.com. Accessed November 19, 2010.
2. Fluconazole can also be taken as a liquid suspension. The cost of one 35 mL bottle (40 mg/mL) is $109.98.
3. Based on AWP listings in *Price Alert* November 15, 2010.

mazole (74%). The rate of mycological cure (30% vs. 27%) and the incidence of relapse by day 35 (26% vs. 28%) was similar in both groups.[5]

ADVERSE EFFECTS — The most common adverse effects reported in clinical trials of buccal miconazole were diarrhea, nausea, upper abdominal pain, vomiting, headache and altered taste. Oral discomfort, burning and pain, mouth ulceration, glossodynia and application site pain were also reported. *Oravig* is classified as category C (risk cannot be ruled out) for use during pregnancy.

DRUG INTERACTIONS — Miconazole is an inhibitor of CYP2C9 and CYP3A4; if absorbed systemically, it could increase serum concentrations of drugs metabolized by these enzymes. Bleeding and bruising have been reported with concomitant use of topical, intra-vaginal or oral miconazole with warfarin (*Coumadin,* and others).

DOSAGE AND ADMINISTRATION — The usual dosage of *Oravig* is one 50-mg buccal tablet applied to the upper gum just above an incisor tooth once daily, alternating sides of the mouth each day, for 14 days. The tablet should be held in place by pressing on the upper lip for 30 seconds to ensure adhesion. It should not be chewed, crushed or swallowed. If the tablet does not adhere for at least 6 hours, it should be reapplied; if it still does not adhere, a new tablet should be used. If the tablet is swallowed within 6 hours, the patient should drink a glass of water and then apply a new tablet. Patients can eat and drink while the tablet is in place, but should not chew gum.

CONCLUSION — The new once-daily buccal tablet formulation of miconazole *(Oravig)* appears to be as effective as 5-times-daily clotrimazole troches for the treatment of oropharyngeal candidiasis, but it costs more.

1. Antifungal drugs. Treat Guidel Med Lett 2009; 7:95.
2. JM Laudenbach and JB Epstein. Treatment strategies for oropharyngeal candidiasis. Expert Opin Pharmacother 2009; 10:1413.
3. N Isham and MA Ghannoum. Antifungal activity of miconazole against recent *Candida* strains. Mycoses 2010; 53:434.
4. RJ Bensadoun et al. Comparison of the efficacy and safety of miconazole 50-mg mucoadhesive buccal tablets with miconazole 500-mg gel in the treatment of oropharyngeal candidiasis: a prospective, randomized, single-blind, multicenter, comparative, phase III trial in patients treated with radiotherapy for head and neck cancer. Cancer 2008; 112:204.
5. JA Vazquez et al. Randomized, comparative, double-blind, double-dummy, multicenter trial of miconazole buccal tablet and clotrimazole troches for the treatment of oropharyngeal candidiasis: study of miconazole Lauriad® efficacy and safety (SMiLES). HIV Clin Trials 2010; 11:186.

DRUGS FOR
HIV Infection

Original publication date – February 2009

New guidelines for use of antiretroviral agents have been published, with a shift towards earlier and more continuous treatment.[1-3] HIV infection is treated with combinations of antiretroviral drugs depending on the patient's HIV RNA levels ("viral load") and CD4 cell count. Increases in viral load while on therapy may indicate development of drug resistance, requiring further testing and a change in treatment regimen. Resistance testing is now recommended when a patient is first seen, regardless of when therapy will be started.[4]

The dosage and cost of drugs for HIV infection are listed in the tables on pages 168 through 175. The regimens of choice are listed on page 179 and drugs that should not be used together on page 181. Antiretroviral drugs interact with each other and with many other drugs; most of these interactions are not included here (for more information on interactions, see *The Medical Letter Adverse Drug Interactions Program*).

NUCLEOSIDE/NUCLEOTIDE REVERSE TRANSCRIPTASE
INHIBITORS (NRTIs)

Nucleoside analogs inhibit HIV reverse transcriptase and decrease or prevent HIV replication in infected cells. Nucleotides are phosphory-lated nucleosides; nucleoside and nucleotide RTIs have similar mechanisms of action.

161

Class Adverse Effects – NRTIs (especially didanosine, stavudine and zidovudine) can cause a potentially fatal syndrome of lactic acidosis with hepatic steatosis. Peripheral lipoatrophy, central fat accumulation and hyperlipidemia can occur with stavudine or zidovudine (peripheral lipoatrophy may be more common when either one of these NRTIs is combined with efavirenz).

Abacavir (ABC, *Ziagen*) – Abacavir is available alone and in a fixed-dose combination with lamivudine *(Epzicom),* which has been used as a dual-NRTI backbone in antiretroviral regimens, and in one with lamivudine and zidovudine *(Trizivir).* A recent clinical trial suggested an increased incidence of virologic failure in treatment-naïve patients with baseline HIV RNA ≥ 100,000 copies/mL being treated with a dual NRTI backbone containing abacavir/lamivudine compared to one containing tenofovir/emtricita- bine.[5]Abacavir should not be used in a triple-NRTI combination with lamivudine (or emtricitabine) and tenofovir because of high rates of virologic failure with this combination.[6]

Adverse Effects – Observational data suggest that there may be an association between abacavir use and myocardial infarction.[7,8] Hypersensitivity reactions, usually with rash, fever and malaise, and sometimes with respiratory or gastrointestinal symptoms are fairly common; they usually develop early in treatment (median of 11 days), but can occur at any time and are strongly associated with the presence of the HLA-B*5701 allele. In one study, a significantly lower incidence of hypersensitivity reactions occurred in patients prospectively screened for HLA-B*5701 compared to unscreened patients (3.4% vs 7.8%).[9] Commercial assays are available, and prospective screening prior to abacavir use is recommended.[10] Patients who screen positive for HLA-B*5701 should not receive abacavir; even those whose screen is negative should be observed carefully because hypersensitivity can still occur rarely. Rechallenges after a hypersensitivity reaction to abacavir have sometimes been fatal.

Didanosine (ddl, *Videx*) – Didanosine is available in enteric-coated capsules (*Videx EC*, and others) and as a pediatric powder for oral solution. Its use is limited now because of its adverse effects.

Adverse Effects – Dose-related peripheral neuropathy, pancreatitis and gastrointestinal disturbances are treatment-limiting toxicities. Gastrointestinal tolerance is better with the enteric-coated capsules than with earlier formulations. Retinal changes and optic neuritis have been reported. The risk of pancreatitis, neuropathy and lactic acidosis is increased when didanosine is combined with stavudine, and this combination is no longer recommended.

Drug Interactions – The pediatric powder formulation of didanosine interferes with absorption of drugs that require gastric acidity, including delavirdine, indinavir and atazanavir. Use of the enteric-coated preparation appears to eliminate this problem. Tenofovir inhibits metabolism of didanosine; if they are used together, the dose of didanosine should be decreased.

Emtricitabine (FTC, *Emtriva*) – Emtricitabine is the 5-fluorinated derivative of lamivudine.[11] It is similar to lamivudine in safety and efficacy, and can be given once daily. Emtricitabine is also available in fixed-dose combinations with tenofovir *(Truvada)* (the preferred NRTI backbone) and with tenofovir and efavirenz *(Atripla)* (the preferred NNRTI-based regimen). Resistance to emtricitabine is conferred by the M184V mutation, which is the main cause of resistance to lamivudine, so cross-resistance is complete.

Adverse Effects – Emtricitabine is among the best tolerated of the NRTIs. It can cause hyperpigmentation of the palms and soles, particularly in dark-skinned patients. Because emtricitabine is also active against hepatitis B virus (HBV), HIV-positive patients with chronic HBV infection may experience a hepatitis flare if emtricitabine is discontinued or if their HBV strain becomes resistant to the drug.

Lamivudine (3TC, *Epivir*) – Lamivudine can be taken once or twice daily. Lamivudine is also available in fixed-dose combinations with abacavir *(Epzicom)*, zidovudine *(Combivir)*, and zidovudine and abacavir *(Trizivir)*. Lamivudine-resistant strains are cross-resistant to emtricitabine, and may have a modest decrease in susceptibility to abacavir and didanosine.

A lower-dose lamivudine tablet is approved for treatment of chronic hepatitis B *(Epivir-HBV)*.

Adverse Effects – Lamivudine, like emtricitabine, is among the best tolerated of the NRTIs. Because lamivudine is also active against hepatitis B virus (HBV), HIV-positive patients with chronic HBV infection may experience a flare of hepatitis if lamivudine is withdrawn or if their HBV strain becomes resistant to the drug. Other adverse effects are uncommon; pancreatitis has been reported rarely in children.

Stavudine (d4T, *Zerit*) – Stavudine is no longer recommended for initial therapy. It is sometimes used after failure of regimens containing other NRTIs, but cross-resistance with zidovudine is virtually complete. Concurrent administration of zidovudine causes antagonism.

Adverse Effects – Fatal lactic acidosis may occur more frequently with stavudine than with other NRTIs. Serum aminotransferase activity may increase with stavudine treatment, and pancreatitis has occurred rarely. Lactic acidosis and pancreatitis are more common when stavudine is combined with didanosine; this combination is not recommended. Stavudine commonly causes peripheral sensory neuropathy, which may persist even if the drug is stopped. Stavudine causes lipoatrophy, raises serum lipid concentrations, and has been associated with development of diabetes.

Zidovudine (AZT, ZDV, *Retrovir*, and others) – Zidovudine is available alone and in fixed-dose combinations with lamivudine *(Combivir)* and with lamivudine and abacavir *(Trizivir)*. It can be given in combination with any other NRTI except stavudine, which causes antagonism. Non-suppressive therapy with a zidovudine-containing regimen results in resistance to zidovudine and cross-resistance to other NRTIs.

Adverse Effects – Adverse effects of zidovudine include anemia, neutropenia, nausea, vomiting, headache, fatigue, confusion, malaise, myopathy, hepatitis, and hyperpigmentation of the oral mucosa and nail beds. It may be better tolerated when taken with food. Zidovudine can cause lipoatrophy, lactic acidosis and hepatic steatosis, but perhaps less frequently than stavudine.

Tenofovir disoproxil fumarate (TDF, *Viread*) – Tenofovir DF is the only nucleotide RTI available for treatment of HIV. It is a prodrug of tenofovir, a potent inhibitor of HIV replication. Tenofovir DF is given once daily. It is effective as part of initial HIV therapy and has activity against some HIV strains that are resistant to other NRTIs. Tenofovir DF is available alone and in fixed-dose combinations with emtri-citabine *(Truvada)* and with emtricitabine and efavirenz *(Atripla)*.

Tenofovir should not be used in triple-NRTI combinations with abacavir/lamivudine or didanosine/lamivudine because of high rates of virologic failure. The combination of tenofovir with didanosine and efavirenz has been associated with early virologic failure and is not recommended for initial antiretroviral therapy.[12]

Tenofovir is also approved for treatment of chronic hepatitis B.[13]

Adverse Effects – Tenofovir is generally well tolerated. Renal toxicity, including a Fanconi-like syndrome and progression to renal failure, has been reported. Tenofovir dosage must be decreased in patients with diminished renal function. HIV-positive patients with chronic HBV infection may experience a hepatitis flare if it is discontinued or if their HBV strain becomes resistant to the drug.

Drug Interactions – If tenofovir is used in combination with didanosine, the dose of didanosine should be decreased. Tenofovir lowers serum concentrations of atazanavir; when the 2 drugs are given in combination ritonavir (100 mg with 300 mg daily of atazanavir) should be added to boost atazanavir levels.

NON-NUCLEOSIDE REVERSE TRANSCRIPTASE INHIBITORS (NNRTIs)

These drugs are direct, non-nucleoside inhibitors of HIV-1 reverse transcriptase. Combinations of an NNRTI with two NRTIs tend to be at least additive in reducing HIV replication *in vitro*. In treatment-naïve patients, NNRTI-based regimens have been at least as effective as protease inhibitor (PI)-based regimens, when each is taken in combination with two NRTIs. Efavirenz and a PI taken together have been associated with increased toxicity (in a 3-class regimen with 1 or 2 NRTIs) and development of resistance.[14,15]

HIV isolates that are resistant to NRTIs and to PIs may remain sensitive to NNRTIs, but cross-resistance is common among NNRTIs, with the exception of etravirine. Resistance to NNRTIs develops rapidly if they are used alone or in combinations that do not completely suppress viral replication. Because of their relatively long plasma half-lives, which are further increased in patients with genetic polymorphisms of CYP450 isoenzymes, discontinuation of NNRTI-based regimens (particularly when efavirenz is the NNRTI) should be approached in a step-wise fashion (some clinicians discontinue the NNRTI first and the NRTIs a week later) or by substituting a PI for up to one month to let the NNRTI "wash out".[16]

Delavirdine (DLV, *Rescriptor*) – Delavirdine is the least potent NNRTI and is given 3 times daily. It is rarely used. Unlike efavirenz and nevirapine, delavirdine inhibits the metabolism and increases serum concentrations of PIs.

Efavirenz (EFV, *Sustiva*) – Efavirenz is the only NNRTI approved for once-daily dosing. In previously untreated patients, the combination of efavirenz with 2 NRTIs has been more effective than lopinavir/ritonavir, indinavir or nelfinavir plus 2 NRTIs in lowering HIV RNA concentrations, even among patients with high baseline viral loads (>100,000 copies/mL), and has been better tolerated. Efavirenz is available alone and in a fixed-dose combination with the NRTIs emtricitabine and tenofovir *(Atripla)*.

Adverse Effects – The most common adverse effects of efavirenz have been rash, dizziness, headache, insomnia and inability to concentrate. Vivid dreams and nightmares can occur. Hallucinations, psychosis, depression and suicidal ideation have been reported. CNS effects tend to occur between 1 and 3 hours after each dose. They may stop within a few days or weeks, but can persist for months or years, and may be associated with high efavirenz serum concentrations.[17,18] When the dose is taken at bedtime, CNS effects may still be present in the morning on awakening and may impair driving; this effect generally wanes with time and can be ameliorated by taking the drug earlier in the evening. Hypertriglyceridemia has occurred. Lipoatrophy induced by stavudine and zidovudine is more common when these drugs are used with efavirenz.

Fetal abnormalities occurred in pregnant monkeys exposed to efavirenz, and neural tube defects have been reported in the offspring of women who took the drug during the first trimester of pregnancy. The drug should not be given to women who are or may become pregnant.

Drug Interactions – Efavirenz is an inducer of CYP3A4. Methadone is metabolized by CYP3A4 and its dosage often needs to be increased if efavirenz is used concurrently. Efavirenz decreases serum concentrations of some PIs. It also decreases serum concentrations of voriconazole *(Vfend)* and may have a similar effect on ketoconazole, itraconazole *(Sporanox)*, and posaconazole *(Noxafil)*; they should generally not be taken together.

NRTIs/NNRTIs FOR HIV INFECTION

Drug	Usual Adult Dosage
NUCLEOSIDE/NUCLEOTIDE REVERSE TRANSCRIPTASE INHIBITORS (NRTIs)	
Abacavir (ABC)	
Ziagen – GlaxoSmithKline*	300 mg bid[2] or 600 mg once/d[2]
Didanosine (ddl)	
generic	400 mg once/d[3,4]
Videx EC – Bristol-Myers Squibb*	
Emtricitabine (FTC)	
Emtriva – Gilead*	200 mg once/d[4,5]
Lamivudine (3TC)	
Epivir – GlaxoSmithKline*	150 mg bid[4,6] or 300 mg once/d[4,6]
Stavudine (d4T)	
Zerit – Bristol-Myers Squibb*	40 mg bid[4,7]
Tenofovir DF (TDF)	
Viread – Gilead	300 mg once/d[4,8]
Zidovudine (AZT, ZDV)	
generic*	300 mg bid[4,9]
Retrovir – GlaxoSmithKline*	
NON-NUCLEOSIDE REVERSE TRANSCRIPTASE INHIBITORS (NNRTIs)	
Delavirdine (DLV)	
Rescriptor – Pfizer	400 mg tid[10]
Efavirenz (EFV)	
Sustiva – Bristol-Myers Squibb	600 mg once/d[11]
Etravirine (ETR)	
Intelence – Tibotec	200 mg bid[12]

* Also available in a liquid or oral powder formulation.
1. Daily cost according to most recent data (November 30, 2008) from retail pharmacies nationwide available from Wolters Kluwer Health.
2. With or without food. Available in 300-mg tablets. Dosage for mild hepatic impairment is 200 mg bid; contraindicated in patients with moderate to severe hepatic impairment.
3. Doses should be taken on an empty stomach. Available in 125- (only *Videx EC*), 200-, 250- and 400-mg capsules; for adults <60 kg, 250 mg once daily, ≥60 kg, 400 mg once daily. The dose of didanosine in adults with CrCl ≥ 60mL/min should be decreased to 250 mg/d for those weighing ≥60 kg and to 200 mg/d for those weighing <60 kg when combined with tenofovir, which increases didanosine serum concentrations.
4. Dosage adjustment required for renal impairment.
5. With or without food. Available in 200-mg capsules.

Total Tablets or Capsules/day	Cost[1]
2	$18.14
1	
1	11.34
	12.88
1	13.47
2	13.52
1	13.49
2	14.50
1	21.66
2	10.74
	15.56
6	9.96
1	19.31
4	25.92

6. With or without food. For patients <50 kg, 2 mg/kg bid. Available in 150- and 300-mg tablets.
7. With or without food. For patients <60 kg, 30 mg bid. Available in 15-, 20-, 30- and 40-mg capsules.
8. May be taken with or without food. Available in 300-mg tablets.
9. With or without food. Available in 100-mg capsules and 300-mg tablets. Can also be given as 200 mg tid. Also available in a parenteral preparation for intrapartum use; the dose during labor and delivery is 2 mg/kg IV over the first hour, and then a continuous IV infusion of 1 mg/kg/hour until clamping of the umbilical cord.
10. With or without food. Available in 100- and 200-mg tablets.
11. Without food. Available in 50- and 200-mg capsules and 600-mg tablets. Take at bedtime for at least the first 2 to 4 weeks.
12. With food. Available in 100-mg tablets.

Continued on next page.

Drug	Usual Adult Dosage
NON-NUCLEOSIDE REVERSE TRANSCRIPTASE INHIBITORS (NNRTIs) (continued)	
Nevirapine (NVP)	
Viramune – Boehringer Ingelheim*	200 mg bid[13]
FIXED-DOSE NRTI COMBINATIONS	
Zidovudine/lamivudine	
Combivir – GlaxoSmithKline	300 mg/150 mg bid[14]
Zidovudine/lamivudine/abacavir	
Trizivir – GlaxoSmithKline	200 mg/150 mg/300 mg bid[15]
Abacavir/lamivudine	
Epzicom – GlaxoSmithKline	600 mg/300 mg once/d[16]
Emtricitabine/tenofovir DF	
Truvada – Gilead	200 mg/300 mg once/d[17]
FIXED-DOSE NNRTI/NRTI COMBINATION	
Efavirenz/emtricitabine/tenofovir DF	
Atripla – Bristol-Myers Squibb/Gilead	600 mg/200 mg/300 mg once/d[18]

13. With or without food. Available in 200-mg tablets. 200 mg once/day for the first 2 weeks of treatment to decrease the risk of rash. Should not be administered to patients with moderate or severe hepatic impairment.
14. Each tablet contains 300 mg of zidovudine and 150 mg of lamivudine.
15. Each tablet contains 300 mg of zidovudine, 150 mg of lamivudine and 300 mg of abacavir.

Etravirine (ETR; *Intelence*) – Etravirine was FDA-approved in 2008. Used in combination with optimized background therapy, it has been effective in achieving virologic control in treatment-experienced patients with documented resistance to both PIs and older NNRTIs.[19] The drug is taken twice daily. The common mutation (K103N) that confers resistance to efavirenz and nevirapine does not reduce the activity of etravirine. Resistance to etravirine has been reported, but the drug appears to have a relatively high genetic barrier to resistance.[20]

Total Tablets or Capsules/day	Cost[1]
2	16.04
2	29.44
2	47.52
1	31.65
1	34.75
1	54.63

16. Each tablet contains 600 mg of abacavir and 300 mg of lamivudine.
17. Each tablet contains 200 mg of emtricitabine and 300 mg of tenofovir DF.
18. Without food. Each tablet contains 600 mg of efavirenz, 200 mg of emtricitabine, and 300 mg tenofovir DF. Taking at bedtime may diminish CNS effects.

Adverse Effects – Etravirine is generally well tolerated. Rash, nausea, peripheral neuropathy and hypertension can occur. Etravirine-induced rash is less frequent than with nevirapine, but it can be severe, and erythema multiforme and Stevens-Johnson syndrome have been reported. Increases in serum transaminases, cholesterol and triglyceride concentrations have also been reported.

Drug interactions – Etravirine is a substrate of CYP3A4, 2C9 and 2C19, an inducer of CYP3A4 and an inhibitor of CYP2C9 and 2C19 and has many drug-drug interactions. Taken with unboosted PIs, etravirine can

PROTEASE, ENTRY, FUSION AND INTEGRASE INHIBITORS FOR HIV INFECTION

Drug	Usual Adult Dosage
PROTEASE INHIBITORS	
Atazanavir (ATV)	
Reyataz – Bristol-Myers Squibb	300 mg/100 mg RTV once/d[2,3,4]
Darunavir (DRV)	800 mg/100 mg RTV once/day or
Prezista – Tibotec	600 mg/100 mg RTV bid[3,5]
Fosamprenavir (FPV)	
Lexiva – GlaxoSmithKline*	1400 mg/100 mg RTV once/d[3,4,6]
Indinavir (IDV)	800 mg q8h or
Crixivan – Merck	800 mg/100 mg RTV bid[3,4,7]
Lopinavir/ritonavir (LPV/RTV)	
Kaletra – Abbott*	400/100 mg bid or 800/200 mg once/d[8]
Nelfinavir (NFV)	
Viracept – Pfizer*	1250 mg bid or 750 mg tid[9]
Saquinavir (SQV)	
Invirase – Roche	1000 mg/100 mg RTV bid[3,10]

* Also available in a liquid or oral powder formulation.
1. Daily cost according to data (November 30, 2008) from retail pharmacies nationwide available from Wolters Kluwer Health.
2. With food. Available in 100-, 150-, 200- and 300-mg capsules. For therapy-experienced patients, the FDA-approved dose is 300 mg/100 mg RTV once/d. For therapy-naïve patients, the FDA-approved dose is 300 mg/100 mg RTV once/d or 400 mg once/d for patients unable to tolerate RTV. The dose with TDF is 300 mg/100 mg RTV and with EFV is 400 mg/100 mg RTV.
3. RTV = Ritonavir (*Norvir* – Abbott). Available as a 100-mg soft-gelatin capsule. The liquid formulation of ritonavir has an unpleasant taste; the manufacturer suggests taking it with chocolate milk or a liquid nutritional supplement.
4. Dosage adjustment required for hepatic impairment.
5. With food. Must be co-administered with RTV. Available in 75-, 300-, 400- and 600-mg tablets. Once-daily dosing in treatment-naïve patients only.

Total Tablets or Capsules/day	Cost[1]
2	$43.03
3	42.46
4	52.94
3	35.98
6	18.00
6	32.52
4	27.96
4	
4 (625-mg tablets)	25.08
9 (250-mg tablets)	22.50
6	50.56

6. With or without food. Available in 700-mg tablets. Can also be given as 1400 mg bid, 1400 mg/200 mg RTV once/day or 700 mg/100 mg RTV bid in treatment-naïve patients and 700 mg/100 mg RTV bid in PI-experienced patients. When taken once daily with efavirenz, the recommended dose is 1400 mg/300 mg RTV.
7. With water or other liquids, 1 hour before or 2 hours after a meal, or with a light meal. Available in 100-, 200-, 333- and 400-mg capsules. Dosage is 600 mg q8h when taken with DLV. Patients should drink at least 48 ounces (1.5 L) of water daily. RTV-boosted dosage is not FDA-approved.
8. With or without food; GI effects are reduced when taken with food. Available in tablets containing 100 or 200 mg lopinavir and 25 or 50 mg ritonavir. The recommended dose is 500/125 mg bid when taken with EFV, NVP, FPV or NFV. Once-daily dosing in treatment-naïve patients only. No refrigeration.
9. With food. Available in 250- and 625-mg tablets.
10. Within 2 hours after a full meal. Available in 200-mg capsules and 500-mg tablets. Dosage is 1000 mg bid (without RTV) when taken with LPV/RTV.

Continued on next page.

Drugs for HIV Infection

PROTEASE, ENTRY, FUSION AND INTEGRASE INHIBITORS FOR
HIV INFECTION (continued)

Drug	Usual Adult Dosage
PROTEASE INHIBITORS (continued)	
Tipranavir (TPV)	
Aptivus – Boehringer Ingelheim	500 mg/200 mg RTV bid[3,11]
ENTRY AND FUSION INHIBITORS	
Enfuvirtide (T20)	
Fuzeon – Roche	90 mg SC bid[12]
Maraviroc (MVC)	
Selzentry – Pfizer	150-300 mg bid[13]
INTEGRASE INHIBITOR	
Raltegravir (RAL)	
Isentress – Merck	400 mg bid[15]

11. With or without food. Must be co-administered with RTV. Available in 250-mg capsules.
12. Available in kits containing a one-month supply of syringes and single-use vials with powder for a 90-mg dose and sterile water for reconstitution.
13. With or without food. Available in 150-mg and 300-mg tablets. It should be dosed at 150 mg bid when given with strong CYP3A4 inhibitors, including PIs (except tipranavir/RTV) and delavirdine. It should be dosed at 600 mg bid when given with strong CYP3A4 inducers including efavirenz. A dose of 300 mg bid can be used with other concomitant medications including nevirapine, tipranavir/RTV, all NRTIs, and enfuvirtide.

increase or decrease the serum concentration of the PIs. Etravirine should not be used with tipranavir/ ritonavir, fosamprenavir/ritonavir or atazanavir/ritonavir, with PIs given without ritonavir, or with other NNRTIs.

Nevirapine (NVP, *Viramune*) – Nevirapine has appeared to be comparable to efavirenz in effectiveness, but unexpected virological failure was reported when it was used with tenofovir/emtricitabine in treatment-naïve patients.[21]

Total Tablets or Capsules/day	Cost[1]
8	78.16
—	86.88
2	34.24[14]
2	34.02

14. Cost is the same for 150 mg and 300 mg bid.
15. With or without food. Available in 400-mg tablets.

Adverse Effects – Nevirapine has a potential for serious adverse effects. It can cause severe hepatotoxicity, hepatic failure and death, particularly in patients with previously elevated transaminases or underlying hepatitis B or C. The manufacturer recommends monitoring all patients treated with the drug for the first 18 weeks of treatment. Fever, nausea and headache can also occur. Rash is common early in treatment with nevirapine and can be more severe than with other NNRTIs; it may progress to Stevens-Johnson syndrome.

To decrease the incidence of both rash and hepatic toxicity, the dose of nevirapine should be 200 mg once daily for the first 2 weeks, and then

200 mg twice daily. Women with baseline CD4 counts >250 cells/mm³ and men with baseline CD4 counts >400 cells/mm³ are at increased risk of nevirapine-associated hepatotoxicity.[22]

Drug Interactions – Like efavirenz, nevirapine is an inducer of CYP3A4. The dose of methadone often needs to be increased if nevirapine is used concurrently. Nevirapine decreases serum concentrations of some PIs. It has also decreased serum concentrations of ketoconazole and may have a similar effect on voriconazole, itraconazole and posaconazole.

FIXED-DOSE COMBINATIONS

NRTIs – Four different fixed-dose NRTI combinations are available (see table on page 170). They offer the advantage of simplifying dosing schedules and reducing pill burden, but they are less flexible in terms of dosage adjustment.

Adverse Effects – Adverse effects are generally similar to those with the drugs taken separately. Some patients with hepatic or renal impairment will not be able to take combinations because the dose cannot be adjusted.

NNRTI/NRTI – *Atripla* is the only fixed-dose combination to contain antiretrovirals from two different classes (1 NNTRI/2 NRTIs). Each tablet contains **efavirenz** 600 mg, **emtricitabine** 200 mg and **tenofovir DF** 300 mg. The dose is one tablet once daily.

An open-label, randomized noninferiority study in 517 treatment-naïve patients compared the combination of efavirenz, emtricitabine and teno fovir once daily with fixed-dose zidovudine and lamivudine *(Combivir)* twice daily plus efavirenz once daily. At week 48, significantly more patients taking emtricitabine/tenofovir/efavirenz achieved and maintained HIV viral loads <400 copies/mL (84% vs. 73%) and <50 copies/mL (80% vs. 70%).[23] At week 96, the percentages of patients with HIV RNA <400 copies/mL were 75% vs. 62%, and with <50 copies/mL were 67%

vs. 61%.[24] After 144 weeks, the percentages of patients with HIV RNA <400 copies/mL were 71% vs. 58%, and with <50 copies/mL were 64% vs. 56%.[25]

Adverse Effects – Adverse effects for *Atripla* are generally similar to those with the drugs taken separately. Patients with moderate or severe renal impairment who require dose adjustments and women who are or might become pregnant should not take *Atripla*.

PROTEASE INHIBITORS (PIs)

Protease inhibitors prevent cleavage of protein precursors essential for HIV maturation, infection of new cells and viral replication. Use of a PI in combination with other drugs has led to marked clinical improvement and prolonged survival even in patients with advanced HIV infection. Most PIs potently suppress HIV replication *in vivo*. Low-dose ritonavir taken with some other PIs inhibits the metabolism and increases serum concentrations of the other PI ("ritonavir boosting"); this technique is recommended for most PIs.

Class Adverse Effects – Many PIs can cause gastrointestinal distress, increased bleeding in hemophiliacs, hyperglycemia, insulin resistance and hyperlipidemia, and have been associated with an increased risk of coronary artery disease.[26] They have also been associated with peripheral lipoatrophy and central fat accumulation. All, especially tipranavir, can cause hepatotoxicity, which may occasionally be severe and is more common in patients who are co-infected with HBV or hepatitis C virus (HCV). All PIs are metabolized by and are inhibitors of hepatic CYP3A4; drug interactions are common and can be severe.[27]

Atazanavir (ATV, *Reyataz*) – Atazanavir is a PI with once-daily dosing.[11] Most clinicians prefer to use boosted atazanavir whenever possible; atazanavir/ritonavir has been comparable to lopinavir/ritonavir in treatment-naïve as well as treatment-experienced patients.[28] Concurrent use of drugs that increase gastric PH, such as proton pump inhibitors, H_2-antihistimines and antacids, may decrease absorption of atazanavir.

Adverse Effects – Atazanavir causes an asymptomatic indirect hyper-bilirubinemia that sometimes produces jaundice; it is reversible when the drug is stopped. Rash occurred in about 20% of patients in clinical trials; it was mostly mild or moderate. Unboosted, atazanavir has had fewer adverse effects than other PIs on lipid profiles. It can cause PR prolongation and should be used with caution in patients with cardiac conduction abnormalities. Atazanavir-containing kidney stones have been reported in patients taking the drug, sometimes years after treatment was started.[29]

Darunavir (DRV, *Prezista*) – Darunavir can now be used in treatment-naïve patients, as well as treatment-experienced patients.[30,31] It is taken twice daily in treatment-experienced and once daily in treatment-naïve patients with ritonavir to achieve adequate bioavailability. It is comparable to lopinavir/ritonavir in treatment-experienced, lopinavir/ritonavir-naïve patients with less emergence of new resistance.[32] In a study of treatment-naïve patients, once-daily darunavir/ritonavir (800 mg/100 mg) was comparable to either once-daily or twice-daily lopinavir/ritonavir, each taken with fixed-dose tenofovir/emtricitabine, after 48 weeks, and was significantly better in patients with baseline HIV RNA $\geq$ 100,000 copies/mL.[33] After 96 weeks, overall virologic response rates with darunavir/ritonavir were superior to those with lopinavir/ritonavir.[34]

Adverse Effects – The incidence of adverse effects with darunavir, including diarrhea, nausea, headache, nasopharyngitis and increased serum transaminases, has been similar to that with other PIs. In one study, gastrointestinal side effects and elevations in total cholesterol and triglycerides were less common with darunavir/ritonavir compared with lopinavir/ritonavir.[33] Rash can occur and severe rash, including erythema multiforme and Stevens-Johnson syndrome, has been reported. Like tipranavir and fosamprenavir, darunavir contains a sulfonamide moiety; it should be used with caution in patients with sulfonamide allergy.

ANTIRETROVIRAL REGIMENS FOR TREATMENT-NAÏVE PATIENTS

NNRTI-BASED (1 NNRTI + 2 NRTIs)

Regimen of Choice

Efavirenz[1] + tenofovir/emtricitabine[2,4,6] (all 3 are also available as a coformulation)

Substitutes

For the NNRTI: nevirapine[6]

For the NRTIs: abacavir[3]/lamivudine[2,4] or zidovudine/lamivudine[2,4] or didanosine + lamivudine[4]

PI-BASED (1 OR 2 PIs + 2 NRTIs)

Regimen of Choice

Lopinavir/ritonavir or atazanavir/ritonavir or fosamprenavir/ritonavir or darunavir/ritonavir + tenofovir/emtricitabine[2,4]

Substitutes

For the PI(s): saquinavir/ritonavir or atazanavir or fosamprenavir

For the NRTIs: abacavir[3]/lamivudine[2,4] or zidovudine/lamivudine[2,4] or didanosine + lamivudine[4]

ALTERNATIVE REGIMENS (generally not recommended)

Quadruple NRTI[5]

Abacavir + lamivudine + zidovudine + tenofovir

1. Except in pregnant women or women who might become pregnant because efavirenz is contraindicated in pregnancy.
2. Available as a coformulation.
3. For patients who test negative for HLA-B*5701.
4. Emtricitabine can be substituted for lamivudine and vice versa.
5. Should only be considered after NNRTI- and PI-based regimens have been excluded and in special circumstances, such as co-administration with tuberculosis therapy. Triple NRTI regimens such as abacavir/zidovudine/lamivudine or tenofovir + zidovudine/lamivudine can also be considered.
6. A regimen containing nevirapine + tenofovir + emtricitabine (or lamivudine) should be used with caution due to reports of early virologic failure.

Fosamprenavir calcium (FPV, *Lexiva*) – Fosamprenavir calcium, a prodrug of amprenavir, is available in 700-mg tablets equivalent to 600 mg of amprenavir. In patients who have not previously been treated with a PI, fosamprenavir can be taken once daily combined with ritonavir, or twice daily with or without ritonavir. In patients who are treatment-experienced, it should be taken twice daily with ritonavir. Fosamprenavir/ritonavir was as effective and as well tolerated as lopinavir/ritonavir, each in combination with abacavir/lamivudine, in treatment-naïve patients.[35] If fosampre-navir/ritonavir once daily is coadministered with efavirenz, the ritonavir dosage should be increased. Fosamprenavir has replaced amprenavir, which is no longer available in the US.

Adverse Effects – The most common adverse effects of fosamprenavir have been nausea, vomiting, perioral paresthesias and rash. Many patients with rash can continue or restart fosamprenavir if the rash is mild or moderate, but about 1% of patients have developed severe rash, including Stevens-Johnson syndrome. Unlike amprenavir, which could not be taken with a fatty meal, fosamprenavir has no food restrictions. The incidence of lipid abnormalities with fosamprenavir is similar to that with lopinavir/ritonavir. Like tipranavir and darunavir, fosamprenavir contains a sulfonamide moiety and should be used with caution in patients with sulfonamide allergy.

Indinavir (IDV, *Crixivan*) – Indinavir taken on an empty stomach has good oral bioavailability. Although labeled for use 3 times daily, it has been effective taken twice daily when combined with low-dose ritonavir. It is used uncommonly, however, because of its toxicity.

Adverse Effects – In addition to adverse effects similar to those of other PIs, indinavir causes asymptomatic elevation of indirect bilirubin, indinavir-containing kidney stones and renal insufficiency, dermatologic changes including alopecia, dry skin and mucous membranes, and paronychia and ingrown toenails. Patients should drink at least 1.5-2 liters of water daily to minimize renal adverse effects. Ritonavir boosting increases the risk of nephrolithiasis. Gallstones have also been reported.[36]

Lopinavir/ritonavir (LPV/RTV, *Kaletra*) – Lopinavir is available in the US only in a fixed-dose combination with ritonavir.[37] Though usually given twice daily, it can be offered once daily to treatment-naïve patients. Lopinavir/ritonavir has been the PI regimen of choice in both treatment-naïve patients and in those with previous HIV treatment and moderate or

SOME ANTIRETROVIRAL DRUGS THAT SHOULD NOT BE USED TOGETHER OR USED WITH CAUTION

Drugs	Effect	Comments
Abacavir + lamivudine (or emtricitabine) + tenofovir	Early virologic failure	Not recommended
Atazanavir (unboosted) + didanosine + emtricitabine (or lamivudine)	Efficacy concerns	Not recommended
Atazanavir + indinavir	Increased risk of hyperbilirubinemia	Not recommended
Didanosine + lamivudine (or emtricitabine) + tenofovir	Early virologic failure	Not recommended
Didanosine + stavudine	Increased risk of peripheral neuropathy, pancreatitis and lactic acidosis	Not recommended for initial therapy or in pregnant women
Didanosine + tenofovir + efavirenz	Early virologic failure	Not recommended for initial therapy
Nevirapine + tenofovir + emtricitabine (or lamivudine)	Early virologic failure	Use with caution
Stavudine + zidovudine	Antagonism	Not recommended

no PI resistance (<5 resistance mutations). Atazanavir/ritonavir appears to be similarly effective in treatment-experienced patients; in treatment-naïve patients, fosamprenavir/ritonavir, atazanavir/ritonavir and saquinavir/ritonavir were non-inferior to lopinavir/ritonavir[28,35,38] and darunavir/ritonavir was superior to lopinavir/ritonavir.[34]

Adverse Effects – Lopinavir/ritonavir is generally well tolerated. The most common adverse effects have been diarrhea, nausea, headache and asthenia. As with other PIs, hyperlipidemia, hyperglycemia, increased serum transaminases and altered body fat distribution have been reported. Fatal pancreatitis has occurred.

Nelfinavir (NFV, *Viracept*) – Nelfinavir once was a commonly used PI, but it appears to be less potent than lopinavir/ritonavir, and cannot be boosted.

Adverse Effects – Nelfinavir is generally well tolerated. Diarrhea, which is nearly universal but may resolve with continued use, is its main adverse effect.

Ritonavir (RTV, *Norvir*) – Ritonavir is well absorbed from the gastrointestinal tract and at full doses potently inhibits HIV, but due to poor tolerability it is now used in doses of 100-200 mg once or twice daily to increase the serum concentrations and decrease the dosage frequency of other PIs.

Adverse Effects – Adverse reactions are common with full doses of ritonavir, but less common with the low doses used for boosting in PI combinations. Ritonavir can cause hypertriglyceridemia, altered taste, nausea, vomiting and, rarely, circumoral and peripheral paresthesias. It interacts with many other drugs.

Saquinavir (SQV, *Invirase*) – Saquinavir is available as a hard-gel capsule or film-coated tablet. Saquinavir/ ritonavir appears to be as effective as and better tolerated than indinavir/ritonavir. In one study in treatment-naïve patients, it was non-inferior to lopinavir/ritonavir.[38]

Adverse Effects – Saquinavir is usually well tolerated, but occasionally causes diarrhea, abdominal discomfort, nausea, glucose intolerance, hyperlipidemia, abnormal fat distribution and increased serum transaminases. It can cause increased bleeding in patients with hemophilia, and rarely causes rash and hyperprolactinemia.

Tipranavir (TPV, *Aptivus*) – Tipranavir is available as a capsule and must be taken with low-dose ritonavir.[39] It can be used in treatment-experienced patients who have ongoing viral replication or in patients with HIV strains known to be resistant to multiple PIs, but darunavir may be better tolerated for the same indication. In clinical studies of patients with extensive treatment experience and drug resistance, tipranavir-containing regimens were more effective than regimens based on some other ritonavir-boosted PIs, including lopinavir/ritonavir, indinavir/ritonavir and saquinavir/ritonavir. Patients on tipranavir who also received the fusion inhibitor enfuvirtide as a part of their background regimen had better response rates.[40]

Adverse Effects – Severe hepatitis, including some fatalities, has been reported in patients taking tipranavir. Careful monitoring of liver function tests is recommended, especially in patients with chronic HBV or HCV infection. Tipranavir may cause diarrhea, nausea, vomiting and abdominal pain. The drug contains a sulfonamide moiety; caution should be used in patients with sulfonamide allergy. Intracranial hemorrhage has been reported among patients taking tipranavir.

ENTRY AND FUSION INHIBITORS

Two drugs are now available that block HIV entry into cells by different mechanisms.

Enfuvirtide (T20, *Fuzeon*) – Enfuvirtide is the only fusion inhibitor currently available. After HIV binds to the host cell surface, a conformational change occurs in the transmembrane glycoprotein subunit (gp41) of the viral envelope, facilitating fusion of the viral and host cell membranes, and entry of the virus into the cell. Enfuvirtide binds to gp41 and prevents the conformational change. It is indicated for treatment-experienced patients with ongoing HIV replication despite current antiretroviral use. It is administered twice-daily by subcutaneous injection. In some clinical trials, patients receiving enfuvirtide as part of optimized background therapy (OBT) had better response rates than those who did not.[41]

Adverse Effects – Almost all patients develop local injection site reactions to enfuvirtide, with mild or moderate pain, erythema, induration, nodules and cysts.[42] Other adverse effects include eosinophilia, systemic hypersensitivity reactions, and possibly an increased incidence of bacterial pneumonia.

Maraviroc (MVC, *Selzentry*) – Maraviroc is the first CCR5 antagonist to receive FDA approval for treatment of HIV infection. CCR5 and CXCR4 are the two major co-receptors used by HIV-1 to gain entry into the host cell. HIV-1 strains can be classified on the basis of which co-receptor they use to gain entry as CCR5 ("R5") tropic, CXCR4 ("X4") tropic, or dual- or mixed-tropic. R5-tropic strains predominate during early stages of infection and remain dominant in 50-60% of late stage disease.[43]

Maraviroc is active against HIV strains resistant to other classes of drugs and is available orally. It is only approved for use in treatment-experienced adults with R5-tropic HIV-1. A commercial assay is available that can determine whether HIV-1 is R5, X4, or dual- or mixed-tropic. Viral resistance to maraviroc has been described, particularly when X4 strains, which tend to emerge as the disease progresses, are present; whether use of maraviroc will increase emergence of X4 is unknown.[44] Approval was based on studies of treatment-experienced patients with R5-tropic HIV-1 who did better with maraviroc and OBT than with placebo and OBT.[45] It has also been studied in treatment-naïve patients, showing non-inferiority to efavirenz, when each was combined with zidovudine/lamivudine in patients with R5 infection.[46]

Adverse Effects – Cough, pyrexia, upper respiratory tract infection, rash, musculoskeletal symptoms, abdominal pain and postural dizziness have been reported with maraviroc use. Hepatotoxicity can occur, sometimes associated with a rash and eosinophilia. Cardiovascular events have also been reported. Increases in infection and malignancy are a theoretical concern because some immune cells have CCR5 receptors.

Drug Interactions – Maraviroc is a substrate of CYP3A and P-glycoprotein. Significant drug-drug interactions occur.[27] The recommended dosage with strong CYP3A inhibitors including PIs is 150 mg bid (except with the combination of tipranavir and ritonavir when the dose is 300 mg bid), and is 600 mg bid when given with CYP3A inducers such as efavirenz. A dose of 300 mg bid can be used with other concomitant medications, including nevirapine, all NRTIs, and enfuvirtide.

INTEGRASE INHIBITOR

Raltegravir (RAL, *Isentress*) – HIV-1 integrase catalyzes the process that results in viral DNA insertion into the host genome. Integrase strand transfer (InST) inhibitors block the enzyme's activity, preventing viral DNA from integrating with cellular DNA. Raltegravir is the first available integrase inhibitor.[43] It is FDA-approved for use in combination therapy of treatment-experienced adults infected with HIV-1 strains resistant to multiple antiretrovirals. Approval was based on studies of treatment-experienced patients who had better virologic outcomes with raltegravir and OBT than with placebo and OBT.[47] This drug was effective even in patients with high baseline viral loads and low CD4 counts.[48] Raltegravir has also been studied in treatment-naïve patients. Two studies compared raltegravir with efavirenz, each combined with tenofovir and either lamivudine or emtricitabine; raltegravir was similar in efficacy to efavirenz, and produced more rapid declines in viral loads.[49,50] Viral resistance to raltegravir has emerged during treatment, especially in patients not taking other fully active drugs, and has been associated with clinical failure.[48] Raltegravir is not metabolized by CYP3A4.

Adverse Effects – Raltegravir is generally well-tolerated. Diarrhea, nausea and headache have been reported, but have been comparable in incidence to placebo. Increases in serum creatinine kinase, myopathy and rhabdomyolysis have occurred in clinical trials.

PREVENTION OF PERINATAL TRANSMISSION

Most perinatal transmission of HIV occurs close to the time of, or during, labor and delivery. **Zidovudine alone**, started at 14-34 weeks of gestation and continued in the infant for the first 6 weeks of life, reduced HIV transmission from 26% to 8%.[51]

Current guidelines recommend combination therapy with **zidovudine and lamivudine plus lopinavir/ritonavir or nevirapine** throughout pregnancy to prevent transmission of HIV to the offspring.[52] Women not already on therapy should consider waiting until after the first trimester to begin. Regardless of the antepartum antiretroviral regimen and the maternal HIV viral load, zidovudine administration is recommended during the intrapartum period and for the newborn for 6 weeks.

Adverse Effects – PI therapy may contribute to development of hyperglycemia in the mother. Some studies suggest that antenatal combination antiretroviral therapy including a PI may be associated with premature birth.[53] However, most clinicians believe that the overwhelming benefit of a potent antiretroviral regimen greatly outweighs the risk.

Already in Labor – For women who are already in labor and have had no antiretroviral therapy, **zidovudine** given to the mother and continued in the infant for 6 weeks beginning within 6-12 hours after birth, can decrease HIV transmission. **Single-dose nevirapine** given in addition to zidovudine, to the mother at the onset of labor and to the infant at 48-72 hours after delivery, may be more effective than zidovudine alone in decreasing the risk of perinatal transmission, but single-dose nevirapine has been associated with emergence of nevirapine-resistant strains, which could compromise future treatment of mother and child. For the mother, adding lamivudine during labor and continuing both lamivudine and zidovudine for 7 days postpartum decreases the risk of nevirapine resistance.[54]

Drugs Not to be Used – Fatal lactic acidosis from the combination of stavudine and didanosine has occurred in pregnant women; this combination should not be used. Efavirenz should be avoided in pregnancy, especially in the first trimester, because of potential teratogenicity. Initiation of nevirapine in pregnancy should be avoided in women with CD4 counts >250 cells/mm^3 because of the increased risk of hepatotoxicity. This restriction does not apply to single-dose nevirapine.

SUMMARY

Over 20 drugs belonging to 6 different mechanistic classes are now available, substantially improving treatment options for HIV infection. Depending on the results of resistance testing, reasonable choices for initial therapy of HIV infection would include an NNRTI, often efavirenz because it has fewer adverse effects than nevirapine, or a boosted PI combination, either combined with 2 NRTIs. For more advanced disease, combinations should be based on resistance testing and include two or more fully active drugs; etravirine, raltegravir, maraviroc, darunavir, tipranavir and enfuvirtide may be particularly helpful in heavily pretreated patients. For all patients, regular monitoring of viral load and CD4 cell count should be used to guide therapy. The CCR5 antagonist maraviroc, NNRTIs and PIs have many adverse interactions with each other and with other drugs.[27]

1. Panel on Antiretroviral Guidelines for Adults and Adolescents. Guidelines for the use of antiretroviral agents in HIV-1-infected adults and adolescents. Department of Health and Human Services. November 3, 2008. Available at www.aidsinfo.nih.gov. Accessed January 14, 2009.
2. SM Hammer et al. Antiretroviral Treatment of Adult HIV Infection: 2008 Recommendations of the International AIDS Society-USA Panel. JAMA 2008;300:555.

3. The Strategies for Management of Antiretroviral Therapy (SMART) Study Group. CD4+ count-guided interruption of antiretroviral treatment. N Engl J Med 2006;355:2283.

4. MS Hirsch et al. Antiretroviral drug resistance testing in adult HIV-1 infection: 2008 recommendations of an International AIDS Society-USA panel. Clin Infect Dis 2008; 47:266.

5. P Sax et al. ACTG 5202: shorter time to virologic failure with abacavir/lamivudine than tenofovir/emtricitabine as part of combination therapy in treatment-naïve subjects with screening HIV RNA 100,000 c/mL. XVII International AIDS Conference, August 3-8, 2008, Mexico City, Mexico; Abstract TUPE0230.

6. JE Gallant et al. Early virological nonresponse to tenofovir, abacavir and lamivudine in HIV-infected antiretroviral-naïve subjects. J Infect Dis 2005; 192:1921.

7. D:A:D Study Group. Use of nucleoside reverse transcriptase inhibitors and risk of myocardial infarction in HIV-infected patients enrolled in the D:A:D study: a multi-cohort collaboration. Lancet 2008; 371:1417.

8. SMART/INSIGHT; DAD Study Groups. Use of nucleoside reverse transcriptase inhibitors and risk of myocardial infarction in HIV-infected patients. AIDS 2008; 22:F17.

9. S Mallal et al. HLA-B*5701 screening for hypersensitivity to abacavir. N Engl J Med 2008; 358:568.

10. FDA Alert 7/24/2008. Information on abacavir (marketed as Ziagen) and abacavir-containing medications. Available at www.fda.gov/cder/drug/infopage/abacavir/default.htm.

11. Atazanavir (Reyataz) and emtricitabine (Emtriva) for HIV infection. Med Lett Drugs Ther 2003; 45:90.

12. D Maitland et al. Early virologic failure in HIV-1 infected subjects on didanosine/tenofovir/efavirenz: 12-week results from a randomized trial. AIDS 2005; 19:1183.

13. P Marcellin et al. Tenofovir disoproxil fumarate versus adefovir dipivoxil for chronic hepatitis B. N Engl J Med 2008; 359:2442.

14. RD MacArthur et al. A comparision of three highly active antiretroviral treatment strategies consisting of non-nucleoside reverse transcriptase inhibitors, protease inhibitors, or both in the presence of nucleoside reverse transcriptase inhibitors as initial therapy (CPCRA 058 First Study): a long-term randomised trial. Lancet 2006;368:2125

15. SA Riddler et al. Class-Sparing Regimens for Initial Treatment of HIV-1 Infection. N Engl J Med 2008;358:2095.

16. HJ Ribaudo et al. Pharmacogenetics of plasma efavirenz exposure after treatment discontinuation: an Adult AIDS Clinical Trials Group Study. Clin Infect Dis 2006; 42:401.

17. DB Clifford et al. Impact of efavirenz on neuropsychological performance and symptoms in HIV-infected individuals. Ann Intern Med 2005; 143:714.

18. F Gutierrez et al. Prediction of neuropsychiatric adverse events associated with long-term efavirenz therapy, using plasma drug level monitoring. Clin Infect Dis 2005; 41:1648.

19. Etravirine (Intelence) for HIV infection. Med Lett Drugs Ther 2008; 50:47.

20. E Poveda et al. Phenotypic impact of resistance mutations on etravirine susceptibility in HIV patients with prior failure to nonnucleoside analogues. AIDS 2008; 22:2395.

21. G Lapadula et al. Risk of early virological failure of once-daily tenofovir-emtricitabine plus twice-daily nevirapine in antiretroviral therapy-naive HIV-infected patients. Clin Infect Dis 2008; 46:1127.

22. BO Taiwo. Nevirapine toxicity. Int J STD AIDS 2006; 17:364.

23. JE Gallant et al. Tenofovir DF, emtricitabine, and efavirenz vs. zidovudine, lamivudine, and efavirenz for HIV. N Engl J Med 2006; 354:251.

24. Al Pozniak et al. Tenofovir disoproxil fumarate, emtricitabine, and efavirenz versus fixed-dose zidovudine/lamivudine and efavirenz in antiretroviral-naive patients: virologic, immunologic, and morphologic changes—a 96-week analysis. J Acquir Immune Defic Syndr 2006; 43:535.

25. JR Arribas et al. Tenofovir disoproxil fumarate, emtricitabine, and efavirenz compared with zidovudine/lamivudine and efavirenz in treatment-naive patients: 144-week analysis. J Acquir Immune Defic Syndr 2008; 47:74.

26. The DAD Study Group. Class of Antiretroviral Drugs and the risk of myocardial infarction. N Engl J Med 2007; 356:1723.

27. The Medical Letter Adverse Drug Interactions Program.

28. JM Molina et al. Once daily atazanavir/ritonavir versus twice-daily lopinavir/ritonavir, each in combination with tenofovir and emtricitabine, for management of antiretroviral-naïve HIV-1-infected patients: 48 week efficacy and safety results of the CASTLE study. Lancet 2008; 372:646.

29. KM Chan-Tack et al. Atazanavir-associated nephrolithiasis: cases from US Food and Drug Administration's Adverse Events Reporting System. AIDS 2007; 21:1215.

30. B Clotet et al. Efficacy and safety of darunavir-ritonavir at week 48 in treatment-experienced patients with HIV-1 infection in POWER 1 and 2: a pooled subgroup analysis of data from two randomised trials. Lancet 2007; 369:1169.

31. JM Molina et al. Safety and efficacy of darunavir (TMC114) with low-dose ritonavir in treatment-experienced patients: 24-week results of POWER 3. J Acquir Immune Defic Syndr 2007; 46:24.

32. JV Madruga et al. Efficacy and safety of darunavir-ritonavir compared with that of lopinavir-ritonavir at 48 weeks in treatment-experienced, HIV-infected patients in TITAN: a randomised controlled phase III trial. Lancet 2007:370:49.

33. R Ortiz et al. Efficacy and safety of once-daily darunavir/ritonavir versus lopinavir/ritonavir in treatment-naïve HIV-1-infected patients at week 48. AIDS 2008; 22:1389.

34. A Mills, et al. Efficacy and safety of darunavir/ritonavir 800/100mg once-daily versus lopinavir/ritonavir in treatment-naïve, HIV-1-infected patients at 96 weeks: ARTEMIS (TMC114-C211). 48th Annual ICAAC/IDSA 46th annual meeting; October 25-28, 2008; Washington, DC. Abstract H-125Oc

35. J Eron Jr et al. The KLEAN study of fosamprenavir-ritonavir versus lopinavir-ritonavir, each in combination with abacavir-lamivudine, for initial treatment of HIV infection over 48 weeks: a randomised non-inferiority trial. Lancet 2006; 368:476.

36. R Verdon et al. Indinavir-induced cholelithiasis in a patient infected with human immunodeficiency virus. Clin Infect Dis 2002; 35:e57.

37. Lopinavir/ritonavir: a protease inhibitor combination. Med Lett Drugs Ther 2001; 43:1.

38. S Walmsley et al. Saquinavir/r (SQV/r) bid versus lopinavir/r (LPV/r) bid, plus emtricitabine/tenofovir (FTC/TDF) qd as initial therapy in HIV-1-infected patients: The Gemini study. 11th European AIDS Conference/EACS, October 24-27, 2007; Madrid, Spain. PS1/4

39. Tipranavir (Aptivus) for HIV. Med Lett Drugs Ther 2005; 47:83.

40. CB Hicks et al. Durable efficacy of tipranavir-ritonavir in combination with an optimised background regimen of antiretroviral drugs for treatment-experienced HIV-1-infected patients at 48 weeks in the Randomized Evaluation of Strategic Intervention in multi-drug reSistant patients with Tipranavir (RESIST) studies: an analysis of combined data from two randomised open-label trials. Lancet 2006; 368:466.

41. P Marr and S Walmsley. Reassessment of enfuvirtide's role in the management of HIV-1 infection. Expert Opin Pharmacother 2008; 9:2349.

42. RA Ball et al. Injection site reactions with the HIV-1 fusion inhibitor enfuvirtide. J Am Acad Dermatol 2003; 49:826.

43. Two new drugs for HIV infection. Med Lett Drugs Ther 2008; 50:2.

44. M Westby et al. Emergence of CXCR4-using human immunodeficiency virus Type 1 (HIV-1) variants in a minority of HIV-1-infected patients following treatment with the CCR5 antagonist maraviroc is from a pretreatment CXCR4-using virus reservoir. J Virol 2006; 80:4909.

45. RM Gulick et al. Maraviroc for previously treated patients with R5 HIV-1 infection. N Engl J Med 2008; 359:1429.

46. M Saag et al. Reanalysis of the MERIT study with enhanced trofile assay (MERIT-ES). 48th Annual ICAAC/IDSA 46th annual meeting; October 25-28, 2008; Washington, DC. Abstract H-1232a.

47. RT Steigbigel et al. Raltegravir with optimized background therapy for resistant HIV-1 infection. N Engl J Med 2008; 359:339.

48. DA Cooper et al. Subgroup and resistance analyses of raltegravir for resistant HIV-1 infection. N Engl J Med 2008; 359:355.

49. M Markowitz et al. Rapid and durable antiretroviral effect of the HIV-1 Integrase inhibitor raltegravir as part of combination therapy in treatment-naive patients with HIV-1 infection: results of a 48-week controlled study. J Acquir Immune Defic Syndr 2007; 46:125.

50. J Lennox et al. First-line raltegravir controls HIV as well as efavirenz for 48 weeks. 48th Annual ICAAC/IDSA 46th annual meeting; October 25-28, 2008; Washington, DC. Abstract H-896a.

51. EM Connor et al. Reduction of maternal-infant transmission of human immunodeficiency virus type 1 with zidovudine treatment. Pediatric AIDS Clinical Trials Group Protocol 076 Study Group. N Engl J Med 1994; 331:1173.

52. Public Health Service Task Force. Recommendations for use of antiretroviral drugs in pregnant HIV-infected women and for maternal health and interventions to reduce perinatal HIV transmission in the United States. Revised July 8, 2008. Available at www.aidsinfo.nih.gov. Accessed on January 14, 2009.

53. AM Cotter et al. Is antiretroviral therapy during pregnancy associated with an increased risk of preterm delivery, low birth weight, or stillbirth? J Infect Dis 2006; 193:1195.

54. ML Chaix et al. Low risk of nevirapine resistance mutations in the prevention of mother-to-child transmission of HIV-1: Agence Nationale de Recherches sur le SIDA Ditrame Plus, Abidjan, Cote d'Ivoire. J Infect Dis 2006; 193:482.

DRUGS FOR
Non-HIV Viral Infections

Original publication date – October 2010

The drugs of choice for treatment of non-HIV viral infections and their dosages are listed in the tables on the pages that follow. Some of the indications and dosages recommended here have not been approved by the FDA. Vaccines used for the prevention of viral infections are discussed on page 301.[1]

DRUGS FOR HERPES SIMPLEX AND VARICELLA-ZOSTER VIRUS

ACYCLOVIR (*Zovirax*, and others) — Available in topical, oral and intravenous (IV) formulations, acyclovir is used to treat herpes simplex virus (HSV) and varicella-zoster virus (VZV) infections. Topical acyclovir cream reduces the duration of orolabial herpes by about 0.5 days. Oral acyclovir can shorten the duration of symptoms in primary orolabial, genital and anorectal HSV infections, and to a lesser extent in recurrent orolabial and genital HSV infections. Long-term oral suppression with acyclovir decreases the frequency of symptomatic genital HSV recurrences and asymptomatic viral shedding. Oral acyclovir begun within 24 hours after the onset of rash decreases the severity of primary varicella infection and can also be used to treat localized zoster. Suppression with acyclovir for one year reduced VZV reactivation in immunocompromised patients. IV acyclovir is the drug of choice for treatment of HSV infections that are visceral, disseminated or involve

191

DRUGS FOR HERPES SIMPLEX VIRUS

Infection	Drug	Usual Adult dosage[1]
OROLABIAL[2]		
Topical		
	Acyclovir – *Zovirax*	5% cream 5x/d x 4d
	Docosanol – *Abreva*[3]	10% cream 5x/d until healing
	Penciclovir – *Denavir*	1% cream applied q2h while awake x 4d
Oral		
	Acyclovir – *Zovirax*, and others	400 mg PO 5x/d q4h x 5d
	Famciclovir – *Famvir*, and others	1500 mg PO single dose
	Valacyclovir – *Valtrex*, and others	2 g PO q12h x 1d
GENITAL		
First episode		
	Acyclovir– *Zovirax*, and others	400 mg PO tid or 200 mg PO 5x/d x 7-10d[4]
	Famciclovir[5] – *Famvir*, and others	250 mg PO tid x 7-10d
	Valacyclovir – *Valtrex*, and others	1 g PO bid x 7-10d
Episodic treatment of recurrences[6]		
	Acyclovir – *Zovirax*, and others	800 mg PO tid x 2d or 400 mg PO tid x 3-5d[7]
	Famciclovir – *Famvir*, and others	1 g PO bid x 1d[8]
	Valacyclovir – *Valtrex*, and others	500 mg PO bid x 3d
Suppression of recurrences[9]		
	Acyclovir – *Zovirax*, and others	400 mg PO bid
	Famciclovir – *Famvir*, and others	250 mg PO bid
	Valacyclovir – *Valtrex*, and others	500 mg - 1 g PO 1x/d[10]
MUCOCUTANEOUS IN IMMUNOCOMPROMISED PATIENTS		
	Acyclovir – *Zovirax*, and others	5 mg/kg IV q8h x 7-14d or 400 mg PO 5x/d x 7-10d

Continued on next page.

DRUGS FOR HERPES SIMPLEX VIRUS (continued)

Infection	Drug	Usual Adult dosage[1]
MUCOCUTANEOUS IN IMMUNOCOMPROMISED PATIENTS (continued)		
	Famciclovir – *Famvir*, and others	500 mg PO bid x 7-10d
	Valacyclovir[5] – *Valtrex*, and others	500 mg-1 g PO bid x 7-10d
ENCEPHALITIS		
	Acyclovir – *Zovirax*, and others	10-15 mg/kg IV q8h x 14-21d
NEONATAL		
	Acyclovir – *Zovirax*, and others	10-20 mg/kg IV q8h x 14-21d
KERATOCONJUNCTIVITIS[11]		
	Trifluridine – *Viroptic*, and others	1% ophth solution 1 drop q2h (max 9 drops/d)[12]
ACYCLOVIR-RESISTANT		
Severe infection, immunocompromised		
	Foscarnet – *Foscavir*, and others	40 mg/kg IV q8h x 14-21d

1. Dosage adjustment may be required for renal insufficiency.
2. Some Medical Letter consultants would treat a first episode of orolabial herpes in the same way as a first episode of genital herpes.
3. Available without a prescription.
4. For severe infection, IV acyclovir (5-10 mg/kg q8h for 5-7d) can be used. Oral acyclovir can be used to complete a 10 day course of therapy.
5. Not approved by the FDA for this indication.
6. Antiviral therapy is variably effective and only if started early.
7. No published data are available to support 3 days' use.
8. For recurrent HSV in HIV-positive patients, 500 mg bid for 7d.
9. Some clinicians discontinue treatment for 1-2 mos/yr to assess the frequency of recurrences.
10. 500 mg once/d in patients with <10 recurrences/yr and 500 mg bid or 1 g/d in patients with ≥10 recurrences/yr.
11. An ophthalmic preparation of acyclovir is available in some countries. Treatment of HSV ocular infections should be supervised by an ophthalmologist; duration of therapy and dosage depend on response.
12. Once the cornea has re-epithelialized, the dose can be decreased to 1 drop q4h x 7d.

the central nervous system (CNS) and for serious or disseminated VZV infections.

Adverse Effects – By any route of administration, acyclovir is generally well tolerated. Gastrointestinal (GI) disturbances and headache can occur. Given IV, the drug may cause phlebitis and inflammation at sites of infusion. IV acyclovir can also cause reversible renal dysfunction due to crystalline nephropathy; rapid infusion, dehydration, renal insufficiency and high dosage increase the risk. IV and, rarely, oral acyclovir have been associated with encephalopathy, including tremors, hallucinations, seizures and coma. Neutropenia and other signs of bone marrow toxicity have been reported rarely.

Pregnancy – Use of acyclovir during pregnancy, even during the first trimester, has not been associated with an increased risk of congenital abnormalities.[2] It is classified as category B (no evidence of risk in humans) for use in pregnancy, and many clinicians prescribe the drug during pregnancy for treatment of genital herpes. Suppression of recurrent genital herpes in pregnant women near term may reduce the need for cesarean sections to avoid neonatal herpes infection.

Resistance – Despite widespread use of acyclovir, the development of HSV resistance in immunocompetent subjects is uncommon (prevalence <1%). Almost all acyclovir-resistant HSV occurs in immunocompromised patients treated with the drug; isolates are usually cross-resistant to famciclovir and valacyclovir. Resistant HSV infection in HIV-positive patients has been associated with progressive mucocutaneous disease and, rarely, visceral involvement. Resistant VZV infection in HIV-positive patients has been associated with chronic cutaneous lesions and, rarely, invasive disease.

Infections with acyclovir-resistant HSV or VZV may respond to foscarnet or cidofovir, which are discussed on pages 200 and 201.

FAMCICLOVIR *(Famvir,* **and others***)* — Famciclovir is rapidly converted to penciclovir after oral administration. It is effective in treating first episodes and recurrences of genital HSV and for chronic suppression. Single-day, patient-initiated famciclovir is similar in efficacy and safety to a 3-day course of valacyclovir;[3] it reduces time to healing of orolabial herpes (1 dose) and genital herpes lesions (2 doses) by about 2 days compared to placebo.[4,5] In patients with herpes zoster, famciclovir begun within 72 hours after onset of rash is effective in speeding the resolution of zoster-associated pain and shortening the duration of postherpetic neuralgia.

Resistance – HSV and VZV strains resistant to acyclovir are generally also resistant to famciclovir.

Adverse Effects – Famciclovir is generally well tolerated. Headache, nausea and diarrhea have been reported.

Pregnancy – Like acyclovir, famciclovir is classified as category B (no evidence of risk in humans) for use in pregnancy.

VALACYCLOVIR *(Valtrex*, and others*)* — Valacyclovir, the L-valyl ester of acyclovir, is metabolized to acyclovir after oral administration, resulting in a 3- to 5-fold increase in bioavailability compared to oral acyclovir. The area under the concentration/time curve (AUC) following high doses of oral valacyclovir resembles that following IV administration of acyclovir.

For orolabial herpes, one day of oral valacyclovir therapy improved time to healing by 1 day and reduced the duration of discomfort by 0.5 days compared to placebo.[6] In first-episode or recurrent genital herpes, valacyclovir twice daily is as effective as acyclovir given 5 times a day. Valacyclovir 500 mg once daily is effective for chronic suppression of genital HSV. Daily suppressive therapy has been shown to reduce clinical and subclinical shedding by 64% and 58%, respectively.[7] One 8-month study of discordant heterosexual couples found that valacyclovir suppressive therapy taken by the infected partner reduced the risk of HSV transmission to the susceptible partner by about 50%.[8] A higher dose (500 mg twice daily or 1 g once daily) may be needed for suppression in patients with frequent recurrences. The results of one study suggested that valacyclovir may be superior to famciclovir for virologic suppression of recur-

DRUGS FOR VARICELLA-ZOSTER VIRUS

Infection	Drug	Usual Adult dosage[1]
VARICELLA		
	Acyclovir – *Zovirax*, and others	20 mg/kg (800 mg max) PO qid x 5d[2]
	Valacyclovir – *Valtrex*, and others	20 mg/kg (1 g max) PO tid x 5d
HERPES ZOSTER		
	Valacyclovir – *Valtrex*, and others	1 g PO tid x 7d
	Famciclovir – *Famvir*, and others	500 mg PO q8h x 7d
	Acyclovir – *Zovirax*, and others	800 mg PO 5x/d x 7-10d
VARICELLA OR ZOSTER IN IMMUNOCOMPROMISED PATIENTS		
	Acyclovir – *Zovirax*, and others	10 mg/kg IV q8h x 7d[3]
ACYCLOVIR-RESISTANT ZOSTER		
	Foscarnet[4] – *Foscavir*, and others	40 mg/kg IV q8-12h x 2-3 wks

1. Dosage adjustment may be required for renal insufficiency.
2. Same dose for children over 40 kg.
3. Pediatric dosage (<12 yrs of age) is 20 mg/kg q8h x 7-10d.
4. Not approved by the FDA for this indication.

rent genital herpes.[9] Suppression with valacyclovir for one year reduced VZV reactivation in immunocompromised patients.[10]

Adverse Effects – Valacyclovir is generally well tolerated; adverse effects are similar to those with acyclovir. GI disturbance, headache and rash are common. CNS effects, such as hallucinations and confusion, nephrotoxicity and seizures can occur. Thrombotic thrombocytopenic purpura/hemolytic uremic syndrome has been reported in some severely immunocompromised patients taking high doses (8 g/day).

Pregnancy – Like acyclovir, using valacyclovir in pregnancy has not been associated with an increased risk of major birth defects, even during the first trimester.[2] It is classified as category B (no evidence of risk in humans) for use during pregnancy.

Resistance – Isolates resistant to acyclovir are generally also resistant to valacyclovir.

OTHER TOPICAL DRUGS — Penciclovir *(Denavir)* – Topical penciclovir 1% cream applied every 2 hours for 4 days while awake decreased the healing time of recurrent orolabial herpes by about 0.7 days in immunocompetent adults.[11]

Docosanol *(Abreva)* – Topical docosanol cream, a long-chain saturated alcohol available without a prescription[12], started within 12 hours of prodromal symptoms, decreases healing time by about 0.5 days in recurrent orolabial herpes. Application site reactions, rash and pruritus are common adverse effects.

Trifluridine (*Viroptic***, and others)** – Trifluridine is a nucleoside analog active against herpes viruses, including acyclovir-resistant strains. Marketed as an ophthalmic preparation, it is FDA-approved for treatment of HSV keratoconjunctivitis and recurrent epithelial keratitis. It is also active against vaccinia virus and has been used to treat accidental ocular infection following smallpox vaccination.[13]

DRUGS FOR CYTOMEGALOVIRUS

GANCICLOVIR (*Cytovene***, and others)** — IV ganciclovir is FDA-approved for both induction and maintenance treatment of cytomegalovirus (CMV) retinitis in immunocompromised patients and for prevention of CMV infection in transplant recipients. It is also used to treat CMV infections at other sites (colon, esophagus, lungs, etc.) and for preemptive treatment of immunosuppressed patients with CMV antigenemia or viremia. Oral ganciclovir is less effective than the IV formulation due to lower bioavailability. It has largely been replaced by oral valganciclovir.

Prophylactic oral ganciclovir, or IV ganciclovir followed by either oral ganciclovir or high-dose oral acyclovir, reduces the risk of CMV in patients who have had liver transplantation, including seronegative recipients of seropositive donors. Limited data in infants with symptomatic congenital CMV disease involving the CNS suggest that treatment with IV ganciclovir may decrease hearing loss and the incidence of developmental delay.[14]

An intraocular implant that releases ganciclovir (*Vitrasert*) has been used to treat CMV retinitis, in combination with systemic therapy with ganciclovir or valganciclovir.

Adverse Effects – In animals, ganciclovir is teratogenic, carcinogenic and mutagenic, and causes asperm-atogenesis. Granulocytopenia, anemia and thrombocytopenia, which are usually reversible, are more common with the IV than with the oral formulation. Severe myelosuppression may occur more frequently when the drug is given concurrently with zidovudine *(Retrovir,* and others*)*, probenecid, azathioprine *(Imuran*, and others) or mycophenolate mofetil *(CellCept,* and others*)*. Granulocyte-colony stimulating factors (GM-CSF; G-CSF) have been used to treat ganciclovir-induced neutropenia. Other adverse effects of systemic ganciclovir include fever, rash, phlebitis, confusion, abnormal liver function, renal dysfunction, headache, GI toxicity and, rarely, psychiatric disturbances and seizures. Intravitreal ganciclovir implants have been associated with loss of visual acuity, vitreous hemorrhage and acute retinal detachment.

Pregnancy – Ganciclovir is classified as category C (risk cannot be ruled out) for use in pregnancy, and men treated with the drug should use barrier contraception during treatment and for at least 90 days afterward.

Resistance – Ganciclovir resistance may be associated with persistent viremia and progressive disease. Ganciclovir-resistant CMV can emerge and cause morbidity when the drug is used for prophylaxis in solid-organ

DRUGS FOR CYTOMEGALOVIRUS

Infection	Drug	Adult dosage[1]
CYTOMEGALOVIRUS (CMV)[2]		
	Valganciclovir – *Valcyte*	900 mg PO bid x 21d followed by 900 mg once/d
or	Ganciclovir – *Cytovene*, and others	5 mg/kg IV q12h x 14-21d followed by 5 mg/kg IV once/d or 6 mg/kg IV 5x/wk or 1 g PO tid
	Vitrasert implant[3]	4.5 mg intraocularly q5-8 mos
or	Foscarnet – *Foscavir*, and others	60 mg/kg IV q8h or 90 mg/kg IV q12h x 14-21d followed by 90-120 mg/kg IV once/d[4]
or	Cidofovir – *Vistide*	5 mg/kg IV once/wk x 2 then 5 mg/kg IV q2wks[5]

1. Dosage adjustment may be required for renal insufficiency.
2. Chronic suppression is recommended in AIDS and in other highly immunocompromised patients with retinitis. Both oral ganciclovir (1g tid) and valganciclovir (900 mg once/d) are approved for prevention of CMV disease in solid organ transplant recipients.
3. Systemic therapy is recommended to prevent CMV disease in the contralateral eye and other organ systems.
4. Higher doses (120 mg/kg/d) may be more effective, but less well tolerated.
5. To minimize renal toxicity patients should receive 1 L of 0.9% saline over 1-2 hrs prior to a 1-hour cidofovir infusion; they should also receive oral probenecid 2 g 3 hours prior to infusion of cidofovir and 1 g 2 and 8 hrs after the infusion. Patients who can tolerate additional fluid should receive a second 1 L of 0.9% saline, started immediately after the cidofovir infusion. Not recommended for patients with serum creatinine >1.5 mg/dL, creatinine clearance ≤55 mL/min or proteinuria ≥100 mg/dL (2+ by dipstick). Dose reduction to 3 mg/kg is recommended for serum creatinine 0.3-0.4 mg/dL above baseline.

transplant recipients taking highly potent immunosuppressive drugs. CMV strains resistant to ganciclovir *in vitro* may be susceptible to foscarnet or cidofovir.

VALGANCICLOVIR *(Valcyte)* — Valganciclovir, an oral prodrug of ganciclovir, achieves plasma concentrations similar to those with IV administration of ganciclovir; it has largely replaced oral ganciclovir.

Valganciclovir is as effective as IV ganciclovir therapy for CMV retinitis. Valganciclovir once daily is at least as effective as oral ganciclovir taken 3 times a day for prevention of CMV disease in high-risk (Donor [D]+, Recipient [R]-) solid organ transplant recipients.[15] Both prophylactic ther-apy and preemptive therapy for CMV detected in blood before development of disease have been shown to be beneficial in those at risk for CMV disease (D+R-, D+R+, D-R+).[16] Valganciclovir is not FDA-approved for use in liver transplant recipients due to data (summarized in the package insert) showing increased tissue-invasive CMV with valganciclovir compared to ganciclovir (14% vs. 3%) in these patients.

Adverse Effects – Adverse effects are similar to those of IV ganciclovir.

Resistance – Isolates that are resistant to ganciclovir are also resistant to valganciclovir.

FOSCARNET (*Foscavir*, and others) — IV foscarnet is FDA-approved for treatment of CMV retinitis in patients with AIDS, including progressive disease due to ganciclovir-resistant strains, and for treatment of acyclovir-resistant HSV infections. It has not been approved, but has been used off-label, for treatment of acyclovir-resistant VZV infections. Foscarnet is more expensive and generally less well tolerated than ganciclovir, and requires controlled infusion rates and large volumes of fluid. In allogeneic stem cell transplant recipients who develop CMV infection, treatment with foscarnet is as effective as IV ganciclovir and causes less hematologic toxicity.[17]

Adverse Effects – Renal dysfunction often develops during treatment with foscarnet and is usually reversible, but renal failure requiring dialysis may occur. Renal toxicity is increased in patients receiving other nephrotoxic drugs; adequate hydration may decrease the risk. Nausea, vomiting, anemia, fatigue, headache, genital ulceration, CNS disturbances, hypocalcemia, hyperphosphatemia, hypokalemia and hypomagnesemia have also occurred. Foscarnet given with zidovudine may increase the risk of anemia. Foscarnet also causes chromosomal damage *in vitro* and *in vivo*. Rapid infusion of the drug has been associated with seizures and arrhythmias.

Pregnancy – Foscarnet is classified as category C (risk cannot be ruled out) for use during pregnancy.

Resistance – HSV, VZV and CMV strains resistant to foscarnet can emerge during treatment. Combined use of foscarnet and ganciclovir may benefit some patients, but CMV strains resistant to both ganciclovir and foscarnet have been reported.

CIDOFOVIR *(Vistide)* — IV cidofovir is used for treatment of CMV retinitis in AIDS patients who have not responded to ganciclovir or foscarnet therapy. Given once weekly for 2 weeks and then once every 2 weeks for maintenance therapy, cidofovir can delay progression of CMV retinitis in patients with AIDS. Cidofovir has been used to treat other CMV infections (pneumonitis, gastroenteritis), acyclovir- or foscarnet-resistant HSV infections, certain forms of human papillomavirus disease, and invasive adenoviral and BK virus infections in transplant populations. IV cidofovir does not have any demonstrable efficacy in the treatment of JC virus-related progressive multifocal leukoencephalopathy (PML).

Adverse Effects – About 25% of patients discontinue cidofovir because of adverse effects such as nephrotoxicity, neutropenia and metabolic acidosis. To decrease the risk of nephrotoxicity, pre-treatment with IV fluids and oral probenecid must be given with each cidofovir dose. Cidofovir is contraindicated in patients taking other nephrotoxic agents. Iritis, uveitis or ocular hypotony can also occur. These ocular adverse effects are more common in patients simultaneously taking antiretroviral drugs. The drug is carcinogenic and teratogenic, and causes hypospermia in animals.

Pregnancy – Cidofovir is classified as category C (risk cannot be ruled out) for use in pregnancy.

Resistance – Although most ganciclovir-resistant CMV isolates remain sensitive to cidofovir, cross-resistance can occur. Acyclovir-resistant HSV or VZV frequently are susceptible to cidofovir.

FOMIVIRSEN *(Vitravene)* — Fomivirsen, an antisense oligonu-cleotide, was FDA-approved for intravitreal treatment of CMV retinitis in HIV-infected patients who cannot tolerate or have not responded to other drugs.[18] It is no longer marketed in the US.

DRUGS FOR INFLUENZA

OSELTAMIVIR *(Tamiflu)* — This oral neuraminidase inhibitor is a prodrug that is rapidly converted to the active antiviral during absorption. Started within 48 hours of symptom onset, it can decrease the severity and duration (by 1-1.5 days) of symptoms caused by either influenza A or B in both children ($\geq$ 1 year old) and adults. In retrospective pooled analyses, treatment of proven influenza infection has been reported to lower the incidence of influenza-related lower respiratory tract complications.[19] A prospective study in patients hospitalized for seasonal influenza found that antiviral treatment was associated with reduced mortality.[20] Taken prophylactically, oseltami-vir has been 70-90% effective in preventing clinical influenza.[21] Prophylaxis is indicated to control institutional influenza outbreaks and protect high-risk patients immunized after or <2 weeks before an epidemic has begun. The drug can also be used as prophylaxis for immunodeficient patients who may respond poorly to influenza vaccine, and in unvaccinated persons who are at high risk for influenza or are caring for high-risk patients.

Adverse Effects – Nausea, vomiting and headache are the most common adverse effects of oseltamivir. Taking the drug with food may decrease the incidence of nausea and vomiting.

Pregnancy – Oseltamivir is classified as category C (risk cannot be ruled out) for use during pregnancy.

Resistance – During treatment with oseltamivir, resistant variants emerge in about 1% of immunocompetent adults and in about 4% of children. Higher levels of resistance have been described during oseltamivir therapy of H5N1 infection. Most (>98%) seasonal A H1N1 isolates prior to 2009 were resistant to oseltamivir, but almost all pandemic 2009 influenza A H1N1 virus strains remained susceptible.[21,22]

ZANAMIVIR *(Relenza)* — Zanamivir is FDA-approved for treatment of acute uncomplicated influenza A or B in patients ≥7 years of age. Started within 2 days after onset of symptoms, this inhaled neuraminidase inhibitor can shorten the duration of illness and may decrease the incidence of lower respiratory tract complications. Once-daily inhaled zanamivir is approved for prophylaxis of influenza in patients ≥5 years of age. Zanamivir has been effective against some avian strains of influenza in animal studies and might be effective for prophylaxis and treatment of H5N1 disease, but human data are lacking.

Adverse Effects – Nasal and throat discomfort and cough can occur. Bronchospasm, sometimes severe, has been reported uncommonly in patients with reactive airway disease; zanamivir should be avoided in such patients. It has rarely caused bronchospasm in previously healthy persons with influenza.

Pregnancy – Zanamivir is classified as category C (risk cannot be ruled out) for use during pregnancy.

Resistance – Zanamivir is active against amantadine/rimantadine-resistant influenza A and most oseltamivir-resistant strains. Emergence of zanamivir resistance during therapy has been described in immunocompromised patients.

DRUGS FOR INFLUENZA A AND B

| Drug[1] | Adult Dosage[2] | |
	Prophylaxis	Treatment
Oseltamivir – Tamiflu[3]	75 mg PO 1x/d[4]	75 mg PO bid[4,5]
Zanamivir – Relenza[6]	2x 5 mg PO inhalations 1x/d	2x 5 mg PO inhalations bid

1. Antiviral drugs may interfere with the efficacy of *FluMist*, the live-attenuated intranasal vaccine (Med Lett Drugs Ther 2009; 51:89); they should be stopped at least 48 hours before and should not be started for ≥2 weeks after *FluMist* administration. Inactivated vaccines *(Fluarix, Fluvirin, Fluzone, FluLaval)* are not affected by antiviral drug therapy.
2. For prophylaxis of exposures in institutions, the drug should be taken for at least 2 weeks, and must be continued for 1 week after the end of the outbreak. For postexposure prophylaxis in households, shorter courses (10 days) may be effective. For treatment of infection, the duration is usually 5 days.

AMANTADINE (*Symmetrel*, **and others**) **and RIMANTADINE** (*Flumadine*, **and others**) — Resistance of influenza A viruses to amantadine or rimantadine can occur spontaneously or emerge rapidly during treatment. Most seasonal A H3N2 and pandemic 2009 A H1N1 isolates are resistant to these agents, but are susceptible to oseltamivir and zanamivir. Due to this resistance, amantadine and rimantidine currently have limited utility in the treatment of influenza.

For susceptible viruses, treatment with oral amantadine or rimantadine begun within 48 hours after the onset of illness can decrease the duration of fever and symptoms by about 1 day. Whether these drugs decrease influenza-related complications or are effective in treating severe influenza pneumonia is unknown. Neither amantadine nor rimantadine is effective against influenza B virus.

| Pediatric Dosage[2] | |
Prophylaxis	Treatment
≥1 yr:	**≥1 yr:**
≤15 kg: 30 mg PO 1x/d[4]	≤15 kg: 30 mg PO bid[4]
16-23 kg: 45 mg PO 1x/d[4]	16-23 kg: 45 mg PO bid[4]
24-40 kg: 60 mg PO 1x/d[4]	24-40 kg: 60 mg PO bid[4]
>40 kg: 75 mg PO 1x/d[4]	>40 kg: 75 mg PO bid[4]
≥5 yrs: 2x 5 mg oral	**≥7 yrs:** 2x 5 mg PO
inhalations 1x/d	inhalations bid

3. Available as capsules (75 mg) or a powder for oral suspension (60 mg/5 mL; 25 mL bottle). Approved for treatment and prophylaxis of influenza in patients ≥1 year old.
4. In patients with CrCl between 10-30 mL/min, doses should be given every other day for prophylaxis and once/d for treatment.
5. Some clinicians have used 150 mg bid for 10 days to treat patients with pneumonia or those in danger of clinical progression (Writing Committee. N Engl J Med 2010; 362:1708).
6. Available as a packet containing 5 rotadisks; each rotadisk contains 4 blisters of drug (5 mg each blister). Approved for treatment of children ≥7 years old and prophylaxis of children ≥5 years.

Adverse Effects – Amantadine may cause anorexia, nausea, peripheral edema and, particularly in the elderly, minor CNS effects such as nervousness, anxiety, insomnia, lethargy, difficulty concentrating and light-headedness. These effects usually diminish after the first week of use and rapidly disappear after the drug is stopped. Serious CNS effects (confusion, hallucinations, seizures) can occur, especially with old age, renal insufficiency, seizure disorders, concomitant CNS stimulant or anticholinergic drug therapy, and underlying psychiatric illness. Amantadine is excreted mainly in urine; the dose must be reduced for creatinine clearance <50 mL/min.

Rimantadine has GI adverse effects similar to those of amantadine, but has a lower risk of CNS effects. It is extensively metabolized by the liver before renal excretion, so dosage reductions are not needed unless the creatinine clearance falls below 10 mL/min.

Pregnancy – Both amantadine and rimantadine are teratogenic in animals and are contraindicated for use during pregnancy.

DRUGS FOR HEPATITIS B AND C

Oral antivirals with more favorable toxicity profiles and better virologic suppression rates have replaced interferon as the first-line treatment for chronic hepatitis B virus infection (HBV). Interferon and ribavirin remain first-line treatment for chronic hepatitis C virus infection (HCV).

HIV/HBV COINFECTION — Resistance to antivirals is more common in HBV patients coinfected with HIV. To minimize resistance, patients who need treatment for both infections should take 2 antiretrovirals that are active against both, such as lamivudine, emtricitabine, tenofovir or entecavir. Coinfected patients who need treatment for HBV but not HIV should not receive monotherapy with HBV drugs that are also active against HIV.

TENOFOVIR *(Viread)* — Tenofovir disoproxil fumarate is a prodrug that requires diester hydrolysis for conversion to tenofovir, a nucleoside analog of adenosine monophosphate. In two double-blind controlled trials, more patients treated with tenofovir had undetectable HBV DNA levels (<400 copies per mL) than those treated with adefovir (71% vs. 49% among HBeAg-negative patients; 67% vs. 12% among HBeAg-positive patients).[23] Results were similar in patients with HIV/HBV coinfection.[24]

Adverse Effects – Rash, headache, nausea, vomiting and diarrhea have been the most common adverse effects of tenofovir. Lactic acidosis and severe hepatomegaly with steatosis can occur in patients with HIV, but are much less likely to occur with monotherapy for treatment of hepatitis B. Stopping tenofovir has been associated with acute hepatitis due to severe acute exacerbations of HBV virus infection.

Pregnancy – Tenofovir is classified as category B (no evidence of risk in humans) for use in pregnancy.

Resistance – Tenofovir has remained active in patients with lamivudine and adefovir resistance from single nucleotide substitutions; cross-resistance can occur with multiple nucleotide substitutions.

ENTECAVIR *(Baraclude)* — Entecavir, a guanosine nucleoside analog, is more potent than lamivudine and has demonstrated efficacy in both treatment-naïve and lamivudine-refractory patients with hepatitis B.[25] Well absorbed after oral administration, its prolonged plasma half-life (128-149 hours) allows once-daily dosing. Compared to lamivudine, entecavir appears to be more efficacious in reducing HBV DNA levels, normalizing serum aminotransferases, and improving histologic abnormalities in HBeAg-positive patients.[26] Higher doses (1 mg daily) are recommended for treatment of lamivudine-resistant infections.

Adverse Effects – Entecavir is generally well tolerated. Adverse effects reported during therapy include headache, fatigue, dizziness, nausea, abdominal pain, rhinitis, fever, diarrhea, cough and myalgia. Lactic acidosis and severe hepatomegaly with steatosis can occur in patients with HIV, but are much less likely to occur with monotherapy for treatment of hepatitis B. Exacerbations of hepatitis due to rebound HBV infection can occur when treatment is stopped.

Pregnancy – Entecavir is classified as category C (risk cannot be ruled out) for use in pregnancy.

Resistance – Entecavir remains active against lamivudine-resistant hepatitis B virus. Development of resistance to entecavir during therapy is uncommon, but is more likely in patients with previous nucleoside analog exposure.

SOME DRUGS FOR HEPATITIS B AND C

Infection	Drug	Usual Adult dosage[1]
HEPATITIS B VIRUS (HBV)		
Chronic	Tenofovir – *Viread*	300 mg/d PO[2]
	Entecavir – *Baraclude*	0.5 mg/d PO x 1-3 yrs[2,3]
	Telbivudine – *Tyzeka*	600 mg/d PO x 1-3 yrs[2]
	Adefovir – *Hepsera*	10 mg PO 1x/d x 1-3 yrs[2]
	Lamivudine[4] – *Epivir HBV*	100 mg PO 1x/d x 1-3 yrs[2,5]
	Emtricitabine[6] – *Emtriva*	200 mg/d PO x48 wks[2,7,8]
	Interferon alfa-2b – *Intron A*	5 million units/d or 10 million units 3x/wk SC or IM x 4 mos
	Peginterferon alfa-2a – *Pegasys*	180 mcg once/wk SC x 48 wks
HEPATITIS C VIRUS (HCV)		
Chronic	Peginterferon alfa-2b – *PegIntron*	1.5 mcg/kg once/wk SC x 48 wks[9]
	plus ribavirin *Rebetol*, and others	800-1400 mg/d PO x 48 wks[9]
or	Peginterferon alfa-2a – *Pegasys*	180 mcg once/wk SC x 48 wks[9]
	plus ribavirin *Copegus*, and others	800-1200 mg/d PO x 48 wks[9]
Acute	Interferon alfa-2b[6] – *Intron A*	5 million units/d x 4 wks, then 3x/wk x 20 wks

1. Dosage adjustment may be required for renal insufficiency.
2. Optimal duration of therapy is uncertain. Some experts recommend that treatment continue for 6 months after anti-HBe seroconversion and negative or stable HBV DNA levels are achieved (EB Keeffe et al. Clin Gastroenterol Hepatol 2008; 6:1315).
3. Dose for nucleoside-naïve patients. The recommended dosage for patients who are refractory to lamivudine is 1 mg/d.
4. In patients coinfected with HIV, use of lamivudine to treat HBV may result in loss of its usefulness in treating the HIV because patients with active HIV replication rapidly develop resistance to lamivudine monotherapy. *Epivir HBV*, which is formulated in a lower dose, cannot be substituted for lamivudine *(Epivir)* in HIV treatment regimens.
5. Pediatric dose (2-17 yrs) is 3 mg/kg/d (maximum 100 mg/dose).
6. Not approved by the FDA for this indication.
7. SG Lim et al. Arch Intern Med 2006; 166:49.
8. Dosage of oral solution is 240 mg (24 mL) 1x/d.
9. Shorter courses (24 rather than 48 wks) and lower ribavirin doses (800 rather than 1000 or 1200 mg/d) appear to be effective for HCV genotypes 2 and 3 but not genotype 1, which is the most common in North America (SJ Hadziyannis et al. Ann Intern Med 2004; 140:346; A Mangia et al. N Engl J Med 2005; 352:2609).

TELBIVUDINE *(Tyzeka)* — Telbivudine, a synthetic thymidine analog, is approved for the treatment of chronic HBV infection in patients ≥16 years old.[27] It is not active against HIV *in vitro*. In the second year of a randomized trial (GLOBE), telbivudine-treated patients had a superior virologic response compared to lamivudine-treated patients: 63% vs 48% in HBeAg-positive patients; 78% vs 66% in HBeAg-negative patients.[28] In an open-label trial, telbivudine also was more effective than adefovir in suppressing HBV DNA in patients with HBeAg-positive chronic hepatitis.[29]

Adverse Effects – Headache and fatigue are common with telbivudine. Nausea and vomiting can occur. Lactic acidosis and severe hepatomegaly with steatosis can occur in patients with HIV, but are much less likely to occur with monotherapy for treatment of hepatitis B. Severe acute exacerbations of hepatitis B have been reported in patients who have stopped taking the drug. Myopathy, manifested by muscle aches and/or weakness with increased CPK has been reported uncommonly.

Pregnancy – Telbivudine is classified as category B (no evidence of risk in humans) for use in pregnancy.

Resistance – After 2 years of treatment, 21.6% of HBeAg-positive and 8.6% of HBeAg-negative telbivudine recipients who responded to telbivudine had a rebound of HBV DNA levels that was associated with resistance mutations.[30] Lamivudine-resistant HBV strains have a high level of cross-resistance to telbivudine and reduced susceptibility to entecavir, but generally remain susceptible to adefovir. Some adefovir-resistant strains remain susceptible to telbivudine.

ADEFOVIR DIPIVOXIL *(Hepsera)* — This phosphonate nucleotide analog inhibits replication of HBV, including variants resistant to lamivudine. It also has activity against HIV (not FDA-approved). In placebo-controlled trials, adefovir treatment of HBeAg-positive or HBeAg-negative chronic hepatitis B was associated with marked reductions in HBV DNA levels, aminotransferase normalization in 48-72% of patients, and histologic improvements in 53-64% at 48 weeks. More prolonged therapy resulted in higher rates of response; anti-HBeAg seroconversion occurred in 23% by 72 weeks.[31,32] Chronic treatment with adefovir for up to 5 years maintained virologic suppression with associated histologic improvement and no increase in toxicity.[33] However, in trials comparing it with tenofovir or telbivudine, patients treated with adefovir had an inferior virologic or histologic response.[23,34] In the treatment of HIV/HBV coinfections, antiretroviral therapy that included adefovir led to less reduction in HBV DNA levels than antiretroviral therapy that included tenofovir.[24] The antiviral effects of adefovir are similar in lamivudine-resistant HBV infections.[35]

Adverse Effects – The doses of adefovir used to treat HBV infection are generally well tolerated, but may be associated with asthenia, headache, diarrhea and abdominal pain. Higher-than-recommended doses (30-60 mg/d) and pre-existing renal impairment are risk factors for azotemia and renal tubular dysfunction. In clinical trials, severe acute exacerbations of hepatitis have been reported in up to 25% of patients who discontinued adefovir.

Pregnancy – Adefovir is classified as category C (risk cannot be ruled out) for use in pregnancy.

Resistance – Adefovir-resistant variants emerge at a low frequency (8% of patients after 3 years of use and 20% after 5 years in HbeAg-negative patients)[31] and have been associated with a rebound in HBV DNA levels; these variants may remain susceptible to lamivudine. Primary resistance has been reported.[36]

LAMIVUDINE *(Epivir; Epivir-HBV)* — This oral antiretroviral nucleoside analog used to treat HIV[37] is also FDA-approved in a lower-dose formulation for treatment of chronic HBV infection. In patients with cirrhosis or advanced fibrosis, treatment for up to 42 months reduced the risk of clinical progression of disease and the development of hepatocellular cancer by about 50%.[38] Lamivudine is active in chronically infected children aged ≥2 years, with 55% showing sustained normalization of aminotransferase levels, 61% HBV DNA suppression, and 22% anti-HBe seroconversion after 1 year of therapy.[39] It also appears to reduce the risk of HBV reinfection in liver transplant recipients. Prenatal lamivudine was effective in preventing vertical transmission of HBV from mother to fetus when given in the last 4 weeks of gestation.

Adverse Effects – Lamivudine is generally well tolerated. Headache, nausea and dizziness are rare. Pancreatitis has been reported in adults and children coinfected with HIV. Severe exacerbations of hepatitis B including fatal liver failure have resulted from sudden discontinuation of lamivudine therapy.

Pregnancy – Lamivudine is classified as category C (risk cannot be ruled out) for use during pregnancy.

Resistance – Resistance emerges in 14-32% of HBV-infected patients receiving lamivudine for one year and increases to 69% at 5 years.[40] Resistant variants have been associated with hepatitis flares, rebound viremia and progressive liver disease.

EMTRICITABINE (*Emtriva*) — Although FDA-approved only for treatment of HIV infection, emtri-citabine has produced histologic, virologic, and biochemical improvement in patients with chronic HBV infection in placebo-controlled trials, particularly in patients coinfected with HIV.[41,42] While current data are inadequate to support using it to treat HBV, emtricitabine may be considered as part of an effective anti-retroviral regimen in HIV/HBV coinfected patients.

INTERFERON ALFA — Interferon alfa is available as alfacon-1 (*Infergen*), alfa-2b (*Intron A*), pegylated alfa-2b (*PegIntron*), and pegylated alfa-2a (*Pegasys*). Currently interferon alfa-2b and pegylated interferon alfa-2a are licensed for hepatitis B, while alfacon-1, interferon alfa-2b, and pegylated interferon alfa-2a and 2b are licensed for hepatitis C. In the treatment of hepatitis B, interferon therapy, while effective, has largely been replaced by oral antiviral agents.

In about one-third of patients with chronic **hepatitis B**, treatment with interferon alfa-2b leads to loss of HBeAg, return to normal aminotransferase activity, sustained histological improvement and, in adults, a lower risk of progressive liver disease. AIDS patients coinfected with HBV, however, generally respond poorly to interferon. Hepatitis D (hepatitis delta virus), which occurs only in patients infected with HBV, may respond to treatment with high doses of interferon alfa, but relapse is common.

The efficacy of peginterferon alfa-2a is similar to or slightly better than that of conventional interferon.[43] Compared to lamivudine, it has been associated with higher rates of sustained response in HBeAg-negative chronic hepatitis B patients[44] and in HBeAg-positive patients.[45] Peginterferon alfa-2b monotherapy has been effective for patients with HBeAg-positive chronic hepatitis B; addition of lamivudine was not superior to monotherapy.

Peginterferon plus ribavirin is the treatment of choice for chronic **hepatitis C**; it provides sustained viral responses (SVRs) in 54-63% of patients. The rate of SVR does not differ significantly between peginterferon alfa-2a or peginterferon alfa-2b. In one study, most of the responses were durable for years after treatment with peginterferon alfa-2a alone or in combination with ribavirin.[46] When used as monotherapy, peginterferons once weekly are more effective than standard interferon 3 times a week, producing SVRs in 30-40%. Genotype 1 infection is most common in the United States and requires 48 weeks of therapy; genotypes 2 and 3 have much higher response rates and may only require 24 weeks of therapy.[47] The combination of peginterferon plus ribavirin is more effective than combinations of standard interferons and ribavirin in patients coinfected with HIV and hepatitis C virus (HCV).[48-50] In one study, interferon alfa-2b treatment of acute hepatitis C prevented chronic infection in most patients.[51]

Adverse Effects – Intramuscular or subcutaneous injection of interferon is commonly associated with an influenza-like syndrome, especially during the first week of therapy. High-dose or chronic therapy may be limited by bone marrow suppression, fatigue, myalgia, weight loss, rash, cough, increased susceptibility to bacterial infections, psychiatric disorders including depression, anxiety, psychosis, mania, agitation and neurocognitive impairment, increased aminotransferase activity, alopecia, hypo- or hyperthyroidism, tinnitus, reversible hearing loss, auto-antibody formation, retinopathy, pneumonitis and possibly cardiotoxicity. Injection-site reactions and dose-related neutropenia and thrombocytopenia have been more common with pegylated interferon. Autoimmune chronic hepatitis and other autoimmune diseases like thyroiditis may be induced or exacerbated by treatment with interferon.

Depression caused by interferon alfa might be treatable with an antidepressant without stopping the interferon; some Medical Letter consultants initiate antidepressant therapy before starting interferon.

Pregnancy – Interferons are classified as category C (risk cannot be ruled out) for use in pregnancy, but are often used together with ribavirin, which is contraindicated for use in pregnancy.

RIBAVIRIN (*Copegus, Rebetol*, and others) — Treatment of HCV with peginterferon alfa and oral ribavirin has produced higher sustained response rates than peginterferon alone and is now considered the regimen of choice for chronic HCV. The standard dose of ribavirin for HCV genotype 1 is weight-based (1000-1200 mg/d); however, the dose is fixed and lower (800 mg/d) for genotypes 2 and 3.[52] Patients relapsing after interferon monotherapy may still respond to the combination. Ribavirin is not effective as monotherapy for HCV.

Adverse Effects – Systemic ribavirin has been associated with hemolytic anemia. Oral ribavirin plus interferon appears to cause a higher incidence of cough, pruritus and rash than interferon alone. Acute deteriora-tion of respiratory function has been reported with use of aerosolized ribavirin *(Virazole)* in infants and in adults with bron-chospastic lung disease. The drug should be used with caution in patients coinfected with HIV who are taking zidovudine because of the risk of severe anemia.

Pregnancy – Ribavirin is teratogenic and embryotoxic in animals, and is contraindicated for use in pregnancy (Pregnancy category X). Both male and female patients exposed to the drug should not conceive children during treatment or for 6 months after stopping it.

DRUGS FOR PAPILLOMAVIRUS, RESPIRATORY SYNCYTIAL VIRUS, AND OTHER VIRUSES

IMIQUIMOD *(Aldara, Zyclara,* **and others***)* — This immunomodula-tor is FDA-approved for topical treatment of external and perianal geni-tal warts, which are caused by human papillomavirus (HPV). Gradual clearance of warts occurs in about 50% of patients over an average of 8-10 weeks. Recurrences are less common than after ablative therapies.

Adverse Effects – Application site reactions (irritation, pruritus, flaking, erosion) are generally mild to moderate in intensity and resolve within 2 weeks of cessation. Pigment changes may persist. Systemic adverse effects including fatigue and influenza-like illness have been reported.

PODOFILOX *(Condylox,* **and others***)* — Also known as podophyllo-toxin, podofilox is the main cytotoxic ingredient of podophyllin, a resin used for many years for topical treatment of warts. The exact mechanism of action is unknown. Podofilox 0.5% solution or gel is similar in effec-tiveness to imiquimod but may have more adverse effects.[53] Systemic adverse reactions have not been reported. Local adverse effects of the

DRUGS FOR HPV AND RSV

Infection	Drug	Adult dosage
PAPILLOMAVIRUS - ANOGENITAL WARTS[1]		
	Imiquimod[2] – *Aldara*, and others	3x/wk (wash off 6-10 hrs after application) x 16 wks max
	Podofilox 0.5%[2] – *Condylox*, and others	2x/d x 3d, followed by 4 days rest, may be repeated up to 4x
RESPIRATORY SYNCYTIAL VIRUS (RSV)[3]		
	Ribavirin – *Virazole*	aerosol treatment 12-18 hrs/d x 3-7d[4]

1. Trichloroacetic acid, bichloroacetic acid, podophyllin and liquid nitrogen are also often used in doctors' offices to treat genital warts.
2. Pregnancy category C.
3. Immunoprophylaxis with IM palivizumab *(Synagis)*, a monoclonal antibody given by monthly injection, can prevent illness in children <24 mos old with bronchopulmonary dysplasia, in infants who were premature (≤35 wks gestation), and in some children ≤24 mos with congenital heart disease (American Academy of Pediatrics. The role of immunoprophylaxis in the reduction of disease attributable to respiratory syncytial virus. Available at: http://www.aap.org/pubiced/RSV-Commentary.pdf. Accessed September 7, 2010).
4. Requires respiratory therapy monitoring for administration and a special aerosol-generating device (*Spag-2* – Viratek) that delivers an aerosol containing 190 mcg/L at a rate of 12.5 L/min.

drug such as pain, burning, inflammation and erosion occur in more than 50% of patients.

TRICHLOROACETIC ACID, PODOPHYLLIN AND CRYO-THERAPY — Trichloroacetic acid, podophyllin and cryotherapy (with liquid nitrogen or a cryoprobe) remain the most widely used treatments for external genital warts, but the response rate is only 60-70%, and at least 20-30% of responders will have a recurrence.

RIBAVIRIN *(Virazole)* — An aerosalized formulation of ribavirin, a synthetic nucleoside, may decrease morbidity in some children hospitalized with respiratory syncytial virus (RSV) bronchiolitis and pneumonia,[54] but because of its potential adverse effects it is not generally recommended for such use. Pregnant women should not directly care for patients receiving aerosolized ribavirin.

Other viruses – IV ribavirin appears to decrease mortality in Lassa fever and in hantavirus hemorrhagic fever with renal syndrome. *In vitro*, high concentrations inhibit West Nile virus, but clinical data are lacking. There are case reports of systemic ribavirin use with some success in cases of LaCrosse encephalitis, Nipah virus encephalitis, and Crimean-Congo hemorrhagic fever, but it is ineffective in severe acute respiratory syndrome (SARS) and hantavirus cardiopulmonary syndrome.[55]

CIDOFOVIR *(Vistide)* — IV and topical cidofovir (3% cream, once daily)[56] have been reported to produce resolution of molluscum contagiosum in immunosuppressed patients.[57] Cidofovir has also been used to treat adenovirus infection in allogeneic stem cell transplant recipients.[58] *In vitro*, cidofovir is active against vaccinia, variola and other pox viruses and has been effective in animal models of lethal infection with these viruses.[59] (For adverse effects, see page 75.)

1. Adult immunization. Treat Guidel Med Lett 2009; 7:27.
2. B Pasternak and A Hviid. Use of acyclovir, valacyclovir and famciclovir in the first trimester of pregnancy and the risk of birth defects. JAMA 2010; 304:859.
3. M Abudalu et al. Single-day, patient-initiated famciclovir therapy versus 3-day valacyclovir regimen for recurrent genital herpes: a randomized, double-blind, comparative trial. Clin Infect Dis 2008; 47:651.
4. SL Spruance et al. Single-dose, patient-initiated famciclovir: a randomized, double-blind, placebo-controlled trial for episodic treatment of herpes labialis. J Am Acad Dermatol 2006; 55:47.
5. FY Aoki et al. Single-day, patient-initiated famciclovir therapy for recurrent genital herpes: a randomized, double-blind, placebo-controlled trial. Clin Infect Dis 2006; 42:8.
6. SL Spruance et al. High-dose, short-duration, early valacyclovir therapy for episodic treatment of cold sores: results of two randomized, placebo-controlled, multicenter studies. Antimicrob Agents Chemother 2003; 47:1072.
7. KH Fife et al. Effect of valacyclovir on viral shedding in immunocompetent patients with recurrent herpes simplex virus 2 genital herpes: a US-based randomized, double-blind, placebo-controlled clinical trial. Mayo Clin Proc 2006; 81:1321.
8. L Corey et al. Once-daily valacyclovir to reduce the risk of transmission of genital herpes. N Engl J Med 2004; 350:11.
9. A Wald et al. Comparative efficacy of famciclovir and valacyclovir for suppression of recurrent genital herpes and viral shedding. Sex Trans Dis 2006; 33:529.

10. V Erard et al. One-year acyclovir prophylaxis for preventing varicella-zoster virus disease after hematopoietic cell transplantation: no evidence of rebound varicella-zoster virus disease after drug discontinuation. Blood 2007; 110:3071.

11. SL Spruance et al. Penciclovir cream for the treatment of herpes simplex labialis. A randomized, multicenter, double-blind, placebo-controlled trial. Topical Penciclovir Collaborative Study Group. JAMA 1997; 277:1374.

12 Docosanol cream (Abreva) for recurrent herpes labialis. Med Lett Drugs Ther 2000; 42:108.

13. JS Pepose et al. Ocular complications of smallpox vaccination. Am J Ophthalmol 2003; 136:343.

14. L Nassetta et al. Treatment of congenital cytomegalovirus infection: implications for further therapeutic strategies. J Antimicrob Chemother 2009; 63:862.

15. C Paya et al. Efficacy and safety of valganciclovir vs. oral ganciclovir for prevention of cytomegalovirus disease in solid organ transplant recipients. Am J Transplant 2004; 4:611.

16. JA Khoury et al. Prophylactic versus preemptive oral valganciclovir for the management of cytomegalovirus infection in adult renal transplant recipients. Am J Transplant 2006; 6:2134.

17. P Reusser et al. Randomized multicenter trial of foscarnet versus ganciclovir for preemptive therapy of cytomegalovirus infection after allogeneic stem cell transplantation. Blood 2002; 99:1159.

18. CM Perry and JA Balfour. Fomivirsen. Drugs 1999; 57:375.

19. L Kaiser et al. Impact of oseltamivir treatment on influenza-related lower respiratory tract complications and hospitalizations. Arch Intern Med 2003; 163:1667.

20. N Lee et al. Outcomes of adults hospitalised with severe influenza. Thorax 2010; 65:510.

21. Antiviral drugs for influenza. Med Lett Drugs Ther 2009; 51:89.

22. Writing Committee of the WHO Consultation on Clinical Aspects of Pandemic (H1N1) 2009 Influenza, E Bautista et al. Clinical aspects of pandemic 2009 influenza A (H1N1) virus. N Engl J Med 2010; 362:1708.

23. P Marcellin et al. Tenofovir disoproxil fumarate versus adefovir dipivoxil for chronic hepatitis B. N Engl J Med 2008; 359:2442.

24. K Lacombe et al. Comparison of the antiviral activity of adefovir and tenofovir on hepatitis B virus in HIV-HBV-coinfected patients. Antivir Ther 2008; 13:705.

25. Entecavir (Baraclude) for chronic hepatitis B. Med Lett Drugs Ther 2005; 47:48.

26. TT Chang et al. A comparison of entecavir and lamivudine for HBeAg-positive chronic hepatitis B. N Engl J Med 2006; 354:1001.

27. Telbivudine (Tyzeka) for chronic hepatitis B. Med Lett Drugs Ther 2007; 49:11.

28. YF Liaw et al. 2-year GLOBE trial results: telbivudine is superior to lamivudine in patients with chronic hepatitis B. Gastroenterology 2009; 136:486.

29. HL Chan et al. Treatment of hepatitis B e antigen-positive chronic hepatitis with telbivudine or adefovir: a randomized trial. Ann Intern Med 2007; 147:745.

30. H Yang et al. Cross-resistance testing of next-generation nucleoside and nucleotide analogues against lamivudine-resistant HBV. Antivir Ther 2005; 10:625.

31. SJ Hadziyannis et al. Adefovir dipivoxil for the treatment of hepatitis B e antigen-negative chronic hepatitis B. N Engl J Med 2003; 348:800.
32. P Marcellin et al. Adefovir dipivoxil for the treatment of hepatitis B e antigen-positive chronic hepatitis B. N Engl J Med 2003; 348:808.
33. SJ Hadziyannis et al. Long-term therapy with adefovir dipivoxil for HBeAg-negative chronic hepatitis B for up to 5 years. Gastroenterology 2006; 131:1743.
34. HL Chan et al. Treatment of hepatitis Be antigen positive chronic hepatitis with telbivudine or adefovir: a randomized trial. Ann Intern Med 2007; 147:745.
35. MG Peters et al. Adefovir dipivoxil alone or in combination with lamivudine in patients with lamivudine-resistant chronic hepatitis B. Gastroenterology 2004; 126:91.
36. O Schildgen et al. Variant of hepatitis B virus with primary resistance to adefovir. N Engl J Med 2006; 354:1807.
37. Drugs for HIV infection. Treat Guidel Med Lett 2009; 7:11.
38. YF Liaw et al. Lamivudine for patients with chronic hepatitis B and advanced liver disease. N Engl J Med 2004; 351:1521.
39. MM Jonas et al. Clinical trial of lamivudine in children with chronic hepatitis B. N Engl J Med 2002; 346:1706.
40. EB Keeffe et al. A treatment algorithm for the management of chronic hepatitis B virus infection in the United States. Clin Gastroenterol Hepatol 2004; 2:87.
41. MS Saag. Emtricitabine, a new antiretroviral agent with activity against HIV and hepatitis B virus. Clin Infect Dis 2006; 42:126.
42. SG Lim et al. A double-blind placebo-controlled study of emtricitabine in chronic hepatitis B. Arch Intern Med 2006; 166:49.
43. E Nevens et al. A randomized, open-label, multicenter study evaluating the efficacy of peginterferon alfa-2a versus interferon alfa-2a, in combination with ribavirin, in naïve and relapsed chronic hepatitis C patients. Acta Gastroenterol Belg 2010; 73:223.
44. P Marcellin et al. Peginterferon alfa-2a alone, lamivudine alone, and the two in combination in patients with HBeAg-negative chronic hepatitis B. N Engl J Med 2004; 351:1206.
45. GK Lau et al. Peginterferon alfa-2a, lamivudine, and the combination for HBeAg-positive chronic hepatitis B. N Engl J Med 2005; 352:2682.
46. MG Swain et al. A sustained virologic response is durable in patients with chronic hepatitis C treated with peginterferon alfa-2a and ribavirin. Gastroenterology 2010; July 14 epub.
47. ML Shiffman et al. ACCELERATE Investigators. Peginterferon alfa-2a and ribavirin for 16 or 24 weeks in HCV genotype 2 or 3. N Engl J Med 2007; 357:124.
48. FJ Torriani et al. Peginterferon alfa-2a plus ribavirin for chronic hepatitis C virus infection in HIV-infected patients. N Engl J Med 2004; 351:438.
49. RT Chung et al. Peginterferon alfa-2a plus ribavirin versus interferon alfa-2a plus ribavirin for chronic hepatitis C in HIV-coinfected persons. N Engl J Med 2004; 351:451.
50. F Carrat et al. Pegylated interferon alfa-2b vs standard interferon alfa-2b, plus ribavirin, for chronic hepatitis C in HIV-infected patients: a randomized controlled trial. JAMA 2004; 292:2839.
51. E Jaeckel et al. Treatment of acute hepatitis C with interferon alfa-2b. N Engl J Med 2001; 345:1452.

52. SJ Hadziyannis et al. PEGASYS International Study Group. Peginterferon alpha-2a and ribavirin combination therapy in chronic hepatitis C: a randomized study of treatment duration and ribavirin dose. Ann Intern Med. 2004; 140:346.

53. J Yan et al. Meta-analysis of 5% imiquimod and 0.5% podophyllotoxin in the treatment of condylomata acuminata. Dermatology 2006; 213:218.

54. American Academy of Pediatrics Committee on Infectious Diseases, Report of the Committee on Infectious Diseases 26th ed, Evanston, III: American Academy of Pediatrics, 2003; page 524.

55. GJ Mertz et al. Placebo-controlled, double-blind trial of intravenous ribavirin for the treatment of hantavirus cardiopulmonary syndrome in North America. Clin Infect Dis 2004; 39:1307.

56. The cream is not marketed commercially, but may be available from some compounding pharmacies.

57. E De Clercq. Clinical potential of the acyclic nucleoside phosphonates cidofovir, adefovir, and tenofovir in treatment of DNA virus and retrovirus infections. Clin Microbiol Rev 2003; 16:569.

58. P Ljungman et al. Cidofovir for adenovirus infections after allogeneic hematopoietic stem cell transplantation: a survey by the Infectious Diseases Working Party of the European Group for Blood and Marrow Transplantation. Bone Marrow Transplant 2003; 31:481.

59. M Bray and CJ Roy. Antiviral prophylaxis of smallpox. J Antimicrob Chemother 2004; 54:1.

DRUGS FOR
Parasitic Infections

Original publication date – June 2010 (Supplement)

With increasing travel, immigration, use of immunosuppressive drugs and the spread of AIDS, physicians anywhere may see infections caused by parasites. The table that begins on the next page lists first-choice and alternative drugs for most parasitic infections. The brand names and manufacturers of the drugs are listed starting on page 429.

TABLE STARTS ON NEXT PAGE.

DRUGS FOR PARASITIC INFECTIONS

Infection		Drug
***ACANTHAMOEBA* keratitis**		
Drug of choice:		See footnote 1
AMEBIASIS *(Entamoeba histolytica)*		
asymptomatic		
Drug of choice:		Iodoquinol[2]
	OR	Paromomycin[3]
	OR	Diloxanide furoate[4]*
mild to moderate intestinal disease		
Drug of choice:[5]		Metronidazole
	OR	Tinidazole[6]
		either followed by
		Iodoquinol[2]
	OR	Paromomycin[3]*
severe intestinal and extraintestinal disease		
Drug of choice:		Metronidazole
	OR	Tinidazole[6]
		either followed by
		Iodoquinol[2]
	OR	Paromomycin[3]*

---

*   Availability problems. See table on page 274.
1.   Keratitis is typically associated with contact lens use (FR Carvalho et al, Cornea 2009; 28:516). Topical 0.02% chlorhexidine and polyhexamethylene biguanide (PHMB, 0.02%), either alone or in combination, have been used successfully in a large number of patients. Treatment with either chlorhexidine or PHMB is often combined with propamidine isethionate *(Brolene)* or hexamidine *(Desmodine)*. None of these drugs is commercially available or approved for use in the US, but they can be obtained from compounding pharmacies (see footnote 4). Leiter's Park Avenue Pharmacy, San Jose, CA (800-292-6773; www.leiterrx.com) is a compounding pharmacy that specializes in ophthalmic drugs. Propamidine is available over the counter in the UK and Australia. Hexamidine is available in France. The combination of chlorhexidine, natamycin (pimaricin) and debridement also has been successful (K Kitagawa et al, Jpn J Ophthalmol 2003; 47:616), as has 0.1% sodium diclofenac (AL Agahan et al, Ann Acad Med Singapore 2009; 38: 175) in a small series of 3 patients. Debridement is most useful during the stage of corneal epithelial infection; keratoplasty in medically unresponsive keratitis was successful in 31 patients (AS Kitzmann et al, Ophthalmology 2009; 116: 864). Most cysts are resistant to neomycin; its use is no longer recommended. Azole antifungal drugs (ketoconazole, itraconazole) have been used as oral or topical adjuncts. Use of corticosteroids is controversial. Prolonged therapy (≥6 months) may be necessary (JK Dart et al, Am J Ophthalmol 2009; 148:487).
2.   Iodoquinol should be taken after meals.

Adult dosage	Pediatric dosage
650 mg PO tid x 20d	30-40 mg/kg/d (max. 2g) PO in 3 doses x 20d
25-35 mg/kg/d PO in 3 doses x 7d	25-35 mg/kg/d PO in 3 doses x 7d
500 mg PO tid x 10d	20 mg/kg/d PO in 3 doses x 10d
500-750 mg PO tid x 7-10d	35-50 mg/kg/d PO in 3 doses x 7-10d
2 g once PO daily x 3d	≥3yrs: 50 mg/kg/d (max. 2g) PO in 1 dose x 3d
650 mg PO tid x 20d	30-40 mg/kg/d (max. 2g) PO in 3 doses x 20d
25-35 mg/kg/d PO in 3 doses x 7d	25-35 mg/kg/d PO in 3 doses x 7d
750 mg PO tid x 7-10d	35-50 mg/kg/d PO in 3 doses x 7-10d
2 g once PO daily x 5d	≥3yrs: 50 mg/kg/d (max. 2g) PO in 1 dose x 5d
650 mg PO tid x 20d	30-40 mg/kg/d (max. 2g) PO in 3 doses x 20d
25-35 mg/kg/d PO in 3 doses x 7d	25-35 mg/kg/d PO in 3 doses x 7d

3. Paromomycin should be taken with a meal.
4. Not available commercially. It may be obtained through compounding pharmacies such as Expert Compounding Pharmacy, 6744 Balboa Blvd, Lake Balboa, CA 91406 (800-247-9767) or Medical Center Pharmacy, New Haven, CT (203-688-7064). Other compounding pharmacies may be found through the National Association of Compounding Pharmacies (800-687-7850) or the Professional Compounding Centers of America (800-331-2498, www.pccarx.com).
5. Nitazoxanide may be effective against a variety of protozoan and helminth infections (DA Bobak, Curr Infect Dis Rep 2006; 8:91; E Diaz et al, Am J Trop Med Hyg 2003; 68:384). It is effective against mild to moderate amebiasis, 500 mg bid x 3d (JF Rossignol et al, Trans R Soc Trop Med Hyg 2007; 101:1025; AE Escobedo et al, Arch Dis Child 2009; 94:478). It is FDA-approved only for treatment of diarrhea caused by *Giardia* or *Cryptosporidium* (Med Lett Drugs Ther 2003; 45:29). Nitazoxanide is available in 500-mg tablets and an oral suspension; it should be taken with food.
6. A nitroimidazole similar to metronidazole, tinidazole appears to be as effective as metronidazole and better tolerated (Med Lett Drugs Ther 2004; 46:70). It should be taken with food to minimize GI adverse effects. For children and patients unable to take tablets, a pharmacist can crush the tablets and mix them with cherry syrup (*Humco*, and others). The syrup suspension is good for 7 days at room temperature and must be shaken before use (HB Fung and TL Doan, Clin Ther 2005; 27:1859). Ornidazole, a similar drug, is also used outside the US.

Continued on next page.

Drugs for Parasitic Infections

Infection	Drug

AMEBIC MENINGOENCEPHALITIS, primary and granulomatous
 Naegleria fowleri
 Drug of choice: Amphotericin B[7,8]

 Acanthamoeba spp.
 Drug of choice: See footnote 9
  Balamuthia mandrillaris
 Drug of choice: See footnote 10
  Sappinia diploidea
 Drug of choice: See footnote 11

* Availability problems. See table on page 274.
7. Not FDA-approved for this indication
8. A *Naegleria fowleri* infection was treated successfully in a 9-year old girl with combination of amphotericin B and miconazole (both drugs given intravenously and intrathecally) plus oral rifampin (JS Seidel et al NEJM 1982; 306:346). While amphotericin B and miconazole appear to have a synergistic effect, Medical Letter consultants believe the rifampin probably had no additional effect (GS Visvesvara et al, FEMS Immunol Med Microbiol 2007; 50:1). Parenteral miconazole is no longer available in the US. Azithromycin (changed to clarithromycin during therapy because of toxicity concerns and for better CNS penetration) has been used in multidrug combination regimens to treat *Balamuthia* infection. *In vitro*, azithromycin is more active than clarithromycin against *Naegleria*, so may be a better choice combined with amphotericin B for treatment of *Naegleria* (TR Deetz et al, Clin Infect Dis 2003; 37:1304; FL Schuster and GS Visvesvara, Drug Resistance Updates 2004; 7:41). Combinations of amphotericin B, ornidazole and rifampin (R Jain et al, Neurol India 2002; 50:470), amphotericin B, fluconazole (IV and PO) and rifampin (J Vargas-Zepeda et al, Arch Med Research 2005;36:83) and amphotericin B, chloramphicol and rifampacin have also been used (R Rai et al, Indian Pediatr 2008; 45:1004). Case reports of other successful therapy have been published (FL Schuster and GS Visvesvara, Int J Parasitol 2004; 34:1001).
9. Several patients with granulomatous amebic encephalitis (GAE) have been successfully treated with combinations of pentamidine, sulfadiazine, flucytosine, and either fluconazole or itraconazole (GS Visvesvara et al, FEMS Immunol Med Microbiol 2007; 50:1). GAE in an AIDS patient was treated successfully with sulfadiazine, pyrimethamine and fluconazole combined with surgical resection of the CNS lesion (M Seijo Martinez et al, J Clin Microbiol 2000; 38:3892). Chronic *Acanthamoeba* meningitis was successfully treated in 2 children with a combination of oral trimethoprim/sulfamethoxazole, rifampin and ketoconazole (T Singhal et al, Pediatr Infect Dis J 2001; 20:623). Disseminated cutaneous infection in an immunocompromised patient was treated successfully with IV pentamidine, topical chlorhexidine and 2% ketoconazole cream, followed by PO itraconazole (CA Slater et al, N Engl J Med 1994; 331:85) and with voriconazole and amphotericin B lipid complex (R Walia et al, Transplant Infect Dis 2007; 9:51). Other reports of successful therapy have been described (FL Schuster and GS Visvesvara, Drug Resistance Updates 2004; 7:41; AC Aichelburg et al, Emerg Infect Dis 2008; 14:1743). Susceptibility testing of *Acanthamoeba* isolates has shown differences in drug sensitivity between species and even among strains of a single species; antimicrobial susceptibility testing is advisable (FL Schuster and GS Visvesvara, Int J Parasitol 2004; 34:1001).

Adult dosage	Pediatric dosage
1.5 mg/kg/d IV in 2 doses x 3d, then 1 mg/kg/d x 6d plus 1.5 mg/d intrathecally x 2d, then 1 mg/d every other day x 8d	1.5 mg/kg/d IV in 2 doses x 3d, then 1 mg/kg/d x 6d plus 1.5 mg/d intrathecally x 2d, then 1 mg/d every other day x 8d

10. *B. mandrillaris* is a free-living ameba that causes subacute to fatal granulomatous amebic encephalitis (GAE) and cutaneous disease (MMWR 2008; 57:768; FL Schuster et al, Clin Infect Dis 2009; 48:879). Three cases of *Balamuthia* encephalitis have been successfully treated with pentamidine, flucytosine, fluconazole and sulfadiazine plus either azithromycin or clarithromycin combined with surgical resection of the CNS lesion; in two cases flucytosine was given as well. Clarithromycin may have less toxicity and better penetration into CSF than azithromycin (TR Deetz et al, Clin Infect Dis 2003; 37:1304; S Jung et al, Arch Pathol Lab Med 2004; 128:466).
11. A free-living ameba that may rarely be pathogenic to humans (GS Visvesvara et al, FEMS Immunol Med Microbiol 2007; 50:1; F Marciano-Cabral, J Infect Dis 2009; 199: 1104). *S. diploidea* has been successfully treated with azithromycin, pentamidine, itraconazole and flucytosine combined with surgical resection of the CNS lesion (BB Gelman et al, J Neuropathol Exp Neurol 2003; 62:990).

Continued on next page.

DRUGS FOR PARASITIC INFECTIONS (continued)

Infection		Drug
ANCYLOSTOMA caninum (Eosinophilic enterocolitis)		
Drug of choice:		Albendazole[7,12]
	OR	Mebendazole
	OR	Endoscopic removal
Ancylostoma duodenale, see HOOKWORM		
ANGIOSTRONGYLIASIS (Angiostrongylus cantonensis, Angiostrongylus costaricensis)		
Drug of choice:		See footnote 13
ANISAKIASIS (Anisakis spp.)		
Treatment of choice:[14]		Surgical or endoscopic removal
ASCARIASIS (Ascaris lumbricoides, roundworm)		
Drug of choice:[5]		Albendazole[7,12]
	OR	Mebendazole
	OR	Ivermectin[7,15]
BABESIOSIS		
Drug of choice:[16]		Atovaquone[7,17]
		plus azithromycin[7]
	OR	Clindamycin[7,18]
		plus quinine[7,19]

---

*   Availability problems. See table on page 274.

12.   Albendazole must be taken with food; a fatty meal increases oral bioavailability.

13.   *A. cantonensis* causes predominantly neurotropic disease (QP Wang et al, Lancet Infect Dis 2008; 8:621). *A. costaricensis* causes gastrointestinal disease. Most patients infected with either species have a self-limited course and recover completely. Analgesics, corticosteroids and periodic removal of CSF can relieve symptoms from increased intracranial pressure (L Ramirez-Avila et al, Clin Infect Dis 2009; 48:322). Treatment of *A. cantonensis* is controversial and varies across endemic areas. No antihelminthic drug is proven to be effective and some patients have worsened with therapy. Mebendazole or albendazole each with or without a corticosteroid appear to shorten the course of infection (K Sawanyawisuth and K Sawanyawisuth, Trans R Soc Trop Med Hyg 2008; 102:990; V Chotmongkol et al. Am J Trop Med Hyg 2009; 81:443).

14.   Gastric anisakiasis can usually be diagnosed and treated by endoscopic removal of the worm. Enteric anisakiasis is more difficult to diagnose; it can be managed without worm removal as the worms eventually die. Surgery may be needed in the event of intestinal obstruction or peritonitis (A Repiso Ortega et al, Gastroenterol Hepatol 2003; 26:341; K Nakaji, Intern Med 2009; 48:573). Successful treatment of anisakiasis with albendazole 400 mg PO bid x 3-5d has been reported, but diagnosis was presumptive (DA Moore et al, Lancet 2002; 360:54; E Pacios et al, Clin Infect Dis 2005; 41:1825).

15.   Safety of ivermectin in young children (<15 kg) and pregnant women remains to be established. Ivermectin should be taken on an empty stomach with water (NM Fox, Curr Opin Infect Dis 2006; 19:588).

Adult dosage	Pediatric dosage
400 mg PO once 100 mg PO bid x 3d	400 mg PO once 100 mg PO bid x 3d
400 mg PO once 100 mg bid PO x 3d or 500 mg once 150-200 mcg/kg PO once	400 mg PO once 100 mg PO bid x 3d or 500 mg once 150-200 mcg/kg PO once

750 mg PO bid x 7-10d
500-1000 mg PO on d1, then
  250-1000 mg PO on d2-10
	40 mg/kg/d PO in 2 doses x 7-10d
	10 mg/kg (max 500 mg/dose) PO
	  on d 1, then 5 mg/kg/d (max 250
	  mg dose) PO on d 2-10

300-600 mg IV qid or 600 mg PO tid x 7-10d	20-40 mg/kg/d PO in 3 doses x 7-10d
650 mg PO tid x 7-10d	30 mg/kg/d PO in 3 doses x 7-10d

16. E Vannier et al, Infect Dis Clin North Am 2008; 22:469; GP Wormser et al, Clin Infect Dis 2006; 43:1089. B. microti is most common in the US. Most disease in Europe is attributed to B. divergens and is generally more severe. Several cases caused by various B. divergens-like agents have also been documented in the US (BL Herwaldt et al, Emerg Infect Dis 2004; 10:622). Exchange transfusion has been used in combination with drug treatment in severely ill patients and those with high (>10%) parasitemia. In non-immunosuppressed patients infected with B. microti who were not severely ill, combination therapy with atovaquone and azithromycin was as effective as clindamycin and quinine and better tolerated (PJ Krause et al, N Engl J Med 2000; 343:1454). Immunosuppressed patients and those with asplenia should be treated a minimum of 6 weeks and at least 2 weeks past the last positive smear. Resistance to azithromycin-atovaquone treatment has been reported in immunocompromised patients (GP Wormser et al. Clin Infect Dis 2010; 50:381). Some patients may be co-infected with the etiologic agents of Lyme disease and human granulocytic anaplasmosis.
17. Atovaquone is available in an oral suspension that should be taken with a meal to increase absorption.
18. Oral clindamycin should be taken with a full glass of water to minimize esophageal ulceration.
19. Quinine should be taken with or after a meal to decrease gastrointestinal adverse effects.

Continued on next page.

Infection	Drug
Balamuthia mandrillaris, see AMEBIC MENINGOENCEPHALITIS, PRIMARY	
BALANTIDIASIS *(Balantidium coli)*	
Drug of choice:	Tetracycline[7,20]
Alternative:	Metronidazole[7]
OR	Iodoquinol[2,7]

BAYLISASCARIASIS *(Baylisascaris procyonis)*	
Drug of choice:	See footnote 21
***BLASTOCYSTIS* spp.** infection	
Drug of choice:	See footnote 22
CAPILLARIASIS *(Capillaria philippinensis)*	
Drug of choice:	Mebendazole[7]
Alternative:	Albendazole[7,12]
Chagas' disease, see TRYPANOSOMIASIS	
Clonorchis sinensis, see FLUKE infection	
CRYPTOSPORIDIOSIS *(Cryptosporidium)*	
Non-HIV infected	
Drug of choice:	Nitazoxanide[5]
HIV infected	
Drug of choice:	See footnote 23

*   Availability problems. See table on page 274.
20. Use of tetracyclines is contraindicated in pregnancy and in children <8 years old. Tetracycline should be taken 1 hour before or 2 hours after meals and/or dairy products.
21. No drug has been demonstrated to be effective. Albendazole 25 mg/kg/d PO x 20d started as soon as possible (up to 3d after possible infection) might prevent clinical disease and is recommended for children with known exposure (ingestion of raccoon stool or contaminated soil) (WJ Murray and KR Kazacos, Clin Infect Dis 2004; 39:1484). Mebendazole, levamisole or ivermectin could be tried if albendazole is not available. Steroid therapy may be helpful, especially in eye and CNS infections (PJ Gavin et al, Clin Microbiol Rev 2005; 18:703). Ocular baylisascariasis has been treated successfully using laser photocoagulation therapy to destroy the intraretinal larvae (CA Garcia et al, Eye (Lond) 2004; 18:624).
22. Blastocystis has been reclassified as a fungus. Clinical significance of these organisms is controversial; metronidazole 750 mg PO tid x 10d, iodoquinol 650 mg PO tid x 20d or trimethoprim/sulfamethoxazole 1 DS tab PO bid x 7d have been reported to be effective (KS Tan, Clin Microbiol Rev 2008; 21:639). Metronidazole resistance may be common in some areas (J Yakoob et al, Br J Biomed Sci 2004; 61:75). Nitazoxanide has been effective in clearing organisms and improving symptoms (E Diaz et al, Am J Trop Med Hyg 2003; 68:384; JF Rossignol, Clin Gastroenterol Hepatol 2005; 3:987).

Adult dosage	Pediatric dosage
500 mg PO qid x 10d	40 mg/kg/d (max. 2 g) PO in 4 doses x 10d
500-750 mg PO tid x 5d	35-50 mg/kg/d PO in 3 doses x 5d
650 mg PO tid x 20d	30-40 mg/kg/d (max 2 g) PO in 3 doses x 20d
200 mg PO bid x 20d	200 mg PO bid x 20d
400 mg PO daily x 10d	400 mg PO daily x 10d
500 mg PO bid x 3d	1-3yrs: 100 mg PO bid x 3d
	4-11yrs: 200 mg PO bid x 3d
	>12yrs: 500 mg PO bid x 3d

23. No drug has proven efficacy against cryptosporidiosis in advanced AIDS (I Abubakar et al, Cochrane Database Syst Rev 2007; 1:CD004932). Potent antiretroviral therapy (ART) is the mainstay of treatment. Nitazoxanide, paromomycin, or a combination of paromomycin and azithromycin may be tried to decrease diarrhea and recalcitrant malabsorption of antimicrobial drugs, which can occur with chronic cryptosporidiosis (B Pantenburg et al, Expert Rev Anti Infect Ther 2009; 7:385).

Continued on next page.

Infection	Drug
CUTANEOUS LARVA MIGRANS (creeping eruption, dog and cat hookworm)	
Drug of choice:[24]	Albendazole[7,12]
OR	Ivermectin[7,15]
CYCLOSPORIASIS (*Cyclospora cayetanensis*)	
Drug of choice:[25]	Trimethoprim/sulfamethoxazole[7]
Alternative:	Ciprofloxacin[7]
CYSTICERCOSIS, see TAPEWORM infection	
CYSTOISOSPORIASIS (*Cystoisospora belli*, formerly known as *Isospora*)	
Drug of choice:[26]	Trimethoprimsulfamethoxazole[7]
DIENTAMOEBA fragilis infection[27]	
Drug of choice:[28]	Iodoquinol[2,7]
OR	Paromomycin[3,7*]
OR	Metronidazole[7]
Diphyllobothrium latum, see TAPEWORM infection	
DRACUNCULUS medinensis (guinea worm) infection	
Drug of choice:	See footnote 29
Echinococcus, see TAPEWORM infection	
Entamoeba histolytica, see AMEBIASIS	
ENTEROBIUS vermicularis (pinworm) infection	
Drug of choice:[30]	Albendazole[7,12]
OR	Mebendazole
OR	Pyrantel pamoate[31*]
Fasciola hepatica, see FLUKE infection	

* Availability problems. See table on page 274.
24. J Heukelbach and H Feldmeier, Lancet Infect Dis 2008; 8:302.
25. CA Warren, Curr Infect Dis Rep 2009; 11:108. In one study of HIV-infected patients with *Cyclospora* infection, ciprofloxacin treatment led to resolution in 87% of patients compared to 100% with TMP/SMX (RI Verdier et al, Ann Intern Med 2000; 132:885). HIV-infected patients may need higher dosage and long-term maintenance. Nitazoxanide (see also footnote 5) has also been used in a few patients (SM Zimmer et al, Clin Infect Dis 2007; 44:466; E Diaz et al, Am J Trop Med Hyg 2003; 68:384).
26. *Isospora belli* has been renamed and included the *Cystoisospora* genus. Usually a self-limited illness in immunocompetent patients. Immunosuppressed patients may need higher doses and longer duration (TMP/SMX qid for up to 3 to 4 weeks (Morbid Mortal Wkly Rep 2009; 58 RR4:1). They may require secondary prophylaxis (TMP/SMX DS tiw). In sulfa-allergic patients, pyrimethamine 50-75 mg daily in divided doses (plus leucovorin 10-25 mg/d) has been effective.

Adult dosage	Pediatric dosage
400 mg PO daily x 3d	400 mg PO daily x 3d
200 mcg/kg PO daily x 1-2d	200 mcg/kg PO daily x 1-2d
TMP 160 mg/SMX 800 mg (1 DS tab) PO bid x 7-10d	TMP 10 mg/kg/SMX 50 mg/kg/d PO in 2 doses x 7-10d
500 mg PO bid x 7d	—
TMP 160 mg/SMX 800 mg (1 DS tab) PO bid x 10d	TMP 10 mg/kg/d/SMX 50 mg/kg/d PO in 2 doses x 10d
650 mg PO tid x 20d	30-40 mg/kg/d (max. 2g) PO in 3 doses x 20d
25-35 mg/kg/d PO in 3 doses x 7d	25-35 mg/kg/d PO in 3 doses x 7d
500-750 mg PO tid x 10d	35-50 mg/kg/d PO in 3 doses x 10d
400 mg PO once; repeat in 2wks	400 mg PO once; repeat in 2wks
100 mg PO once; repeat in 2wks	100 mg PO once; repeat in 2wks
11 mg/kg base PO once (max. 1 g); repeat in 2wks	11 mg/kg base PO once (max. 1 g); repeat in 2wks

27. DJ Stark et al, Trends Parasitol 2006; 22:92; O Vandenberg et al, Pediatr Infect Dis J 2007; 26:88.
28. In one study, single-dose ornidazole, a nitroimidazole similar to metronidazole that is available in Europe, was effective and better tolerated than 5 days of metro-nidazole (O Kurt, Clin Microbiol Infect 2008; 14:601).
29. No drug is curative against *Dracunculus*. A program for monitoring local sources of drinking water to eliminate transmission has dramatically decreased the number of cases worldwide. The treatment of choice is slow extraction of worm combined with wound care and pain management (Morbid Mortal Wkly Rep 2009; 58:1123).
30. Since family members are usually infected, treatment of the entire household is recommended; retreatment after 14-21d may be needed.
31. Pyrantel pamoate suspension can be mixed with milk or fruit juice.

Continued on next page.

DRUGS FOR PARASITIC INFECTIONS (continued)

Infection	Drug
FILARIASIS[32, 33]	
Wuchereria bancrofti, Brugia malayi, Brugia timori	
Drug of choice:[34]	Diethylcarbamazine*
Loa loa	
Drug of choice:[37]	Diethylcarbamazine*
Mansonella ozzardi	
Drug of choice:	See footnote 38
Mansonella perstans	
Drug of choice[39]	Albendazole[7,12]
OR	Mebendazole[7]
Mansonella streptocerca	
Drug of choice:[40]	Diethylcarbamazine*
OR	Ivermectin[7,15]
Tropical Pulmonary Eosinophilia (TPE)[41]	
Drug of choice:	Diethylcarbamazine*

* Availability problems. See table on page 274.

32. Antihistamines or corticosteroids may be required to decrease allergic reactions to components of disintegrating microfilariae that result from treatment, especially in infection caused by *Loa loa*.

33. Endosymbiotic *Wolbachia* bacteria, which are present in most human filariae except *Loa loa*, are essential to filarial growth, development, embryogenesis and survival and represent an additional target for therapy. Doxycycline 100 or 200 mg/d PO x 6-8wks in lymphatic filariasis, onchocercia-sis, and *Mansonella perstans* has resulted in substantial loss of *Wolbachia* and decrease in both micro- and macrofilariae (MJ Bockarie et al, Expert Rev Anti Infect Ther 2009; 7:595; A Hoerauf, Curr Opin Infect Dis 2008; 21:673; YI Coulibaly et al, N Engl J Med 2009; 361:1448). Use of tetra-cyclines is contraindicated in pregnancy and in children <8 yrs old.

34. Most symptoms are caused by adult worm. A single-dose combination of albendazole (400 mg PO) with either ivermectin (200 mcg/kg PO) or diethylcarbamazine (6 mg/kg PO) is effective for reduc-tion or suppression of *W. bancrofti* microfilaria; none of these drug combinations kills all the adult worms (D Addiss et al, Cochrane Database Syst Rev 2004; CD003753).

35. For patients with microfilaria in the blood, Medical Letter consultants start with a lower dosage and scale up: d1: 50 mg; d2: 50 mg tid; d3: 100 mg tid; d4-14: 6 mg/kg/d in 3 doses (for *Loa Loa* d4-14: 9 mg/kg/d in 3 doses). Multi-dose regimens have been shown to provide more rapid reduction in microfilaria than single-dose diethylcarbamazine, but microfilaria levels are similar 6-12 months after treatment (A Hoerauf et al, Trans R Soc Trop Med Hyg 1995; 89:319; PE Simonsen et al, Am J Trop Med Hyg 1995; 53:267). A single dose of 6 mg/kg is used in endemic areas for mass treatment, but there are no studies directly comparing the efficacy of the single-dose regimen to a 12-day course. It should be used cautiously in geographic regions where *O. volvulus* coexists with other filariae. One review concluded that the 12-day regimen did not have a higher macrofilaricidal effect than single dose (A Hoerauf, Curr Opin Infect Dis 2008; 21: 673; J Figueredo-Silva et al, Trans R Soc Trop Med Hyg 1996; 90:192; J Noroes et al, Trans R Soc Trop Med Hyg 1997; 91:78).

36. Diethylcarbamazine should not be used for treatment of *Onchocerca volvulus* due to the risk of increased ocular side effects (including blindness) associated with rapid killing of the worms. It should be used cautiously in geographic regions where *O. volvulus* coexists with other filariae. Diethylcarbamazine is contraindicated during pregnancy. See also footnote 42.

Adult dosage	Pediatric dosage
6 mg/kg/d PO in 3 doses x 12d[35,36]	6 mg/kg/d PO in 3 doses x 12d[35,36]
9 mg/kg/d PO in 3 doses x 12d[35,36]	9 mg/kg/d PO in 3 doses x 12d[35,36]
400 mg PO bid x 10d 100 mg PO bid x 30d	400 mg PO bid x 10d 100 mg PO bid x 30d
6 mg/kg/d PO in 3 doses x 12d[36] 150 mcg/kg PO once	6 mg/kg/d PO in 3 doses x 12d[36] 150 mcg/kg PO once
6 mg/kg/d in 3 doses x 12-21d[36]	6 mg/kg/d in 3 doses x 12-21d[36]

37. In heavy infections with *Loa loa*, rapid killing of microfilariae can provoke encephalopathy. Apheresis has been reported to be effective in lowering microfilarial counts in patients heavily infected with *Loa loa* (EA Ottesen, Infect Dis Clin North Am 1993; 7:619). Albendazole may be useful for treatment of loiasis when diethylcarbamazine is ineffective or cannot be used, but repeated courses may be necessary (AD Klion et al, Clin Infect Dis 1999; 29:680; TE Tabi et al, Am J Trop Med Hyg 2004; 71:211). Ivermectin has also been used to reduce microfilaremia, but albendazole is preferred because of its slower onset of action and lower risk of precipitating encephalopathy (AD Klion et al, J Infect Dis 1993; 168:202; M Kombila et al, Am J Trop Med Hyg 1998; 58:458). Diethylcarbamazine, 300 mg PO once/wk, has been recommended for prevention of loiasis (TB Nutman et al, N Engl J Med 1988; 319:752).
38. Diethylcarbamazine has no effect. A single dose of ivermectin 200 mcg/kg PO reduces microfilaria densities and provides both short- and long-term reductions in *M. ozzardi* microfilaremia (AA Gonzalez et al, W Indian Med J 1999; 48:231).
39. One small study compared single-dose ivermectin to albendazole alone or the two together although the combination reduced microfilaremia 1 and 3 months post treatment, the effect was not significant at 6 and 12 months (SM Asio et al, Ann Trop Med Parasitol 2009; 103:31).
40. Diethylcarbamazine is potentially curative due to activity against both adult worms and microfilariae. Ivermectin is active only against microfilariae.
41. VK Vijayan, Curr Opin Pulm Med 2007; 13:428. Relapses occur and can be treated with a repeated course of diethylcarbamazine.

Continued on next page.

DRUGS FOR PARASITIC INFECTIONS (continued)

Infection	Drug
FILARIASIS[32, 33] (continued)	
Onchocerca volvulus (River blindness)	
Drug of choice:	Ivermectin[15,42]
FLUKE, hermaphroditic, infection	
Clonorchis sinensis (Chinese liver fluke)[43]	
Drug of choice:	Praziquantel[44]
OR	Albendazole[7,12]
Fasciola hepatica (sheep liver fluke)[43]	
Drug of choice:[45]	Triclabendazole*
Alternative:	Bithionol*
OR	Nitazoxanide[5,7]
Fasciolopsis buski, Heterophyes heterophyes, Metagonimus yokogawai (intestinal flukes)	
Drug of choice:	Praziquantel[7,44]
Metorchis conjunctus (North American liver fluke)	
Drug of choice:	Praziquantel[7,44]
Nanophyetus salmincola	
Drug of choice:	Praziquantel[7,44]
Opisthorchis viverrini (Southeast Asian liver fluke)[43]	
Drug of choice:	Praziquantel[44]

---

* Availability problems. See table on page 274.

42. Diethylcarbamazine should not be used for treatment of this disease because rapid killing of the worms can lead to blindness. Periodic treatment with ivermectin (every 3-12 months), 150 mcg/kg PO, can prevent blindness due to ocular onchocerciasis (DN Udall, Clin Infect Dis 2007; 44:53). Skin reactions after ivermectin treatment are often reported in persons with high microfilarial skin densities. Ivermectin has been inadvertently given to pregnant women during mass treatment programs; the rates of congenital abnormalities were similar in treated and untreated women. Because of the high risk of blindness from onchocerciasis, the use of ivermectin after the first trimester is considered acceptable according to the WHO. Addition of 6-8 weeks of doxycycline to ivermectin is increasingly common. Doxycycline (100 mg/day PO for 6 weeks), followed by a single 150 mcg/kg PO dose of ivermectin, resulted in up to 19 months of amicrofilaridermia and 100% elimination of *Wolbachia* species (A Hoerauf et al, Lancet 2001; 357:1415).

Adult dosage	Pediatric dosage
150 mcg/kg PO once, repeated every 6-12mos until asymptomatic	150 mcg/kg PO once, repeated every 6-12mos until asymptomatic
75 mg/kg/d PO in 3 doses x 2d 10 mg/kg/d PO x 7d	75 mg/kg/d PO in 3 doses x 2d 10 mg/kg/d PO x 7d
10 mg/kg PO once or twice 30-50 mg/kg on alternate days x 10-15 doses 500 mg PO bid x 7d	10 mg/kg PO once or twice 30-50 mg/kg on alternate days x 10-15 doses 1-3yrs: 100 mg PO bid x 7d 4-11yrs: 200 mg PO bid x 7d >12yrs: 500 mg PO bid x 7d
75 mg/kg/d PO in 3 doses x 1d	75 mg/kg/d PO in 3 doses x 1d
75 mg/kg/d PO in 3 doses x 1d	75 mg/kg/d PO in 3 doses x 1d
60 mg/kg/d PO in 3 doses x 1d	60 mg/kg/d PO in 3 doses x 1d
75 mg/kg/d PO in 3 doses x 2d	75 mg/kg/d PO in 3 doses x 2d

43. LA Marcos, Curr Opin Infect Dis 2008; 21:523.
44. Praziquantel should be taken with liquids during a meal.
45. Unlike infections with other flukes, *Fasciola hepatica* infections may not respond to praziquantel. Triclabendazole (*Egaten* - Novartis) appears to be safe and effective, but data are limited (J Keiser et al, Expert Opin Investig Drugs 2005; 14:1513). It is available from Victoria Pharmacy, Zurich, Switzerland (www.pharmaworld.com; 011-4143-344-60-60) and should be given with food for better absorption. Nitazoxanide also appears to have efficacy in treating fascioliasis in adults and in children (L Favennec et al, Aliment Pharmacol Ther 2003; 17:265; JF Rossignol et al, Trans R Soc Trop Med Hyg 1998; 92:103; SM Kabil et al, Curr Ther Res 2000; 61:339).

Continued on next page.

Infection		Drug

FLUKE, hermaphroditic, infection (continued)
  Paragonimiasis (*P. westermani, P. miyazaki, P. skrjabini, P. hueitungensis,*
  ***P. heterotrema, P. utcerobilaterus, P. Africanus, P. Mexicanus, P. Kellicotti,*)**
  (lung fluke)

Drug of choice:		Praziquantel[7,44]
Alternative:		Triclabendazole[46*]
		Bithionol[*]

GIARDIASIS (*Giardia duodenalis*)

Drug of choice:		Metronidazole[7]
	OR	Tinidazole[6]
	OR	Nitazoxanide[5]
Alternative:[47]		Paromomycin[3,7,48*]
	OR	Furazolidone[*]
	OR	Quinacrine[4,49*]

GNATHOSTOMIASIS (*Gnathostoma spinigerum*) [50]

Treatment of choice:		Albendazole[7,12]
	OR	Ivermectin[7,15]
		either
	±	Surgical removal

GONGYLONEMIASIS (*Gongylonema* sp.) [51]

Treatment of choice:		Surgical removal
	OR	Albendazole[7,12]

---

*   Availability problems. See table on page 274.
46. J Keiser et al, Expert Opin Investig Drugs 2005; 14:1513. See footnote 45 for availability.
47. Additional option: albendazole (400 mg/d PO x 5d in adults and 10 mg/kg/d PO x 5d in children) (K Yereli et al, Clin Microbiol Infect 2004; 10:527; O Karabay et al, World J Gastroenterol 2004; 10:1215). Refractory disease: standard doses of metronidazole plus quinacrine x 3wks (TE Nash et al, Clin Infect Dis 2001; 33:22). In one study, nitazoxanide was used successfully in high doses (1.5 g PO bid x 30d) to treat a case of *Giardia* resistant to metronidazole and albendazole (P Abboud et al, Clin Infect Dis 2001; 32:1792).

Adult dosage	Pediatric dosage
75 mg/kg/d PO in 3 doses x 2d	75 mg/kg/d PO in 3 doses x 2d
10 mg/kg PO once or twice	10 mg/kg PO once or twice
30-50 mg/kg on alternate days x 10-15 doses	30-50 mg/kg on alternate days x 10-15 doses
250 mg PO tid x 5-7d	15 mg/kg/d PO in 3 doses x 5-7d
2 g PO once	≥3yrs: 50 mg/kg PO once (max. 2 g)
500 mg PO bid x 3d	1-3yrs: 100 mg PO bid x 3d
	4-11yrs: 200 mg PO bid x 3d
	>12yrs: 500 mg PO bid x 3d
25-35 mg/kg/d PO in 3 doses x 5-10d	25-35 mg/kg/d PO in 3 doses x 5-10d
100 mg PO qid x 7-10d	6 mg/kg/d PO in 4 doses x 7-10d
100 mg PO tid x 5d	6 mg/kg/d PO in 3 doses x 5d (max 300 mg/d)
400 mg PO bid x 21d	400 mg PO bid x 21d
200 mcg/kg/d PO x 2d	200 mcg/kg/d PO x 2d
400 mg/d PO x 3d	400 mg/d PO x 3d

48. Poorly absorbed; may be useful for treatment of giardiasis in pregnancy.
49. Quinacrine should be taken with liquids after a meal. It is not available in the US but can be compounded by Gallipot Pharmacy (www.gallipot.com; 800-423-6967).
50. All patients should be treated with medication whether surgery is attempted or not. JS Herman and PL Chiodini, Clin Microbiol Rev 2009; 22:484; L Ramirez-Avila et al, Clin Infect Dis 2009; 48:322.
51. S Pasuralertsakul et al, Am Trop Med Parasitol 2008; 102:455; G Molavi et al, J Helminth 2006; 80:425.

Continued on next page.

DRUGS FOR PARASITIC INFECTIONS (continued)

Infection		Drug
HOOKWORM infection *(Ancylostoma duodenale, Necator americanus)*		
Drug of choice:		Albendazole[7,12]
	OR	Mebendazole
	OR	Pyrantel pamoate[7,31]*
Hydatid cyst, see TAPEWORM infection		
Hymenolepis nana, see TAPEWORM infection		
Isospora belli, see *Cystoisospora*		
LEISHMANIASIS		
Visceral[52,53]		
Drug of choice:		Liposomal amphotericin B[54]
	OR	Sodium stibogluconate*
	OR	Meglumine antimonate*
	OR	Miltefosine[56,57]*
Alternative:	OR	Amphotericin B[7]
	OR	Paromomycin[3,7,58]* sulfate

*   Availability problems. See table on page 274.
52.   To maximize effectiveness and minimize toxicity, the choice of drug, dosage and duration of thera-
      py should be individualized based on the region of disease acquisition, likely infecting species, and
      host factors such as immune status (BL Herwaldt, Lancet 1999; 354:1191). Some of the listed
      drugs and regimens are effective only against certain *Leishmania* species/strains and only in cer-
      tain areas of the world (J Arevalo et al, J Infect Dis 2007; 195:1846). Medical Letter consultants rec-
      ommend consultation with physicians experienced in management of this disease.
53.   Visceral infection is most commonly due to the Old World species *L. donovani* (kala-azar) and
      L. infantum (referred to as *L. chagasi* in the New World).
54.   Liposomal amphotericin B *(AmBisome)* is the only lipid formulation of amphotericin B FDA-approved
      for treatment of visceral leishmania, largely based on clinical trials in patients infected with *L. infan-
      tum* (A Meyerhoff, Clin Infect Dis 1999; 28:42). In one open-label study one 10 mg/kg dose of lipo-
      somal amphotericin B was as effective as 15 infusions of amphotericin B (1 mg/kg/d) on alternate
      days (S Sundar et al, N Engl J Med 2010; 362:504). It is the drug of choice for visceral leishmania
      in pregnancy. Two other amphotericin B lipid formulations, amphotericin B lipid complex *(Abelcet)*
      and amphotericin B cholesteryl sulfate *(Amphotec)* have been used, but are considered investiga-
      tional for this condition and may not be as effective (C Bern et al, Clin Infect Dis 2006; 43:917).
55.   The FDA-approved dosage regimen for immunocompromised patients (e.g., HIV infected) is
      4 mg/kg/d IV on days 1-5, 10, 17, 24, 31 and 38. The relapse rate is high; maintenance therapy
      (secondary prevention) may be indicated, but there is no consensus as to dosage or duration.

Adult dosage	Pediatric dosage
400 mg PO once	400 mg PO once
100 mg PO bid x 3d or 500 mg once	100 mg PO bid x 3d or 500 mg once
11 mg/kg (max. 1g) PO daily x 3d	11 mg/kg (max. 1g) PO daily x 3d
3 mg/kg/d IV d 1-5, 14 and 21[55]	3 mg/kg/d IV d 1-5, 14 and 21[55]
20 mg Sb/kg/d IV or IM x 28d	20 mg Sb/kg/d IV or IM x 28d
20 mg Sb/kg/d IV or IM x 28d	20 mg Sb/kg/d IV or IM x 28d
2.5 mg/kg/d PO (max 150 mg/d) x 28d	2.5 mg/kg/d PO (max 150 mg/d) x 28d
1 mg/kg IV daily x 15-20d or every second day for up to 8 wks (total usually 15-20 mg/kg)	1 mg/kg IV daily x 15-20d or every second day for up to 8 wks (total usually 15-20 mg/kg)
15 mg/kg/d IM x 21d	15 mg/kg/d IM x 21d

56. Miltefosine *(Impavido)* is manufactured in 10- or 50-mg capsules by Paladin (Montreal, Canada) and is not available in the US. The drug is contraindicated in pregnancy; a negative pregnancy test before drug initiation and effective contraception during and for 2 months after treatment is recommended (HW Murray et al, Lancet 2005; 366:1561).

57. Miltefosine is effective for both antimony-sensitive and -resistant *L. donovani* (Indian).

58. Paromomycin IM has been effective against *Leishmania* in India; it has not yet been tested in South America or the Mediterranean and there are insufficient data to support its use in pregnancy (S Sundar et al, N Engl J Med 2007; 356:2571; S Sundar and J Chakravarty, Expert Opin Investig Drugs 2008; 17:787). One study in India used a 14-day course of paromomycin (S Sundar et al, Clin Infect Dis 2009; 49:914). Topical paromomycin should be used only in geographic regions where cutaneous leishmaniasis species have low potential for mucosal spread. A formulation of 15% paromomycin/12% methylbenzethonium chloride *(Leshcutan)* in soft white paraffin for topical use has been reported to be partially effective against cutaneous leishmaniasis due to *L. major* in Israel and *L. mexicana* and *L. (V.) braziliensis* in Guatemala, where mucosal spread is very rare (BA Arana et al, Am J Trop Med Hyg 2001; 65:466; DH Kim et al, PLoS Negl Trop Dis 2009; 3:e381). The methylbenzethonium is irritating to the skin; lesions may worsen before they improve.

Continued on next page.

DRUGS FOR PARASITIC INFECTIONS (continued)

Infection		Drug
LEISHMANIASIS (continued)		
Cutaneous[52,59]		
Drugs of choice:		Sodium stibogluconate*
	OR	Meglumine antimonate*
	OR	Miltefosine[56,60]*
Alternative:[61]		Paromomycin[3,7,58]*
	OR	Pentamidine[7]
Mucosal[52,63]		
Drug of choice:		Sodium stibogluconate*
	OR	Meglumine antimonate*
	OR	Amphotericin B[7]
	OR	Miltefosine[56,64]*

---

*   Availability problems. See table on page 274.

59. Cutaneous infection is most commonly due to the Old World species *L. major* and *L. tropica* and the New World species *L. mexicana*, *L. (Vianna) braziliensis*, *L. (V.) panamensis* and others.

60. In a placebo-controlled trial in patients ≥12 years old, miltefosine was effective for treatment of cutaneous leishmaniasis due to *L.(V.) panamensis* in Colombia, but not *L.(V.) braziliensis* or *L. mexicana* in Guatemala (J Soto et al, Clin Infect Dis 2004; 38:1266). For forms of disease that require long periods of treatment, such as diffuse cutaneous leishmaniasis and post kala-azar dermal leishmaniasis, miltefosine might be a useful treatment (JJ Berman, Expert Opin Drug Metab Toxicol 2008; 4:1209).

61. Although azole drugs (fluconazole, ketoconazole, itraconazole) have been used to treat cutaneous disease, they are not reliably effective and have very limited if any efficacy against mucosal disease (JA Blum and CS Hatz, J Travel Med 2009; 16:123). For treatment of *L. major* cutaneous lesions, a study in Saudi Arabia found that oral fluconazole, 200 mg once/d x 6wks appeared to modestly accelerate the healing process (AA Alrajhi et al, N Engl J Med 2002; 346:891). Thermotherapy may be an option for some cases of cutaneous *L. tropica* infection (R Reithinger et al, Clin Infect Dis 2005; 40:1148). A device that generates focused and controlled heating of the skin is being marketed (*ThermoMed* – ThermoSurgery Technologies Inc., Phoenix, AZ, 602-264-7300; www.thermosurgery.com). In one small study after 12 months of followup localized thermal heat was as effective as 10 doses of sodium stibogluconate with less toxicity (NE Aronson et al, PLOS Negl Trop Dis 2010; 4:e628).

Adult dosage	Pediatric dosage
20 mg Sb/kg/d IV or IM x 20d	20 mg Sb/kg/d IV or IM x 20d
20 mg Sb/kg/d IV or IM x 20d	20 mg Sb/kg/d IV or IM x 20d
2.5 mg/kg/d PO (max 150 mg/d) x 28d	2.5 mg/kg/d PO (max 150 mg/d) x 28d
Topically 2x/d x 10-20d	Topically 2x/d x 10-20d
2-3 mg/kg IV or IM daily or every second day x 4-7 doses[62]	2-3 mg/kg IV or IM daily or every second day x 4-7 doses[62]
20 mg Sb/kg/d IV or IM x 28d	20 mg Sb/kg/d IV or IM x 28d
20 mg Sb/kg/d IV or IM x 28d	20 mg Sb/kg/d IV or IM x 28d
0.5-1 mg/kg IV daily or every second day for up to 8wks	0.5-1 mg/kg IV daily or every second day for up to 8wks
2.5 mg/kg/d PO (max 150 mg/d) x 28d	2.5 mg/kg/d PO (max 150 mg/d) x 28d

62. At this dosage pentamidine has been effective in Colombia predominantly against *L. (V.) panamensis* (J Soto-Mancipe et al, Clin Infect Dis 1993; 16:417; J Soto et al, Am J Trop Med Hyg 1994; 50:107). Activity against other species is not well established.
63. Mucosal infection (espundia) is most commonly due to New World species *L. (V.) braziliensis*, *L. (V.) panamensis*, or *L. (V.) guyanensis*.
64. Miltefosine has been effective for mucosal leishmania due to *L.(V.) braziliensis* in Bolivia (J Soto et al, Clin Infect Dis 2007; 44:350; J Soto et al, Am J Trop Med Hyg 2009; 81:387).

Continued on next page.

DRUGS FOR PARASITIC INFECTIONS (continued)

Infection	Drug
LICE infestation *(Pediculus humanus, P. capitis, Phthirus pubis)* [65]	
Drug of choice:	Pyrethrins with piperonyl butoxide[66]
OR	1% Permethrin[66]
OR	5% Benzyl alcohol lotion[67]
OR	0.5% Malathion[68]
Alternative:	Ivermectin[7,15,69]
Loa loa, see FILARIASIS	

*   Availability problems. See table on page 274.

65.   Pediculocides should not be used for infestations of the eyelashes. Such infestations are treated with petrolatum ointment applied 2-4x/d x 8-10d. Oral TMP/SMX has also been used (TL Meinking and D Taplin, Curr Probl Dermatol 1996; 24:157). For pubic lice, treat with 5% permethrin or ivermectin as for scabies (see page 10). TMP/SMX has also been effective when used together with permethrin for head lice (RB Hipolito et al, Pediatrics 2001; 107:E30).

66.   Permethrin and pyrethrin are pediculocidal; retreatment in 7-10d is needed to eradicate the infestation. Some lice are resistant to pyrethrins and permethrin (TL Meinking et al, Arch Dermatol 2002; 138:220). Medical Letter consultants prefer pyrethrin products with a benzyl alcohol vehicle.

67.   FDA-approved to treat head lice in 2009, benzyl alcohol prevents lice from closing their respiratory spiracles and the lotion vehicle then obstructs their airway causing them to asphyxiate. It is not ovicidal. Two applications at least 7d apart are needed. Resistance, which is a problem with other drugs, is unlikely to develop (Med Lett Drugs Ther 2009; 51:57).

Adult dosage	Pediatric dosage
Topically, 2 x at least 7d apart	Topically, 2 x at least 7d apart
Topically, 2 x at least 7d apart	Topically, 2 x at least 7d apart
Topically, 2 x at least 7d apart	Topically, 2 x at least 7d apart
Topically, 2 x at least 7d apart	Topically, 2 x at least 7d apart
200 or 400 mcg/kg PO	≥15kg: 200 or 400 mcg/kg PO

68. Malathion is both ovicidal and pediculocidal; 2 applications at least 7d apart are generally necessary to kill all lice and nits.
69. Ivermectin is pediculocidal, but not ovicidal; more than one dose is generally necessary to eradicate the infestation (KN Jones and JC English 3rd, Clin Infect Dis 2003; 36:1355). The number of doses and interval between doses has not been established. In one study for treatment of head lice, 2 doses of ivermectin (400 mcg/kg) 7 days apart was more effective than treatment with topical malathion (O Chosidow et al, N Engl J Med 2010; 362:896). In one study for treatment of body lice, 3 doses of ivermectin (12 mg each) administered at 7d intervals were effective (C Fouault et al, J Infect Dis 2006; 193:474).

Continued on next page.

DRUGS FOR PARASITIC INFECTIONS (continued)

Infection	Drug
MALARIA, Treatment of *(Plasmodium falciparum,*[70] *P. vivax,*[71] *P. ovale, P. malariae*[72] *and P. knowlesi*[73]*)*	
ORAL (Uncomplicated or mild infection)[74]	
P. falciparum or unidentified species[75] acquired in areas of chloroquine-resistant *P. falciparum*[70]	
Drug of choice:	Atovaquone/proguanil[76]

---

*   Availability problems. See table on page 274.

70. Chloroquine-resistant *P. falciparum* occurs in all malarious areas except Central America (including Panama north and west of the Canal Zone), Mexico, Haiti, the Dominican Republic, Paraguay, northern Argentina, North and South Korea, Georgia, Armenia, most of rural China and some countries in the Middle East (chloroquine resistance has been reported in Yemen, Saudi Arabia and Iran). For treatment of multiple-drug-resistant *P. falciparum* in Southeast Asia, especially Thailand, where mefloquine resistance is frequent, atovaquone/proguanil, quinine plus either doxycycline or clindamycin, or artemether/lumefantrine may be used.

71. *P. vivax* with decreased susceptibility to chloroquine is a significant problem in Papua-New Guinea and Indonesia. There are also reports of resistance from Myanmar, Vietnam, Korea, India, the Solomon Islands, Vanuatu, Indonesia, Guyana, Brazil, Colombia and Peru (JK Baird, Clin Microbiol Rev 2009; 22:508).

72. Chloroquine-resistant *P. malariae* has been reported from Sumatra (JD Maguire et al, Lancet 2002; 360:58).

73. Human infection with the simian species, *P. knowlesi* has been reported in Malaysia where it was initially misdiagnosed as *P. malariae.* Additional cases have been reported from Thailand, Myanmar, Singapore, the Thai-Burma border, and the Philippines (J Cox-Singh et al, Clin Infect Dis 2008; 46:165; MMWR 2009; 58:229). Treatment with the usual antimalarials, such as chloroquine and atovaquone/proguanil appear to be effective.

74. Uncomplicated or mild malaria may be treated with oral drugs. Severe malaria (e.g. impaired consciousness, parasitemia >5%, shock, etc.) should be treated with parenteral drugs (KS Griffin et al, JAMA 2007; 297:2264).

Adult dosage	Pediatric dosage
4 adult tabs PO once/d or 2 adult tabs PO bid[77] x 3d	<5kg: not indicated 5-8kg: 2 peds tabs PO once/d x 3d 9-10kg: 3 peds tabs PO once/d x 3d 11-20kg: 1 adult tab PO once/d x 3d 21-30kg: 2 adult tabs PO once/d x 3d 31-40kg: 3 adult tabs PO once/d x 3d >40kg: 4 adult tabs PO once/d x 3d[77]

75. Primaquine is given as part of primary treatment to prevent relapse after infection with *P. vivax* or *P. ovale*. Some experts also prescribe primaquine phosphate 30 mg base/d (0.6 mg base/kg/d for children) for 14d after departure from areas where these species are endemic (Presumptive Anti-Relapse Therapy [PART], "terminal prophylaxis"). Since this is not always effective as prophylaxis (E Schwartz et al, N Engl J Med 2003; 349:1510), others prefer to rely on surveillance to detect cases when they occur, particularly when exposure was limited or doubtful. See also footnote 87.

76. Atovaquone/proguanil is available as a fixed-dose combination tablet: adult tablets (*Malarone*; atovaquone 250 mg/proguanil 100 mg) and pediatric tablets (*Malarone Pediatric*; atovaquone 62.5 mg/proguanil 25 mg). To enhance absorption and reduce nausea and vomiting, it should be taken with food or a milky drink. Safety in pregnancy is unknown; in a few small studies; outcomes were normal in women treated with the combination in the 2nd and 3rd trimester (AK Boggild et al, Am J Trop Med Hyg 2007; 76:208). The drug should not be given to patients with severe renal impairment (creatinine clearance <30mL/min). There have been isolated case reports of resistance in *P. falciparum* in Africa, but Medical Letter consultants do not believe there is a high risk for acquisition of *Malarone*-resistant disease (E Schwartz et al, Clin Infect Dis 2003; 37:450; A Farnert et al, BMJ 2003; 326:628; S Kuhn et al, Am J Trop Med Hyg 2005; 72:407; CT Happi et al, Malaria Journal 2006; 5:82).

77. Although approved for once-daily dosing, Medical Letter consultants usually divide the dose in two to decrease nausea and vomiting.

Continued on next page.

DRUGS FOR PARASITIC INFECTIONS (continued)

Infection	Drug
MALARIA, Treatment of (continued)	
ORAL (continued)	
P. falciparum or unidentified species[75] acquired in areas of chloroquine-resistant *P. falciparum*[70] (continued)	
	OR Artemether/lumefantrine[78,79]
	OR Quinine sulfate **plus** doxycycline[7,20,81] **or plus** tetracycline[7,20] **or plus** clindamycin[7,18,82]

---

*   Availability problems. See table on page 274.

78.   The artemisinin-derivatives, artemether and artesunate, are both frequently used globally in combination regimens to treat malaria. Both are available in oral, parenteral and rectal formulations, but manufacturing standards are not consistent (HA Karunajeewa et al, JAMA 2007; 297:2381; EA Ashley and NJ White, Curr Opin Infect Dis 2005; 18:531). Oral artesunate is not available in the US; the IV formulation is available through the CDC Malaria branch (M-F, 8am-4:30pm ET, 770-488-7788, or after hours, 770-488-7100) under an IND for patients with severe disease who do not have timely access, cannot tolerate, or fail to respond to IV quinidine (Med Lett Drugs Ther 2008; 50:37). To avoid development of resistance, monotherapy should be avoided (PE Duffy and CH Sibley, Lancet 2005; 366:1908). Reduced susceptibility to artesunate characterized by slow parasitic clearance has been reported in Cambodia (WO Rogers et al, Malaria J 2009; 8:10; AM Dundorp et al, N Engl J Med 2009; 361:455). Based on the few studies available, artemesin have been relatively safe during pregnancy (I Adam et al, Am Trop Med Parisitol 2009; 103; 205), but some experts would not prescribe them in the 1st trimester (RL Clark, Reprod Toxicol 2009; 28:285).

79.   Artemether/lumefantrine is available as a fixed-dose combination tablet (*Coartem* in the US and in countries with endemic malaria, *Riamet* in Europe and countries without endemic malaria); each tablet contains artemether 20 mg and lumefantrine 120 mg. It is FDA-approved for treatment of uncomplicated malaria and should not be used for severe infection or for prophylaxis. It is contraindicated during the 1st trimester of pregnancy; safety during the 2nd and 3rd trimester is not known. The tablets should be taken with fatty food (tablets may be crushed and mixed with 1-2 tsp water, and taken with milk). Artemether/lumefantrine should not be used in patients with cardiac arrhythmias, bradycardia, severe cardiac disease or QT prolongation. Concomitant use of drugs that prolong the QT interval or are metabolized by CYP2D6 is contraindicated (Med Lett Drugs Ther 2009; 51:75).

Adult dosage	Pediatric dosage
6 doses over 3d (4 tabs/dose at 0, 8, 24, 36, 48 and 60 hours)	6 doses over 3d at same intervals as adults; 5-15kg: 1 tab/dose ≥15-25kg: 2 tabs/dose ≥25-35kg: 3 tabs/dose ≥35kg: 4 tabs/dose
650 mg PO q8h x 3 **or** 7d[80]	30 mg/kg/d PO in 3 doses x 3 **or** 7d[80]
100 mg PO bid x 7d	4 mg/kg/d PO in 2 doses x 7d
250 mg PO qid x 7d	25 mg/kg/d PO in 4 doses x 7d
20 mg/kg/d PO in 3 doses x 7d[83]	20 mg/kg/d PO in 3 doses x 7d[83]

80. Available in the US in a 324-mg capsule; 2 capsules suffice for adult dosage. In Southeast Asia, relative resistance to quinine has increased and treatment should be continued for 7d. Quinine should be taken with or after meals to decrease gastrointestinal adverse effects. It is generally considered safe in pregnancy.
81. Doxycycline should be taken with adequate water to avoid esophageal irritation. It can be taken with food to minimize gastrointestinal adverse effects.
82. For use in pregnancy and in children <8 yrs.
83. B Lell and PG Kremsner, Antimicrob Agents Chemother 2002; 46:2315; M Ramharter et al, Clin Infect Dis 2005; 40:1777.

Continued on next page.

DRUGS FOR PARASITIC INFECTIONS (continued)

Infection	Drug
MALARIA, Treatment of (continued) **ORAL** (continued) *P. falciparum* or unidentified species[75] acquired in areas of chloroquine-resistant *P. falciparum*[70] (continued)	
Alternative:	Mefloquine[84,85]
OR	Artesunate[78]* **plus** see footnote 86
P. vivax acquired in areas of chloroquine-resistant *P. vivax*[71]	
Drug of choice:	Artemether/lumefantrine[78,79]
OR	Atovaquone/proguanil[76]

---

* Availability problems. See table on page 274.

84. At this dosage, adverse effects include nausea, vomiting, diarrhea and dizziness. Disturbed sense of balance, toxic psychosis and seizures can also occur. Mefloquine should not be used for treatment of malaria in pregnancy unless there is not another treatment option (F Nosten et al, Curr Drug Saf 2006; 1:1). It should be avoided for treatment of malaria in persons with active depression or with a history of psychosis or seizures and should be used with caution in persons with any psychiatric illness. Mefloquine should not be used in patients with conduction abnormalities; it can be given to patients taking β-blockers if they do not have an underlying arrhythmia. Mefloquine should not be given together with quinine or quinidine, and caution is required in using quinine or quinidine to treat patients with malaria who have taken mefloquine for prophylaxis. Mefloquine should not be taken on an empty stomach; it should be taken with at least 8 oz of water.

Adult dosage	Pediatric dosage
750 mg PO followed 12 hrs later by 500 mg 4 mg/kg/d PO x 3d	15 mg/kg PO followed 12 hrs later by 10 mg/kg 4 mg/kg/d PO x 3d
6 doses over 3d (4 tabs/dose at 0, 8, 24, 36, 48 and 60 hours)	6 doses over 3d at same intervals as adults; 5-15kg: 1 tab/dose ≥15-25kg: 2 tabs/dose ≥25-35kg: 3 tabs/dose ≥35kg: 4 tabs/dose
4 adult tabs PO once/d or 2 adult tabs bid[77] x 3d	<5kg: not indicated 5-8kg: 2 peds tabs PO once/d x 3d 9-10kg: 3 peds tabs PO once/d x 3d 11-20kg: 1 adult tab PO once/d x 3d 21-30kg: 2 adult tabs PO once/d x 3d 31-40kg: 3 adult tabs PO once/d x 3d >40kg: 4 adult tabs PO once/d x 3d[77]

85. *P. falciparum* with resistance to mefloquine is a significant problem in the malarious areas of Thailand and in areas of Myanmar and Cambodia that border on Thailand. It has also been reported on the borders between Myanmar and China, Laos and Myanmar, and in Southern Vietnam. In the US, a 250-mg tablet of mefloquine contains 228 mg mefloquine base. Outside the US, each 275-mg tablet contains 250 mg base.

86. Adults treated with artesunate should also receive oral treatment doses of either atovaquone/proguanil, doxycycline, clindamycin or mefloquine; children should take either atovaquone/proguanil, clindamycin or mefloquine (F Nosten et al, Lancet 2000; 356:297; M van Vugt, Clin Infect Dis 2002; 35:1498; F Smithuis et al, Trans R Soc Trop Med Hyg 2004; 98:182). If artesunate is given IV, oral medication should be started when the patient is able to tolerate it (SEAQUAMAT group, Lancet 2005; 366:717).

Continued on next page.

DRUGS FOR PARASITIC INFECTIONS (continued)

Infection	Drug
MALARIA, Treatment of (continued)	
ORAL (continued)	
P. vivax acquired in areas of chloroquine-resistant *P. vivax*[71] (continued)	
OR	Quinine sulfate
	plus
	doxycycline[7,20,81]
ALL PLUS	primaquine phosphate[75,87]
Alternative:	Mefloquine[84]
	Chloroquine phosphate[88,89]
	plus
	doxycycline[7,20,81]
ALL PLUS	primaquine phosphate[75,87]
All *Plasmodium* species except chloroquine-resistant *P. falciparum*[70] and chloroquine-resistant *P. vivax*[71]	
Drug of choice:[75]	Chloroquine phosphate[88]

* Availability problems. See table on page 274.

87. Primaquine phosphate can cause hemolytic anemia, especially in patients whose red cells are deficient in G-6-PD. This deficiency is most common in African, Asian and Mediterranean peoples. Patients should be screened for G-6-PD deficiency before treatment. Primaquine should not be used during pregnancy. It should be taken with food to minimize nausea and abdominal pain. Primaquine-tolerant *P. vivax* can be found globally. Relapses of primaquine-resistant strains may be retreated with 30 mg (base) x 28d.

Adult dosage	Pediatric dosage
650 mg PO q8h x 3-7d[80]	30 mg/kg/d PO in 3 doses x 3-7d[80]
100 mg PO bid x 7d	4 mg/kg/d PO in 2 doses x 7d
30 mg base/d PO x 14d	0.5 mg/kg/d PO x 14d
750 mg PO followed 12 hrs later by 500 mg	15 mg/kg PO followed 12 hrs later by 10 mg/kg
25 mg base/kg PO in 3 doses over 48 hrs	25 mg base/kg PO in 3 doses over 48 hrs
100 mg PO bid x 7d	4 mg/kg/d PO in 2 doses x 7d
30 mg base/d PO x 14d	0.5 mg/kg/d PO x 14d
1 g (600 mg base) PO, then 500 mg (300 mg base) 6 hrs later, then 500mg (300 mg base) at 24 and 48 hrs	10 mg base/kg (max. 600 mg base) PO, then 5 mg base/kg 6 hrs later, then 5 mg base/kg at 24 and 48 hrs

88. Chloroquine should be taken with food to decrease gastrointestinal adverse effects. If chloroquine phosphate is not available, hydroxychloroquine sulfate is as effective; 400 mg of hydroxychloroquine sulfate is equivalent to 500 mg of chloroquine phosphate.
89. Chloroquine combined with primaquine was effective in 85% of patients with *P. vivax* resistant to chloroquine and could be a reasonable choice in areas where other alternatives are not available (JK Baird et al, J Infect Dis 1995; 171:1678).

Continued on next page.

DRUGS FOR PARASITIC INFECTIONS (continued)

Infection	Drug
MALARIA, Treatment of (continued)	
PARENTERAL (severe infection)[74]	
All *Plasmodium* species (Chloroquine-sensitive and resistant)	
Drug of choice:[75,90]	Quinidine gluconate[91]
	OR Quinine dihydrochloride[91*]
	OR Artesunate[78*]
	plus see footnote 86

---

*   Availability problems. See table on page 274.
90. Exchange transfusion is controversial, but has been helpful for some patients with high-density (>10%) parasitemia, altered mental status, pulmonary edema or renal complications (PJ Van Genderen et al, Transfusion 2009; Nov 20 epub).

Adult dosage	Pediatric dosage
10 mg/kg IV loading dose (max. 600 mg) in normal saline over 1-2 hrs, followed by continuous infusion of 0.02 mg/kg/min until PO therapy can be started	10 mg/kg IV loading dose (max. 600 mg) in normal saline over 1-2 hrs, followed by continuous infusion of 0.02 mg/kg/min until PO therapy can be started
20 mg/kg IV loading dose in 5% dextrose over 4 hrs, followed by 10 mg/kg over 2-4 hrs q8h (max. 1800 mg/d) until PO therapy can be started	20 mg/kg IV loading dose in 5% dextrose over 4 hrs, followed by 10 mg/kg over 2-4 hrs q8h (max. 1800 mg/d) until PO therapy can be started
2.4 mg/kg/dose IV x 3d at 0, 12, 24, 48 and 72 hrs	2.4 mg/kg/dose IV x 3d at 0, 12, 24, 48 and 72 hrs

91. Continuous EKG, blood pressure and glucose monitoring are recommended. Quinine IV is not available in the US. Quinidine may have greater antimalarial activity than quinine. The loading dose should be decreased or omitted in patients who have received quinine or mefloquine. If more than 48 hours of parenteral treatment is required, the quinine or quinidine dose should be reduced by 30-50%. Intrarectal quinine has been tried for the treatment of cerebral malaria in children (J Achan et al, Clin Infect Dis 2007; 45:1446).

Continued on next page.

DRUGS FOR PARASITIC INFECTIONS (continued)

Infection	Drug
MALARIA, Prevention of[92]	
All *Plasmodium* species in chloroquine-resistant areas[70-73]	
Drug of choice:[75]	Atovaquone/proguanil[76]
	OR Doxycycline[20,81]
	OR Mefloquine[85,95]
Alternative:[97]	Primaquine[7,87] phosphate
All *Plasmodium* species in chloroquine-sensitive areas[70-73]	
Drug of choice:[75,99]	Chloroquine phosphate[88,100]

---

*   Availability problems. See table on page 274.

92. Beginning 1-2 d before travel and continuing for the duration of stay and for 1wk after leaving malarious zone. In one study of malaria prophylaxis, atovaquone/proguanil was better tolerated than mefloquine in nonimmune travelers (D Overbosch et al, Clin Infect Dis 2001; 33:1015). The protective efficacy of *Malarone* against *P. vivax* is variable ranging from 84% in Indonesian New Guinea (J Ling et al, Clin Infect Dis 2002; 35:825) to 100% in Colombia (J Soto et al, Am J Trop Med Hyg 2006; 75:430). Some Medical Letter consultants prefer alternate drugs if traveling to areas where *P. vivax* predominates.

94. Beginning 1-2 d before travel and continuing for the duration of stay and for 4wks after leaving malarious zone. Doxycycline can cause gastrointestinal disturbances, vaginal moniliasis and photosensitivity reactions.

95. Mefloquine has not been approved for use during pregnancy. However, it has been reported to be safe for prophylactic use during the second and third trimester of pregnancy and possibly during early pregnancy as well (CDC Health Information for International Travel, 2010, page 141). Not recommended for use in travelers with active depression or with a history of psychosis or seizures and should be used with caution in persons with psychiatric illness. Mefloquine should not be used in patients with conduction abnormalities; it can be given to patients taking β-blockers if they do not have an underlying arrhythmia.

Adult dosage	Pediatric dosage
1 adult tab/d[93]	5-8kg: ½ peds tab/d[76,93]
	9-10kg: ¾ peds tab/d[76,93]
	11-20kg: 1 peds tab/d[76,93]
	21-30kg: 2 peds tabs/d[76,93]
	31-40kg: 3 peds tabs/d[76,93]
	>40kg: 1 adult tab/d[76,93]
100 mg PO daily[94]	2 mg/kg/d PO, up to 100 mg/d[94]
250 mg PO once/wk[96]	≤ 9kg: 5 mg/kg salt once/wk[96]
	9-19kg: ¼ tab once/wk[96]
	>19-30kg: ½ tab once/wk[96]
	>31-45kg: ¾ tab once/wk[96]
	>45kg: 1 tab once/wk[96]
30 mg base PO daily[98]	0.5 mg/kg base PO daily[98]
500 mg (300 mg base) PO once/wk[101]	5 mg/kg base PO once/wk, up to adult dose of 300 mg base[101]

96. Beginning 1-2 wks before travel and continuing weekly for the duration of stay and for 4wks after leaving malarious zone. Most adverse events occur within 3 doses. Some Medical Letter consultants favor starting mefloquine 3 weeks prior to travel and monitoring the patient for adverse events, this allows time to change to an alternative regimen if mefloquine is not tolerated. Mefloquine should not be taken on an empty stomach; it should be taken with at least 8 oz of water. For pediatric doses <½ tablet, it is advisable to have a pharmacist crush the tablet, estimate doses by weighing, and package them in gelatin capsules. There is no data for use in children <5 kg, but based on dosages in other weight groups, a dose of 5 mg/kg can be used.

97. The combination of weekly chloroquine (300 mg base) and daily proguanil (200 mg) is recommended by the World Health Organization (www.WHO.int) for use in selected areas; this combination is no longer recommended by the CDC. Proguanil (*Paludrine* – AstraZeneca, United Kingdom) is not available alone in the US but is widely available in Canada and Europe. Prophylaxis is recommended during exposure and for 4 weeks afterwards. Proguanil has been used in pregnancy without evidence of toxicity (PA Phillips-Howard and D Wood, Drug Saf 1996; 14:131).

98. Studies have shown that daily primaquine beginning 1d before departure and continued until 3-7 d after leaving the malarious area provides effective prophylaxis against chloroquine-resistant *P. falciparum* (DR Hill et al, Am J Trop Med Hyg 2006; 75:402). Nausea and abdominal pain can be diminished by taking with food.

99. Alternatives for patients who are unable to take chloroquine include atovaquone/proguanil, mefloquine, doxycycline or primaquine dosed as for chloroquine-resistant areas.

100. Has been used extensively and safely for prophylaxis in pregnancy.

101. Beginning 1-2wks before travel and continuing weekly for the duration of stay and for 4 wks after leaving malarious zone.

Continued on next page.

DRUGS FOR PARASITIC INFECTIONS (continued)

Infection	Drug
MALARIA, Prevention of relapses: *P. vivax* and *P. ovale*[75]	
Drug of choice:	Primaquine phosphate[87]
MALARIA, Self-Presumptive Treatment[102]	
Drug of Choice:	Atovaquone/proguanil[7,76]
OR	Artemether/lumefantrine[7,78,79]
OR	Quinine sulfate **plus** doxycycline[7,20,81]
OR	Artesunate[78*] **plus** see footnote 86

---

* Availability problems. See table on page 274.
102. A traveler can be given a course of medication for presumptive self-treatment of febrile illness. The
     drug given for self-treatment should be different from that used for prophylaxis. This approach
     should be used only in very rare circumstances when a traveler would not be able to get medical
     care promptly.

Adult dosage	Pediatric dosage
30 mg base/d PO x 14d	0.5 mg base/kg/d PO x 14d
4 adult tabs once/d or 2 adult tabs bid x 3d[77]	<5kg: not indicated 5-8kg: 2 peds tabs once/d x 3d 9-10kg: 3 peds tabs once/d x 3d 11-20kg: 1 adult tab once/d x 3d 21-30kg: 2 adult tabs once/d x 3d 31-40kg: 3 adult tabs once/d x 3d >40kg: 4 adult tabs once/d x 3d[77]

6 doses over 3d (4 tabs/dose at
  0, 8, 24, 36, 48 and 60 hours)
	6 doses over 3d at same intervals
	  as adults;
	5-15kg: 1 tab/dose
	15-25kg: 2 tabs/dose
	25-35kg: 3 tabs/dose
	>35kg: 4 tabs/dose

650 mg PO q8h x 3 or 7d[70]	30 mg/kg/d PO in 3 doses x 3 or 7d[70]
100 mg PO bid x 7d 4 mg/kg/d PO x 3d	4 mg/kg/d PO in 2 doses x 7d 4 mg/kg/d PO x 3d

Continued on next page.

DRUGS FOR PARASITIC INFECTIONS (continued)

Infection	Drug
MICROSPORIDIOSIS	
Ocular *(Encephalitozoon hellem, E. cuniculi, Vittaforma [Nosema] corneae)*	
Drug of choice:	Fumagillin[103]*
	plus
	albendazole[7,12]
Intestinal *(E. bieneusi, E. [Septata] intestinalis)*	
E. bieneusi	
Drug of choice:	Fumagillin[104]*
E. intestinalis	
Drug of choice:	Albendazole[7,12]
Disseminated *(E. hellem, E. cuniculi, E. intestinalis, Pleistophora sp., Trachipleistophora sp. and Anncaliia [Brachiola] vesicularum)*	
Drug of choice:[105]	Albendazole[7,12]
Mites, see SCABIES	
MONILIFORMIS *moniliformis* infection	
Drug of choice:	Pyrantel pamoate[7,31]*
***Naegleria* species**, see AMEBIC MENINGOENCEPHALITIS, PRIMARY	
Necator americanus, see HOOKWORM infection	
***OESOPHAGOSTOMUM* bifurcum**	
Drug of choice:	See footnote 106
Onchocerca volvulus, see FILARIASIS	
Opisthorchis viverrini, see FLUKE infection	

* Availability problems. See table on page 274.
103. CM Chan et al, Ophthalmology 2003; 110:1420. Ocular lesions due to *E. hellem* in HIV-infected patients have responded to fumagillin eyedrops prepared from *Fumidil-B* (bicyclohexyl ammonium fumagillin) used to control a microsporidial disease of honey bees (MJ Garvey et al, Ann Pharmacother 1995; 29:872), available from Leiter's Park Avenue Pharmacy (see footnote 1). For lesions due to *V. corneae*, topical therapy is generally not effective and keratoplasty may be required (RM Davis et al, Ophthalmology 1990; 97:953).
104. Oral fumaagillin *(Flisint* – Sanofi-Aventis, France) has been effective in treating *E. bieneusi* in patients with HIV or solid organ transplants (J-M Molina et al, N Engl J Med 2002; 346:1963; F Lanternier et al, Transpl Infect Dis 2009; 11:83), but has been associated with thrombocytopenia and neutropenia. Potent anti retroviral therapy (ART) may lead to microbiologic and clinical response in HIV-infected patients with microsporidial diarrhea. Octreotide *(Sandostatin)* has provided symptomatic relief in some patients with large-volume diarrhea.

Adult dosage	Pediatric dosage
400 mg PO bid	15 mg/kg/d in 2 doses (max 400 mg/dose)
20 mg PO tid x 14d	
400 mg PO bid x 21d	15 mg/kg/d in 2 doses (max 400 mg/dose)
400 mg PO bid	15 mg/kg/d in 2 doses (max 400 mg/dose)
11 mg/kg PO once, repeat twice, 2wks apart	11 mg/kg PO once, repeat twice, 2wks apart

105. J-M Molina et al, J Infect Dis 1995; 171:245. There is no established treatment for *Pleistophora*. For disseminated disease due to *Trachipleistophora* or *Anncaliia*, itraconazole 400 mg PO once/d plus albendazole may also be tried (CM Coyle et al, N Engl J Med 2004; 351:42).
106. Albendazole or pyrantel pamoate may be effective (JB Ziem et al, Ann Trop Med Parasitol 2004; 98:385).

Continued on next page.

DRUGS FOR PARASITIC INFECTIONS (continued)

Infection	Drug
Paragonimus westermani, see FLUKE infection	
Pediculus capitis, humanus, Phthirus pubis, see LICE	
Pinworm, see ENTEROBIUS	
PNEUMOCYSTIS JIROVECII (formerly *carinii*) pneumonia (PCP)[107]	
Moderate to severe disease[108]	
Drug of choice:	Trimethoprim/sulfamethoxazole
Alternative:	Pentamidine
	OR Primaquine[7,87]
	plus clindamycin[7,18]

---

* Availability problems. See table on page 274.
107. Pneumocystis has been reclassified as a fungus.
108. In severe disease with room air PO_2 ≤70 mmHg or Aa gradient ≥35 mmHg, prednisone or its IV equivalent should also be used. For adults: d 1-5: 40 mg PO bid; d 6-10: 40 mg PO daily; d 11-21: 20 mg PO daily. For children: d 1-5: 2 mg/kg/d PO in 2 doses; d 6-10: 1 mg/kg/d PO in 2 doses; d 11-21: 0.5 mg/kg/d PO daily (JE Kaplan et al, Morbid Mortal Wkly Rep 2009; 58(RR04):1; Morbid Mortal Wkly Rep 2009; 58(RR11):1).

Adult dosage	Pediatric dosage
TMP 15-20 mg/kg/d SMX 75-100 mg/kg/d PO or IV in 3 or 4 doses (change to PO after clinical improvement) x 21d 3-4 mg/kg IV daily x 21d 30 mg base PO daily x 21d	TMP 15-20 mg/kg/d SMX 75-100 mg/kg/d PO or IV in 3 or 4 doses (change to PO after clinical improvement) x 21d 3-4 mg/kg IV daily x 21d 0.3 mg/kg base PO (max. 30 mg) daily x 21d
600-900 mg IV tid or qid x 21d, or 300-450 mg PO tid or qid x 21d (change to PO after clinical improvement)	15-25 mg/kg IV tid or qid (max 600 mg/dose) x 21 d, or 10 mg/kg PO tid or qid (max 300-450 mg/dose)x 21d (change to PO after clinical improvement)

Continued on next page.

DRUGS FOR PARASITIC INFECTIONS (continued)

Infection	Drug
PNEUMOCYSTIS JIROVECII (formerly *carinii*) pneumonia (PCP)[107] (continued)	
Mild to moderate disease	
Drug of Choice:	Trimethoprim/sulfamethoxazole
Alternative:	Dapsone[7]
	plus
	Trimethoprim[7]
OR	Primaquine[7,87]
	plus
	clindamycin[7,18]
OR	Atovaquone[17]
Primary and secondary prophylaxis[109]	
Drug of Choice:	Trimethoprim/sulfamethoxazole
Alternative:	Dapsone[7]
OR	Dapsone[7]
	plus pyrimethamine[110]
OR	Atovaquone[7,17]
OR	Pentamidine

River Blindness, see FILARIASIS

Roundworm, see ASCARIASIS

Sappinia diploidea, See AMEBIC MENINGOENCEPHALITIS, PRIMARY

---

*   Availability problems. See table on page 274.
109. Primary/secondary prophylaxis in patients with HIV can be discontinued after CD4 count increases
       to >200 x 10⁶/L for >3mos.

Adult dosage	Pediatric dosage
2 DS tablets (160 mg/800 mg) PO tid x 21d	TMP 15-20 mg/kg/SMX 75-100 mg/kg/d PO in 3 or 4 doses x 21d
100 mg PO daily x 21d	2 mg/kg/d (max. 100 mg) PO x 21d
15 mg/kg/d PO in 3 doses 30 mg base PO daily x 21d	15 mg/kg/d PO in 3 doses 0.3 mg/kg base PO daily (max. 30 mg) x 21d
300-450 mg PO tid or qid x 21 d	10 mg/kg PO tid or qid (max 300-450 mg/dose) x 21d
750 mg PO bid x 21d	1-3 mos: 30 mg/kg/d PO x 21d 4-24 mos: 45 mg/kg/d PO x 21d >24 mos: 30 mg/kg/d PO x 21d
1 tab (SS or DS) daily or 1 DS tab PO 3d/wk	TMP 150 mg/SMX 750 mg/m²/d PO in 2 doses 3d/wk
50 mg PO bid or 100 mg PO daily	≥ 1 mos: 2 mg/kg/d (max. 100 mg) PO or 4 mg/kg (max. 200 mg) PO each wk
50 mg PO daily or 200 mg PO each wk	
50 mg PO daily or 75 mg PO each wk	
1500 mg/d PO in 1 or 2 doses	1-3mos: 30 mg/kg/d PO 4-24mos: 45 mg/kg/d PO >24mos: 30 mg/kg/d PO
300 mg aerosol inhaled monthly via *Respirgard II* nebulizer	≥5yrs: 300 mg inhaled monthly via *Respirgard II* nebulizer

110. Plus leucovorin 25 mg with each dose of pyrimethamine. Pyrimethamine should be taken with food to minimize gastrointestinal adverse effects.

Continued on next page.

DRUGS FOR PARASITIC INFECTIONS (continued)

Infection	Drug
SARCOCYSTIS spp. (intestinal and muscular), see footnote 111	
SCABIES *(Sarcoptes scabiei)*[112]	
Drug of choice:	5% Permethrin
Alternative:[113]	Ivermectin[7,15]
	10% Crotamiton
SCHISTOSOMIASIS *(Bilharziasis)*	
S. haematobium	
Drug of choice:	Praziquantel[44,115]
S. intercalatum[116]	
Drug of Choice:	Praziquantel[44,115]
S. japonicum	
Drug of choice:	Praziquantel[44,115]
S. mansoni	
Drug of choice:	Praziquantel[44,115]
Alternative:	Oxamniquine[117]*
S. mekongi	
Drug of choice:	Praziquantel[44,115]
Sleeping sickness, see TRYPANOSOMIASIS	
STRONGYLOIDIASIS *(Strongyloides stercoralis)*	
Drug of choice:[119]	Ivermectin[15]
Alternative:	Albendazole[7,12]

* Availability problems. See table on page 274.
111. Sarcocystis in humans is acquired by ingesting sporocysts in infected meat, infections characterized by nausea, abdominal pain and diarrhea. Muscular infections are usually mild or subclinical (R Fayer, Clin Microbiol Rev 2004; 17:894). Albendazole was reported to be efficacious (MK Arness et al, Am J Trop Med Hyg 1999; 61:548).
112. TL Meinking et al, Infestations in LA Schachner and RA Hansen, eds. *Pediatric Dermatology*. 3rd ed. St Louis: Mosby; 2003, page 1291.
113. Lindane (γ-benzene hexachloride) should be reserved for treatment of patients who fail to respond to other drugs. The FDA has recommended it not be used for immunocompromised patients, young children, the elderly, pregnant and breast-feeding women, and patients weighing <50 kg.
114. BJ Currie and JS McCarthy, N Engl J Med 2010; 362:717. A second ivermectin dose taken 2 weeks later increased the cure rate to 95%, which is equivalent to that of 5% permethrin (V Usha et al, J Am Acad Dermatol 2000; 42:236). Ivermectin, either alone or in combination with a topical scabicide, is the drug of choice for crusted scabies in immunocompromised patients (P del Giudice, Curr Opin Infect Dis 2004; 15:123).
115. MJ Doenhoff et al, Curr Opin Infect Dis 2008; 21:659.

Adult dosage	Pediatric dosage
Topically, 2x at least 7 d apart 200 mcg/kg PO 2x at least 7 d apart[114] Topically overnight on days 1, 2, 3, 8	Topically, 2x at least 7 d apart 200 mcg/kg PO, 2x at least 7 d apart[114] Topically overnight on days 1, 2, 3, 8
40 mg/kg/d PO in 1 or 2 doses x 1d	40 mg/kg/d PO in 2 doses x 1d
40 mg/kg/d PO in 1 or 2 doses x 1d	40 mg/kg/d PO x 1d
60 mg/kg/d PO in 2 or 3 doses x 1d	60 mg/kg/d PO in 3 doses x 1d
40 mg/kg/d PO in 1 or 2 doses x 1d 15 mg/kg PO once[118]	40 mg/kg/d PO in 2 doses x 1d 20 mg/kg/d PO in 2 doses x 1d[118]
60 mg/kg/d PO in 2 or 3 doses x 1d	60 mg/kg/d PO in 3 doses x 1d
200 mcg/kg/d PO x 2d 400 mg PO bid x 7d	200 mcg/kg/d PO x 2d 400 mg PO bid x 7d

116. Geographically restricted to Central Western Africa and the island of São Tomé. Usually a disease of the lower GI tract; there are also case reports of complications including central nervous system, liver and cardiopulmonary involvement (A Murinello et al, GE - J Port Gastrenterol 2006; 13:97).
117. Oxamniquine, which is not available in the US, is generally not as effective as praziquantel. It has been useful, however, in some areas in which praziquantel is less effective (ML Ferrari et al, Bull World Health Organ 2003; 81:190; A Harder, Parasitol Res 2002; 88:395). Oxamniquine is contraindicated in pregnancy. It should be taken after food.
118. In East Africa, the dose should be increased to 30 mg/kg PO, and in Egypt and South Africa to 30 mg/kg/d PO x 2d. Some experts recommend 40-60 mg/kg PO over 2-3d in all of Africa (KC Shekhar, Drugs 1991; 42:379).
119. In immunocompromised patients or disseminated disease, it may be necessary to prolong or repeat therapy, or to use other agents. Veterinary parenteral and enema formulations of ivermectin have been used in severely ill patients with hyperinfection who were unable to take or reliably absorb oral medications (FM Marty et al, Clin Infect Dis 2005; 41:e5; P Lichtenberger et al, Transpl Infect Dis 2009; 11:137). In disseminated strongyloidiasis, combination therapy with albendazole and ivermectin has been suggested (M Seqarra, Ann Pharmacother 2007; 41:1992).

Continued on next page.

DRUGS FOR PARASITIC INFECTIONS (continued)

Infection	Drug
TAPEWORM infection	
— **Adult** (intestinal stage)	
Diphyllobothrium latum **(fish),** *Taenia saginata* **(beef),** *Taenia solium* **(pork),**	
Dipylidium caninum **(dog)**	
Drug of choice:	Praziquantel[7,44]
Alternative:	Niclosamide[120]*
Hymenolepis nana **(dwarf tapeworm)**	
Drug of choice:	Praziquantel[7,44]
Alternative:[121]	Niclosamide[120]*
— **Larval** (tissue stage)	
Echinococcus granulosus **(hydatid cyst)**	
Drug of choice:[122]	Albendazole[12]
Echinococcus multilocularis	
Treatment of choice: See footnote 123	
Taenia solium (Cysticercosis)	
Treatment of choice: See footnote 124	
Alternative:	Albendazole[12]
OR	Praziquantel[7,44]

---

*   Availability problems. See table on page 274.

120. Niclosamide must be thoroughly chewed or crushed and swallowed with a small amount of water.

121. Nitazoxanide may be an alternative (JJ Ortiz et al, Trans R Soc Trop Med Hyg 2002; 96:193; JC Chero et al, Trans R Soc Trop Med Hyg 2007; 101:203; E Diaz et al, Am J Trop Med Hyg 2003; 68:384).

122. Patients may benefit from surgical resection or percutaneous drainage of cysts. Praziquantel is useful preoperatively or in case of spillage of cyst contents during surgery. Percutaneous aspiration-injection-reaspiration (PAIR) with ultrasound guidance plus albendazole therapy has been effective for management of hepatic hydatid cyst disease (P Moro and PM Schantz, Int J Infect Dis 2009; 13:125.).

123. Surgical excision is the only reliable means of cure. Reports have suggested that in nonresectable cases use of albendazole (400 mg bid) can stabilize and sometimes cure infection (P Moro and PM Schantz, Int J Infect Dis 2009; 13:125).

Adult dosage	Pediatric dosage
5-10 mg/kg PO once 2 g PO once	5-10 mg/kg PO once 50 mg/kg PO once
25 mg/kg PO once 2 g PO daily x 7 d	25 mg/kg PO once 11-34 kg: 1 g PO on d 1 then 500 mg/d PO x 6 days > 34 kg: 1.5 g PO on d 1 then 1 g/d PO x 6 days
400 mg PO bid x 1-6mos	15 mg/kg/d (max. 800 mg) PO in 2 doses x 1-6mos
400 mg PO bid x 8-30d; can be repeated as necessary	15 mg/kg/d (max. 800 mg) PO in 2 doses x 8-30d; can be repeated as necessary
100 mg/kg/d PO in 3 doses x 1 day then 50 mg/kg/d in 3 doses x 29 days	100 mg/kg/d PO in 3 doses x 1 day then 50 mg/kg/d in 3 doses x 29 days

124. Advances in neuroimaging using CT and MRI have facilitated the ability to make an accurate diagnosis (AC White Jr, J Infect Dis 2009; 199:1261). Initial therapy for patients with inflamed parenchymal cysticercosis should focus on symptomatic treatment with anti-seizure medication (S Sinha and BS Sharma, J Clin Neurosci 2009; 16:867). Patients with live parenchymal cysts who have seizures should be treated with albendazole together with steroids and an anti-seizure medication (HH Garcia et al, N Engl J Med 2004; 350:249). Patients with subarachnoid cysts or giant cysts in the fissures should be treated for at least 30d (JV Proaño et al, N Engl J Med 2001; 345:879). Surgical intervention (especially neuroendoscopic removal) or CSF diversion followed by albendazole and steroids is indicated for obstructive hydocephalus. Arachnoiditis, vasculitis or cerebral edema is treated with albendazole or praziquantel plus prednisone (60 mg/d) or examethasone (4-6 mg/d). Any cysticercocidal drug may cause irreparable damage when used to treat ocular or spinal cysts, even when corticosteroids are used. An ophthalmic exam should always precede treatment to rule out intraocular cysts.

Continued on next page.

DRUGS FOR PARASITIC INFECTIONS (continued)

Infection	Drug
Toxocariasis, see VISCERAL LARVA MIGRANS	
TOXOPLASMOSIS (Toxoplasma gondii)	
CNS disease[125]	
Drug of choice:	Pyrimethamine[126]
	plus sulfadiazine[127]
OR	**plus** clindamycin[7,128]
OR	**plus** atovaquone[7,17,128]
Alternative:	Trimethoprim/sulfamethoxazole[7]
Primary infection in pregnancy	
Treatment of choice: See footnote 129	
TRICHINELLOSIS (Trichinella spiralis)	
Drug of choice:[130]	Steroids for severe symptoms, e.g. prednisone 30-60 mg PO daily x10-15 d **plus** Albendazole[7,12]
Alternative:	Mebendazole[7]

* Availability problems. See table on page 274.
125. Treatment is followed by chronic suppression with lower dosage regimens of the same drugs. For primary prophylaxis in HIV patients with CD4 <100 x 10^6 cells/L, either trimethoprim-sulfamethoxazole, pyrimethamine with dapsone, or atovaquone with or without pyrimethamine can be used. Primary or secondary prophylaxis may be discontinued when the CD4 count increases to >200 x 10^6 cells/L for >3mos (MMWR Morb Mortal Wkly Rep 2009; 58 [RR4]:1). In ocular toxoplasmosis with macular involvement, corticosteroids are recommended in addition to antiparasitic therapy (JG Montoya and O Liesenfeld, Lancet 2004; 363:1965).
126. Plus leucovorin 10-25 mg with each dose of pyrimethamine. Pyrimethamine should be taken with food to minimize gastrointestinal adverse effects.
127. Sulfadiazine should be taken on an empty stomach with adequate water.
128. Clindamycin has been used in combination with pyrimethamine to treat CNS toxoplasmosis in HIV infected patients who developed sulfonamide sensitivity while on sulfadiazine (G Beraud et al, Am J Trop Med Hygiene 2009; 80:583). Atovaquone has also been used to treat sulfonamide-intolerant patients (K Chirgwin et al, Clin Infect Dis 2002; 34:1243).

Adult dosage	Pediatric dosage
200 mg PO x 1 then 50-75 mg/d PO x 3-6 wks	2 mg/kg/d PO x 2d, then 1 mg/kg/d (max. 25 mg/d) x 3-6 wks
1-1.5 g PO qid x 3-6 wks	100-200 mg/kg/d PO x 3-6 wks
1.8-2.4 g/d IV or PO in 3 or 4 doses	5-7.5 mg/kg/d IV or PO in 3 or 4 doses (max 600 mg/dose)
1500 mg PO bid	1500 mg PO bid
15-20 mg/kg/SMX 75-100 mg/kg/d PO or IV in 3 or 4 doses	15-20 mg/kg/SMX 75-100 mg/kg/d PO or IV in 3 or 4 doses
400 mg PO bid x 8-14d	400 mg PO bid x 8-14d
200-400 mg PO tid x 3d, then 400-500 mg tid x 10d	200-400 mg PO tid x 3d, then 400-500 mg tid x 10d

129. Women who develop toxoplasmosis during the first trimester of pregnancy should be treated with spiramycin (3-4 g/d). After the first trimester, if there is no documented transmission to the fetus, spiramycin can be continued until term. Spiramycin is not currently available in the US but can be obtained at no cost from Palo Alto Medical Foundation Toxoplasma Serology Laboratory (PAMF-TSL, 650-853-4828), US National Collaborative Treatment Trials Study (773-834-4152), or the FDA (301-796-1600). If transmission has occurred *in utero*, therapy with pyrimethamine and sulfadiazine should be started. Pyrimethamine is a potential teratogen and should be used only after the first trimester (JG Montoya and JS Remington, Clin Infect Dis 2008; 47:554). Congenitally infected new borns should be treated with pyrimethamine every 2 or 3 days and a sulfonamide daily for about one year (JS Remington and G Desmonts in JS Remington and JO Klein, eds, *Infectious Disease of the Fetus and Newborn Infant*, 6th ed, Philadelphia:Saunders, 2006, page 1038).
130. B Gottstein et al. Clin Microbiol Rev 2009; 22:127.

Continued on next page.

DRUGS FOR PARASITIC INFECTIONS (continued)

Infection		Drug
TRICHOMONIASIS (*Trichomonas vaginalis*)		
Drug of choice:[131]		Metronidazole
	OR	Tinidazole[6]
TRICHOSTRONGYLUS infection		
Drug of choice:		Pyrantel pamoate[7, 31]*
Alternative:		Mebendazole[7]
	OR	Albendazole[7,12]
TRICHURIASIS (*Trichuris trichiura*, whipworm)		
Drug of choice:		Albendazole[7,12]
Alternative:		Mebendazole
	OR	Ivermectin[7,15]
TRYPANOSOMIASIS		
T. cruzi (American trypanosomiasis, Chagas' disease)[132]		
Drug of choice:		Nifurtimox*
	OR	Benznidazole[133]*

* Availability problems. See table on page 274.
131. Sexual partners should be treated simultaneously with same dosage. If treatment failure occurs and reinfection is excluded, treat with metronidazole 500 mg PO bid x7d, or tinidazole 2 g PO once (MMWR Morb Mortal Wkly Rep 2006; 55 [RR11]:1).
132. Treatment of chronic or indeterminate Chagas' disease with benznidazole has been associated with reduced progression and increased negative seroconversion (C Bern et al, JAMA 2007; 298:2171; JA Perez-Molina et al, J Antimicrob Chemother 2009; 64:1139).

Adult dosage	Pediatric dosage
2 g PO once	15 mg/kg/d PO in 3 doses x 7d
2 g PO once	50 mg/kg once (max. 2 g)
11 mg/kg base PO once (max. 1 g)	11 mg/kg PO once (max. 1 g)
100 mg PO bid x 3d	100 mg PO bid x 3d
400 mg PO once	400 mg PO once
400 mg PO x 3d	400 mg PO x 3d
100 mg PO bid x 3d	100 mg PO bid x 3d
200 mcg/kg/d PO x 3d	200 mcg/kg/d PO x 3d
8-10 mg/kg/d PO in 3-4 doses x 90-120d	1-10yrs: 15-20 mg/kg/d PO in 4 doses x 90-120d
	11-16yrs: 12.5-15 mg/kg/d PO in 4 doses x 90-120d
5-7 mg/kg/d PO in 2 doses x 60-90d	≤12yrs: 10 mg/kg/d PO in 2 doses x 60-90d
	>12 yrs: 5-7 mg/kg/d PO in 2 doses x 60-90d

133. Benznidazole should be taken with meals to minimize gastrointestinal adverse effects. It is contraindicated during pregnancy.

Continued on next page.

DRUGS FOR PARASITIC INFECTIONS (continued)

Infection	Drug

TRYPANOSOMIASIS (continued)
T. brucei gambiense (West African trypanosomiasis, sleeping sickness)[134]
  Hemolymphatic stage

Drug of choice:[135]	Pentamidine[7]
Alternative:	Suramin*

  Late disease with CNS involvement

Drug of Choice:[136]		Eflornithine[137]*
	OR	Eflornithine[137]*
		plus
		Nitfurtimox
	OR	Melarsoprol[138]

T. b. rhodesiense (East African trypanosomiasis, sleeping sickness)[134]
  Hemolymphatic stage

Drug of choice:	Suramin*

  Late disease with CNS involvement

Drug of choice:	Melarsoprol[138]

VISCERAL LARVA MIGRANS[139] (*Toxocariasis*)

Drug of choice:		Albendazole[7,12]
	OR	Mebendazole[7]

Whipworm, see TRICHURIASIS
Wuchereria bancrofti, see FILARIASIS

---

* Availability problems. See table on page 274.
134. PG Kennedy, Ann Neurol 2008; 64:116.
135. Pentamidine and suramin have equal efficacy, but pentamidine is better tolerated.
136. In one study eflornithine for 7 days combined with nifurtimox x 10 d was more effective and less toxic than eflornithine x 14 d (G Priotto et al, Lancet 2009; 374:56).
137. Eflornithine is highly effective in *T.b. gambiense*, but not in *T.b. rhodesiense* infections. In one study of treatment of CNS disease due to *T.b. gambiense*, there were fewer serious complications with eflornithine than with melarsoprol (PG Kennedy, Ann Neurol 2008; 64:116). Eflornithine is available in limited supply only from the WHO. It is contraindicated during pregnancy.

Adult dosage	Pediatric dosage
4 mg/kg/d IM x 7d 100-200 mg (test dose) IV, then 1 g IV on days 1,3,7,14 and 21	4 mg/kg/d IM x 7d 20 mg/kg on d 1,3,7,14 and 21
400 mg/kg/d IV in 4 doses x 14d 400 mg/kg IV in 2 doses x 7d	400 mg/kg/d IV in 4 doses x 14d
15 mg/kg/d PO in 3 doses x 10d 2.2 mg/kg/d IV x 10d	2.2 mg/kg/d IV x 10d
100-200 mg (test dose) IV, then 1 g IV on days 1,3,7,14 and 21	20 mg/kg IV on d 1,3,7,14 and 21

2-3.6 mg/kg/d IV x 3d; after 7d
  3.6 mg/kg/d x 3d; repeat again
  after 7d
	2-3.6 mg/kg/d IV x 3d; after 7d
	  3.6 mg/kg/d x 3d; repeat again
	  after 7d

400 mg PO bid x 5d 100-200 mg PO bid x 5d	400 mg PO bid x 5d 100-200 mg PO bid x 5d

138. E Schmid et al, J Infect Dis 2005; 191:1922. Corticosteroids have been used to prevent arsenical encephalopathy (J Pepin et al, Trans R Soc Trop Med Hyg 1995; 89:92). Up to 20% of patients with *T.b.gambiense* fail to respond to melarsoprol (MP Barrett, Lancet 1999; 353:1113). In one study, a combination of low-dose melarsoprol (1.2 mg/kg/d IV) and nifurtimox (7.5 mg/kg PO bid) x 10 d was more effective than standard-dose melarsoprol alone (S Bisser et al, J Infect Dis 2007; 195:322).

139. Optimum duration of therapy is not known; some Medical Letter consultants would treat x 20 d. For severe symptoms or eye involvement, corticosteroids can be used in addition (D Despommier, Clin Microbiol Rev 2003; 16:265).

MANUFACTURERS OF DRUGS USED TO TREAT
PARASITIC INFECTIONS

A-200 (Hogil) – pyrethrins and piperonyl butoxide

albendazole – *Albenza* (GlaxoSmithKline)

Albenza (GlaxoSmithKline) – albendazole

Alinia (Romark) – nitazoxanide

AmBisome (Gilead) – amphotericin B, liposomal

amphotericin B – *Fungizone* (Apothecon), others

amphotericin B, liposomal – *AmBisome* (Gilead)

Ancobon (Valeant) – flucytosine

§ *Antiminth* (Pfizer) – pyrantel pamoate

• *Aralen* (sanofi-aventis) – chloroquine HCl and chloroquine phosphate

§ artemether – *Artenam* (Arenco, Belgium)

artemether/lumefantrine – *Coartem, Riamet* (Novartis)

§ *Artenam* (Arenco, Belgium) – artemether

• † artesunate – (Guilin No. 1 Factory, People's Republic of China)

atovaquone – *Mepron* (GlaxoSmithKline)

atovaquone/proguanil – *Malarone* (GlaxoSmithKline)

azithromycin – *Zithromax* (Pfizer), others

• *Bactrim* (AR Scientific) – TMP/Sulfa

Benzyl alcohol lotion – *Ulesfia* (Sciele)

§ benznidazole – *Rochagan* (Brazil)

• *Biaxin* (Abbott) – clarithromycin

Biltricide (Bayer) – praziquantel

† bithionol – *Bitin* (Tanabe, Japan)

† *Bitin* (Tanabe, Japan) – bithionol

§ *Brolene* (Aventis, Canada) – propamidine isethionate

chloroquine HCl and chloroquine phosphate – *Aralen* (sanofi-aventis), others

• clarithromycin – *Biaxin* (Abbott), others

• *Cleocin* (Pfizer) – clindamycin

clindamycin – *Cleocin* (Pfizer), others

Coartem (Novartis) – artemether/lumefantrine

crotamiton – *Eurax* (Ranbaxy)

dapsone – (Jacobus)

§ *Daraprim* (GlaxoSmithKline) – pyrimethamine USP

† diethylcarbamazine citrate (DEC) – *Hetrazan*

• *Diflucan* (Pfizer) – fluconazole

§ diloxanide furoate – *Furamide*

---

§ Not available in the US; may be available through a compounding pharmacy (see footnote 4 on page 223).

† Available from the CDC Drug Service, Centers for Disease Control and Prevention, Atlanta, Georgia 30333; 404-639-3670 (evenings, weekends, or holidays: 770-488-7100).

• Also available generically.

Continued on next page.

MANUFACTURERS OF DRUGS USED TO TREAT
PARASITIC INFECTIONS (continued)

doxycycline – *Vibramycin* (Pfizer), others

§ eflornithine (Difluoromethylornithine, DFMO) – *Ornidyl* (Aventis)

§ *Egaten* (Novartis) – triclabendazole

Elimite (Allergan) – permethrin

Eurax (Ranbaxy) – crotamiton

• *Flagyl* (Pfizer) – metronidazole

§ *Flisint* (Sanofi-Aventis, France) – fumagillin

fluconazole – *Diflucan* (Pfizer), others

flucytosine – *Ancobon* (Valeant)

§ fumagillin – *Flisint* (Sanofi-Aventis, France)

• *Fungizone* (Apothecon) – amphotericin

§ *Furamide* – diloxanide furoate

§ furazolidone – *Furoxone* (Roberts)

§ *Furoxone* (Roberts) – furazolidone

† *Germanin* (Bayer, Germany) – suramin sodium

§ *Glucantime* (Aventis, France) – meglumine antimonate

† *Hetrazan* – diethylcarbamazine citrate (DEC)

§ *Impavido* (Paladin, Montreal, Canada) – miltefosine

iodoquinol – *Yodoxin* (Glenwood), others

itraconazole – *Sporanox* (Ortho-McNeil-Janssen), others

ivermectin – *Stromectol* (Merck)

ketoconazole – *Nizoral* (Janssen), others

† *Lampit* (Bayer, Germany) – nifurtimox

§ *Leshcutan* (Teva, Israel) – topical paromomycin

lumefantrine/artemether – *Coartem*, *Riamet* (Novartis)

Malarone (GlaxoSmithKline) – atovaquone/proguanil

malathion – *Ovide* (Taro)

mebendazole

mefloquine

§ meglumine antimonate – *Glucantime* (Aventis, France)

† melarsoprol – *Mel-B*

† *Mel-B* – melarsoprol

Mepron (GlaxoSmithKline) – atovaquone

metronidazole – *Flagyl* (Pfizer), others

§ miconazole – *Monistat i.v.*

§ miltefosine – *Impavido* (Paladin, Montreal, Canada)

§ *Monistat i.v.* – miconazole

NebuPent (Fujisawa) – pentamidine isethionate

Neutrexin (US Bioscience) – trimetrexate

---

§ Not available in the US; may be available through a compounding pharmacy (see footnote 4 on page 223).
† Available from the CDC Drug Service, Centers for Disease Control and Prevention, Atlanta, Georgia 30333; 404-639-3670 (evenings, weekends, or holidays: 770-488-7100).
• Also available generically.

Continued on next page.

MANUFACTURERS OF DRUGS USED TO TREAT
PARASITIC INFECTIONS (continued)

§ niclosamide – *Yomesan* (Bayer, Germany)

† nifurtimox – *Lampit* (Bayer, Germany)

nitazoxanide – *Alinia* (Romark)

• *Nizoral* (Janssen) – ketoconazole

Nix (GlaxoSmithKline) – permethrin

§ ornidazole – *Tiberal* (Roche, France)

Ornidyl (Aventis) – eflornithine (Difluoromethylornithine, DFMO)

Ovide (Taro) – malathion

§ oxamniquine – *Vansil* (Pfizer)

§ *Paludrine* (AstraZeneca, United Kingdom) – proguanil

§ paromomycin – Oral generics; *Leshcutan* (Teva, Israel; (topical formulation not available in US)

Pentam 300 (Fujisawa) – pentamidine isethionate

pentamidine isethionate – *Pentam 300* (Fujisawa), *NebuPent* (Fujisawa)

† *Pentostam* (GlaxoSmithKline, United Kingdom) – sodium stibogluconate

permethrin – *Nix* (GlaxoSmithKline), *Elimite* (Allergan)

praziquantel – *Biltricide* (Bayer)

primaquine phosphate USP

§ proguanil – *Paludrine* (AstraZeneca, United Kingdom)

proguanil/atovaquone – *Malarone* (GlaxoSmithKline)

§ propamidine isethionate – *Brolene* (Aventis, Canada)

§ pyrantel pamoate – *Antiminth* (Pfizer)

pyrethrins and piperonyl butoxide – *A-200* (Hogil), others

§ pyrimethamine USP – *Daraprim* (GlaxoSmithKline)

Qualaquin – quinine sulfate (AR Scientific)

quinidine gluconate

§ quinine dihydrochloride

quinine sulfate – *Qualaquin* (AR Scientific)

Riamet (Novartis) – artemether/lumefantrine

• *Rifadin* (sanofi-aventis) – rifampin

rifampin – *Rifadin* (sanofi-aventis), others

§ *Rochagan* (Brazil) – benznidazole

* *Rovamycine* (Aventis) – spiramycin

† sodium stibogluconate – *Pentostam* (GlaxoSmithKline, United Kingdom)

* spiramycin – *Rovamycine* (Aventis)

---

§ Not available in the US; may be available through a compounding pharmacy (see footnote 4 on page 223).
† Available from the CDC Drug Service, Centers for Disease Control and Prevention, Atlanta, Georgia 30333; 404-639-3670 (evenings, weekends, or holidays: 770-488-7100).
• Also available generically.

Continued on next page.

MANUFACTURERS OF DRUGS USED TO TREAT
PARASITIC INFECTIONS (continued)

- *Sporanox* (Ortho-McNeil-Janssen) – itraconazole
  Stromectol (Merck) – ivermectin sulfadiazine
† suramin sodium – *Germanin* (Bayer, Germany)
§ *Tiberal* (Roche, France) – ornidazole
  Tindamax (Mission) – tinidazole
  tinidazole – *Tindamax* (Mission)
  TMP/Sulfa – *Bactrim* (AR Scientific), others

§ triclabendazole – *Egaten* (Novartis)
  trimetrexate – *Neutrexin* (US Bioscience)
  Ulesfia – benzyl alcohol
§ *Vansil* (Pfizer) – oxamniquine
- *Vibramycin* (Pfizer) – doxycycline
- *Yodoxin* (Glenwood) – iodoquinol
§ *Yomesan* (Bayer, Germany) – niclosamide
- *Zithromax* (Pfizer) – azithromycin

---

§ Not available in the US; may be available through a compounding pharmacy (see footnote 4 on page 223).
† Available from the CDC Drug Service, Centers for Disease Control and Prevention, Atlanta, Georgia 30333; 404-639-3670 (evenings, weekends, or holidays: 770-488-7100).
- Also available generically.

DRUGS FOR
Sexually Transmitted Infections

Original publication date – July 2010

Many infections can be transmitted during sexual contact. The text and tables that follow are limited to management of sexually transmitted infections (STIs) other than HIV, viral hepatitis and enteric infections. The drugs of choice, their dosages and alternatives are listed in a table that begins on page 282. A table listing the adverse effects of some of these antimicrobials begins on page 294.

PARTNER TREATMENT — Management of STIs should include evaluation and, for bacterial STIs and trichomoniasis, treatment of the sex partners of infected persons. Ideally, partners should themselves be examined and tested for STIs, but that may be difficult to accomplish. For gonorrhea or chlamydia, an alternate approach is to treat sex partners without direct examination or counseling, either by prescription or by giving the medication for the partner to the index patient, a practice called expedited partner treatment (EPT).[1,2]

CHLAMYDIA — A single 1-g dose of azithromycin (*Zithromax,* and others) or 7 days' treatment with doxycycline (*Vibramycin*, and others) is effective for treatment of uncomplicated urethral or cervical infection caused by *Chlamydia trachomatis*. Levofloxacin *(Levaquin)* for 7 days is an effective alternative. Erythromycin (*Ery-Tab*, and others) is also effective, but frequently causes gastrointestinal (GI) adverse effects.

In Pregnancy – Azithromycin is the treatment of choice for chlamydial infection during pregnancy.[3-5] Erythromycin is another alternative, but is often poorly tolerated, and erythromycin estolate is contraindicated in pregnancy because of an increased risk of cholestatic jaundice. Doxycycline, other tetracyclines and the fluoroquinolones should not be used during pregnancy.

In Infancy – Children born to untreated women with cervical *C. trachomatis* infection are at risk for neonatal conjunctivitis and pneumonia. Ophthalmic antibiotics used for gonococcal prophylaxis do not prevent ocular chlamydial infection in the newborn. For treatment of newborns with conjunctivitis or pneumonia caused by *C. trachomatis,* some clinicians have used systemic erythromycin for 14 days, but an association has been reported between hypertrophic pyloric stenosis and use of systemic erythromycin. In one study in 8 infants, a short course of oral azithromycin was effective for treatment of chlamydial conjunctivitis.[6]

Lymphogranuloma Venereum – Infections with the strains of *C. trachomatis* that cause lymphogranuloma venereum, manifested primarily by acute proctitis, have been reported in several urban areas worldwide among men who have sex with men (MSM).[7] A 3-week course of doxycycline is recommended.

NONGONOCOCCAL NONCHLAMYDIAL URETHRITIS AND CERVICITIS — *Mycoplasma genitalium* causes 10-25% of nongonococcal urethritis (NGU). Other causes include *Ureaplasma urealyticum, Trichomonas vaginalis*, herpes simplex virus or adenovirus, but the etiology of NGU is often unknown.[8] Most cases respond to treatment with azithromycin or doxycycline; azithromycin is more effective for *M. genitalium*. Persistent or recurrent NGU should be treated with azithromycin if doxycycline was used initially, and vice versa.

Mucopurulent cervicitis has been characterized as the female counterpart of NGU in men. Like NGU, cervicitis generally responds to azithromycin or doxycycline. Empiric treatment for *Neisseria gonorrhoeae* should also be given to women in population groups with high rates of gonorrhea.

GONORRHEA — Resistance of gonococci to fluoroquinolones has increased markedly in recent years, and these drugs are no longer recommended to treat gonorrhea. A single intramuscular (IM) injection of ceftriaxone (*Rocephin*, and others) is the treatment of choice for urethral, anogenital and pharyngeal gonorrhea, including infection with penicillin-, fluoroquinolone-, and tetracycline-resistant strains of *N. gonorrhoeae*. The recommended dose of ceftriaxone has been increased from 125 mg to 250 mg. Cefixime *(Suprax)* is an oral alternative that is effective for anogenital gonorrhea and is 75-95% effective against pharyngeal infection. Cefpodoxime (*Vantin*, and others) is another option for oral therapy, but is less effective than cefixime for pharyngeal infection.

Patients with gonorrhea should also be treated for presumptive chlamydial infection, usually with a single 1-g dose of azithromycin or 7 days of doxycycline. Although azithromycin 2 g orally is generally effective against both gonorrhea and *C. trachomatis*, it is expensive and may be poorly tolerated; it is recommended for such use only in pregnant women who are allergic to beta-lactam antibiotics. Emergence of gonococcal resistance to macrolides has, however, been reported.[9]

Gonococcal ophthalmia, bacteremia, arthritis or meningitis in adults, and all gonococcal infections in children are best treated with appropriate doses of a parenteral third-generation cephalosporin such as ceftriaxone.

In Pregnancy – There are no well-studied options for treatment of gonorrhea in pregnant women who are truly allergic to beta-lactam antibiotics. Spectinomycin is no longer available in the US. Azithromycin 2 g appears to be the best option,[4] but the 2-g dose has not been studied in pregnancy and GI intolerance may be a problem. Some experts believe

DRUGS OF CHOICE FOR SOME SEXUALLY TRANSMITTED INFECTIONS

Type or Stage		Drugs of Choice
CHLAMYDIAL INFECTION AND RELATED CLINICAL SYNDROMES[1]		
Urethritis, cervicitis, conjunctivitis, or proctitis (except lymphogranuloma venereum)		
		Azithromycin[2]
	OR	Doxycycline[2,4,6,7]
Infection in Pregnancy		
		Azithromycin
Neonatal Ophthalmia or Pneumonia		
		Erythromycin[9]
Lymphogranuloma venereum		
		Doxycycline[4,6]
GONORRHEA[10]		
Urethral, cervical or rectal		Ceftriaxone
	OR	Cefixime
Pharyngeal		Ceftriaxone
EPIDIDYMITIS		
		Ceftriaxone
		plus
		doxycycline[6]

1. Related clinical syndromes include nonchlamydial nongonococcal urethritis (NGU) and cervicitis.
2. For cases of persistent or recurrent nonchlamydial NGU, azithromycin should be used if initial treatment was with doxycycline. Some experts add tinidazole or metronidazole as recommended against trichomoniasis.
3. Should be used only if fluoroquinolone-resistant *Neisseria gonorrhoeae* has been excluded.
4. Not recommended in pregnancy.
5. Not FDA-approved for chlamydial infections.
6. Or oral tetracycline 500 mg qid (contraindicated in pregnancy).
7. Less effective than azithromycin against NGU associated with *Mycoplasma genitalium*.

Dosage	Some Alternatives
1 g PO once	Levofloxacin[3,4,5] 500 mg PO once/d x 7d
100 mg PO bid x 7d	Erythromycin[8] 500 mg PO qid x 7d
1 g PO once	Erythromycin[8] 500 mg PO qid x 7d
12.5 mg/kg PO qid x 14d	Azithromycin 20 mg/kg PO once/d x 3d
100 mg PO bid x 21d	Erythromycin[8] 500 mg PO qid x 21d
250 mg IM once[11]	Cefpodoxime 400 mg PO once[12]
400 mg PO once	Azithromycin 2 g PO once[13]
250 mg IM once[11]	
250 mg IM once	Ofloxacin[3] 300 mg PO bid x 10d
	Levofloxacin[3,14] 500 mg PO once/d x 10d
100 mg PO bid x 10d	

8. Erythromycin ethylsuccinate 800 mg may be substituted for erythromycin base 500 mg; erythromycin estolate is contraindicated in pregnancy.
9. Pyloric stenosis has been associated with use of erythromycin in newborns.
10. All patients should also receive a course of treatment effective for chlamydia.
11. 125 mg is effective, but the smallest marketed dose is 250 mg and some experts use the larger dose.
12. Efficacy uncertain for pharyngeal infection.
13. Use of azithromycin is recommended only for pregnant women allergic to beta-lactam drugs.
14. Not FDA-approved for acute epididymitis.

Continued on next page.

DRUGS OF CHOICE FOR SOME SEXUALLY TRANSMITTED INFECTIONS (continued)

Type or Stage		Drugs of Choice
PELVIC INFLAMMATORY DISEASE		
Parenteral		Cefotetan
	OR	Cefoxitin[16]
		followed by
		doxycycline[4]
	OR	Clindamycin
		plus
		gentamicin
		followed by
		doxycycline[4]
Oral		Ceftriaxone
		followed by
		doxycycline[4,19]
		+/- metronidazole
BACTERIAL VAGINOSIS		
		Metronidazole
	OR	Tinidazole
	OR	Metronidazole 0.75% gel
	OR	Clindamycin 2% cream

15. Parenteral therapy is continued until clinical improvement occurs, and then oral doxycycline is substituted to complete 14 days' total therapy.
16. Cefoxitin has been in short supply.
17. Or clindamycin 450 mg oral qid to complete 14 days.

Dosage	Some Alternatives
2 g IV q12h[15]	Ampicillin/sulbactam 3 g IV q6h
2 g IV q6h[15]	**plus** doxycycline[4] 100 mg PO or IV q12h
	followed by doxycycline[4] 100 mg PO
100 mg PO bid to complete 14d total[17]	bid to complete 14d[17]
900 mg IV q8h[15]	
2 mg/kg IV once, then 1.5 mg/kg IV q8h[15,18]	
100 mg PO bid to complete 14d total[17]	
250 mg IM once	Cefoxitin 2g IM once
	plus probenecid 1g PO once
100 mg PO bid x 14d	**followed by** doxycycline[4,19]
500 mg PO bid x 14d	100 mg PO bid x 14d
	+/- metronidazole 500 mg PO bid x 14d

500 mg PO bid x 7d	Metronidazole ER 750 mg PO once/d x 7d
2 g PO once/d x 2-3d	Tinidazole 1 g PO once/d x 5d
5 g intravaginally once or twice daily x 5d	Clindamycin 300 mg PO bid x 7d
	Clindamycin ovules 100 mg intravaginally at
5 g intravaginally at bedtime x 3-7d	bedtime x 3d

18. A single daily dose of 3 mg/kg is likely to be effective, but has not been studied in pelvic inflammatory disease.
19. Some experts would add metronidazole 500 mg bid.

Continued on next page.

DRUGS OF CHOICE FOR SOME SEXUALLY TRANSMITTED INFECTIONS (continued)

Type or Stage		Drugs of Choice
TRICHOMONIASIS		
		Metronidazole[20]
	OR	Tinidazole
SYPHILIS		
Early (Primary, secondary, or latent less than one year)		
		Penicillin G benzathine
Late (more than one year's duration, cardiovascular, gumma, late-latent)		
		Penicillin G benzathine
Neurosyphilis, incuding ocular syphilis		Penicillin G[22]
Congenital		Penicillin G
	OR	Penicillin G procaine
CHANCROID[24]		
		Azithromycin
	OR	Ceftriaxone
GENITAL WARTS[25]		
Provider-applied		Trichloroacetic acid
	OR	Bichloroacetic acid 80-90%
	OR	Podophyllin resin 10-25%[4]
	OR	Cryotherapy with liquid nitrogen or cryoprobe
Patient-applied		Imiquimod 5%[4]
	OR	Podofilox 0.5%[4]
	OR	Sinecatechins 15% ointment

20. Limited data support efficacy against trichomoniasis in men.
21. Some experts recommend a repeat dose after 7 days, especially in patients with HIV infection or pregnant women.
22. Patients allergic to penicillin should be desensitized and treated with penicillin.
23. Dose for neonates <7 days old is 50,000 units/kg q12h; dose is q8h for those >7 days old.

Dosage	Some Alternatives
2 g PO once	Metronidazole 250 mg PO tid x 7d
2 g PO once	
2.4 MU IM once[21]	Doxycycline[4] 100 mg PO bid x 14 d
2.4 MU IM wkly x 3wks	Doxycycline[4] 100 mg PO bid x 4wks
3 to 4 MU IV q4h	Penicillin G procaine 2.4 MU IM 1x/d
or 24 MU	**plus** probenecid 500 mg PO qid,
continuous IV infusion	both x 10-14d
x 10-14d	Ceftriaxone 2 g IV 1x/d x 10-14d
50,000 units/kg IV	
q8-12h[23] for 10-14d	
50,000 units/kg IM 1x/d	
for 10-14d	
1 g PO once	Ciprofloxacin[4] 500 mg PO bid x 3d
250 mg IM once	Erythromycin[7] 500 mg PO tid x 7d
1-2x/wk until resolved	Surgical removal
	Laser surgery
3x/wk x 16wks	
bid x 3d, 4 days rest, then	
repeated up to 4x	
tid up to 16 weeks	

24. All regimens, especially single-dose ceftriaxone, are less effective in HIV-infected patients.
25. Recommendations for external genital warts. Liquid nitrogen can also be used for vaginal, urethral, and oral warts. Podofilox or imiquimod can be used for urethral meatus warts. Trichloroacetic or bichloroacetic acid can be used for anal warts.

Continued on next page.

DRUGS OF CHOICE FOR SOME SEXUALLY TRANSMITTED INFECTIONS (continued)

Type or Stage		Drugs of Choice
GENITAL HERPES		
First Episode		Acyclovir
	OR	Famciclovir[26]
	OR	Valacyclovir
Severe (hospitalized patients)		Acyclovir
Suppression[27]		Acyclovir
	OR	Famciclovir
	OR	Valacyclovir
Episodic Treatment[29]		Acyclovir
	OR	Famciclovir
	OR	Valacyclovir

26. Not FDA-approved for treatment of initial episodes of genital herpes.
27. Some Medical Letter consultants discontinue preventive treatment for 1 to 2 months once a year to reassess the frequency of recurrence.
28. Use 500 mg once daily in patients with <10 recurrences per year and 500 mg bid or 1 g daily in patients with ≥10 recurrences per year. For HIV-infected patients, 500 mg bid.

that many patients with a history of rash after receiving a penicillin can tolerate a third-generation cephalosporin.

Neonatal Ocular Prophylaxis – Ocular prophylaxis can prevent gonococcal ophthalmia and is required by law in most states in the US. Erythromycin 0.5% ophthalmic ointment is the only FDA-approved formulation available for this indication in the US. Its use is recommended for all infants, whether delivered vaginally or by caesarean section. If it is not available and the infant is at risk for gonorrhea, ceftriaxone 25-50 mg/kg (max 125 mg) can be given IV or IM.

Dosage	Some Alternatives
400 mg PO tid x 7-10d	Acyclovir 200 mg PO 5x/d x 7-10d
250 mg PO tid x 7-10d	
1g PO bid x 7-10d	
5-10 mg/kg IV q8h x 5-7d	
400 mg PO bid	Acyclovir 200 mg PO 4-5x/d
250 mg PO bid	
500 mg-1g PO once/d[28]	
800 mg PO tid x 2-5d	
or 400 mg PO tid x 3-5d[30]	
1 g PO bid x 1d[31]	
or 125mg bid x 5d	
or 500 mg x1 then 250 mg	
bid x 2d	
500 mg PO bid x 3d	
or 1 g PO 1x/d x 5d	

29. Antiviral therapy is variably effective for episodic treatment of recurrences; only effective if started early.
30. No published data are available to support 3 days' use.
31. For recurrent HSV in HIV-positive patients, 500 mg bid for 7d.

FOLLOW-UP — Early retesting to document cure of gonorrhea or chlamydia (3-4 weeks after treatment) is not recommended except in pregnant women, or when adherence is in doubt. Rescreening to detect reinfection has been recommended 3 months after treatment for all men and women with gonorrhea or chlamydial infection.[10]

EPIDIDYMITIS — Acute epididymitis in men <35 years old is usually caused by *C. trachomatis* or, less frequently, *N. gonorrhoeae*. Older men or those who have had urinary tract instrumentation may have epididymitis due to enteric gram-negative bacilli or *Pseudomonas*. Gram-negative bacilli may also cause urethritis or epididymitis in men who practice insertive anal intercourse. When sexually acquired epididymitis is suspected, epididymitis should be treated with ceftriaxone plus doxycycline, which together are effective against gonorrhea and chlamydial infection. Ofloxacin (*Floxin*, and others) or levofloxacin (*Levaquin*) should be used if gonorrhea and chlamydia are unlikely.

PELVIC INFLAMMATORY DISEASE — *C. trachomatis* or *N. gonorrhoeae* is frequently the cause of acute, nonrecurrent pelvic inflammatory disease (PID), but *M. genitalium, M. hominis* and various facultative and anaerobic bacteria may also be involved. Treatment regimens should include antimicrobial agents active against all of these pathogens. Parenteral regimens include cefotetan (*Cefotan*, and others) or cefoxitin (*Mefoxin,* and others) plus doxycycline, or clindamycin *(Cleocin,* and others) plus an aminoglycoside. Parenteral therapy is continued until clinical improvement occurs, and then oral doxycycline is substituted to complete 14 days' total therapy. An oral alternative is doxycycline, with or without metronidazole (*Flagyl*, and others), after an initial IM dose of a cephalosporin such as ceftriaxone. Levofloxacin or ofloxacin should not be used unless infection with *N. gonorrhoeae* has been excluded.

BACTERIAL VAGINOSIS — The role of sexual transmission is unclear in bacterial vaginosis, in which normal H_2O_2-producing *Lactobacillus* sp. are replaced by overgrowth with *Gardnerella vaginalis, Mobiluncus*, various anaerobic bacteria and *M. hominis*.[11] Bacterial vaginosis has also been associated with an increased risk of PID. Oral metronidazole for 7 days or tinidazole *(Tindamax)* for 3 or 5 days[12] is usually effective. Vaginal metronidazole, or oral or vaginal clindamycin, also is usually effective. With any regimen, recurrence is common; retreatment with the same agent or an alternative is usually effective in the short term, but symptomatic second recurrence is common. Maintenance suppressive therapy with metronidazole gel reduces the recurrence rate.[13] No male counterpart has been identified and treatment of patients' male sex partners does not reduce the frequency of recurrence.

In Pregnancy – Symptomatic bacterial vaginosis in pregnancy should be treated. Bacterial vaginosis has been associated with premature labor and complications of delivery, but whether treatment of asymptomatic bacterial vaginosis in pregnant women reduces the frequency of adverse pregnancy outcomes is uncertain.

VULVOVAGINAL CANDIDIASIS — Vulvovaginal candidiasis, typically caused by *Candida albicans*, is not sexually transmitted, but is common in women being evaluated for STIs. Many remedies are available. Uncomplicated candidiasis of mild to moderate severity in immunocompetent women responds well to intravaginal butoconazole (*Gynazole*), clotrimazole (*Gyne-Lotrimin*, and others), miconazole (*Monistat*, and others), terconazole (*Terazol*, and others) or tioconazole (*Vagistat* and others).[14] A single oral dose of fluconazole (*Diflucan*, and others) 150 mg is as effective as 7 days of intravaginal clotrimazole or miconazole and is preferred by many patients; severe episodes may require additional doses of fluconazole.

Complicated vulvovaginal candidiasis (defined as recurrent or clinically severe episodes) due to azole-resistant *C. glabrata* or other nonalbicans species, or infection in immunodeficient women, those with poorly controlled diabetes, or pregnant women, often require more aggressive or more prolonged treatment. Six months of prophylaxis with oral fluconazole 150 mg once weekly has been reported to reduce the number of recurrences.[15]

ALTERNATIVE TREATMENTS FOR VAGINAL INFECTIONS — "Broad-spectrum" vaginal preparations and currently available preparations of *Lactobacillus* sp. or dairy products are not effective for treatment or prevention of any vaginal infection. Douching is not effective for prevention or treatment of vaginal infection; it may lead to upper genital tract infection, is unnecessary for hygiene and should be discouraged.

TRICHOMONIASIS — Oral metronidazole has been the treatment of choice for trichomoniasis. Intravaginal treatment with metronidazole gel is not effective. Resistance to metronidazole, especially high-grade resistance, remains rare. Tinidazole *(Tindamax)*, a nitroimidazole similar to metronidazole, is also effective and may be better tolerated; it is often effective against metronidazole-resistant vaginal infections.

In Pregnancy – Trichomoniasis in pregnancy has been associated with adverse pregnancy outcomes.[16] Metronidazole is believed to be safe during all stages of pregnancy and should be used to treat symptomatic trichomoniasis in pregnancy.

SYPHILIS — Parenteral penicillin G remains the drug of choice for treating all stages of syphilis. Primary, secondary or latent syphilis known to be of less than one year's duration (early syphilis) should be treated with a single IM injection of penicillin G benzathine, a repository formulation. Doxycycline is also usually effective if compliance is assured. For late syphilis (more than one year's duration) other than neurosyphilis, treatment with 3 weekly doses of IM penicillin G benzathine is recommended.

Azithromycin 2 g in a single dose was as effective as benzathine penicillin against early syphilis in a randomized controlled trial in Tanzania.[17] However, in several locations in North America and Europe, strains of *Treponema pallidum* resistant to azithromycin are common. Routine use of azithromycin is not recommended for treatment of syphilis in the US.[18]

Neurosyphilis – Symptomatic neurosyphilis, including ophthalmic infection, requires treatment with high doses of IV aqueous penicillin G or IM procaine penicillin G with probenecid.

Syphilis and HIV – The majority of HIV-infected patients with syphilis respond to standard benzathine penicillin regimens appropriate to syphilis stage. Cerebrospinal fluid abnormalities are common in patients with syphilis and HIV, but the clinical significance of these findings in asymptomatic patients is unclear.[19]

IV ceftriaxone for 10 days may be as effective as IV penicillin G for treatment of neurosyphilis in HIV-infected patients.[20]

Syphilis in Pregnancy – Syphilis in pregnant women should be treated with penicillin in doses appropriate to the stage of the disease. When pregnant women with syphilis are allergic to penicillin, most experts recommend hospitalization, desensitization and treatment with penicillin. However, some experts believe that many patients with a history of rash after receiving a penicillin can tolerate a third-generation cephalosporin. Retreatment in subsequent pregnancies is unnecessary in the absence of clinical or serological evidence of new or persistent infection.

Congenital Syphilis – A positive serological test for syphilis in a newborn without stigmata of syphilis may be due either to passive transfer of maternal antibodies or to prenatal infection. If there is no definite evidence of adequate treatment of the mother with penicillin during the pregnancy, Medical Letter consultants recommend prompt treatment of such infants rather than waiting 3-6 months to see if the antibody titer falls.

CHANCROID — Chancroid, caused by *Haemophilus ducreyi,* is uncommon in the US. A single dose of azithromycin or ceftriaxone is usually effective, but more prolonged therapy may be required in HIV-infected patients.

PEDICULOSIS AND SCABIES — *Phthirus pubis* (pubic lice), which can be found on eyelashes and on back, axillary and leg hairs as well as pubic areas, and *Sarcoptes scabiei* (scabies) can both be transmitted by intimate exposure and are common in persons at risk for STIs. The drug

ADVERSE EFFECTS OF SOME DRUGS FOR SEXUALLY TRANSMITTED INFECTIONS

Drug	Adverse Effects
Acyclovir (*Zovirax*, and others)	**Frequent**: local irritation at infusion site **Occasional**: local reactions with topical use; rash, nausea, diarrhea, headache, vertigo and arthralgias with oral use; decreased renal function sometimes progressing to renal failure; metabolic encephalopathy; bone marrow depression; abnormal hepatic function in immunocompromised patients **Rare**: lethargy or agitation; tremor, disorientation; hallucinations; transient hemiparesthesia
Ampicillin/sulbactam (*Unasyn*)	**Frequent**: pain at injection site **Occasional**: diarrhea; rash **Rare**: itching; nausea; vomiting; candidiasis; fatigue; malaise; headache; chest pain; flatulence; abdominal distension; glossitis; urine retention; dysuria; edema; facial swelling; erythema; chills; tightness in throat; substernal pain; epistaxis; mucosal bleeding
Azithromycin (*Zithromax*, and others)	**Occasional**: nausea; diarrhea; abdominal pain; headache; dizziness; vaginitis **Rare**: angioedema; cholestatic jaundice; photosensitivity; reversible dose-related hearing loss; QTc prolongation
Bichloroacetic acid	**Frequent**: local irritation at infusion site
Clindamycin (*Cleocin*, and others)	**Frequent**: diarrhea; allergic reactions **Occasional**: *Clostridium difficile* infection, sometimes severe, can occur even with topical use **Rare**: hematologic abnormalities; esophageal ulceration; hepatotoxicity

Continued on next page.

ADVERSE EFFECTS OF SOME DRUGS FOR SEXUALLY
TRANSMITTED INFECTIONS (continued)

Drug	Adverse Effects
Doxycycline (*Vibramycin*, and others)	**Frequent**: GI disturbance; bone lesions and staining and deformity of teeth in children up to 8 years old, and in the newborn when given to pregnant women after the fourth month of pregnancy **Occasional**: malabsorption; enterocolitis; photosensitivity reactions; exacerbation of renal failure; hepatitis; parenteral doses may cause serious liver damage, especially in pregnant women and patients with renal disease receiving $\geq$ 1 gram/day; esophageal ulcerations; cutaneous and mucosal hyperpigmentation **Rare**: hypersensitivity reactions, including serum sickness and anaphylaxis; *Clostridium difficile* infection; hemolytic anemia and other hematologic abnormalities; autoimmune hepatitis; increased intracranial pressure; transient acute myopia; blurred vision, diplopia, papilledema
Erythromycin (*Ery-Tab*, and others)	**Frequent**: GI disturbance **Occasional**: stomatitis; cholestatic hepatitis especially with erythromycin estolate in adults; QTc prolongation **Rare**: allergic reactions, including severe respiratory distress; pseudomembranous colitis; hemolytic anemia; hepatic pancreatitis; transient hearing loss with high doses, prolonged use, or in patients with renal insufficiency; ventricular arrhythmias and torsades de pointes; aggravation of myasthenia gravis; hypothermia; hypertrophic pyloric stenosis following treatment of infants

Continued on next page.

ADVERSE EFFECTS OF SOME DRUGS FOR SEXUALLY TRANSMITTED INFECTIONS (continued)

Drug	Adverse Effects
Famciclovir (*Famvir*)	**Occasional**: headache; nausea; diarrhea
Gentamicin (*Garamycin*)	**Occasional**: vestibular damage; renal damage; rash **Rare**: auditory damage; neuromuscular blockade and apnea, reversible with calcium or neostigmine; neurotoxicity; polyneuropathy; anaphylaxis
Imiquimod (*Aldara*, and others)	**Frequent**: hyperbilirubinemia; dysuria; kidney stones; flank pain; hematuria; crystalluria
Metronidazole (*Flagyl*, and others)	**Frequent**: nausea; headache; anorexia; metallic taste **Occasional**: vomiting; diarrhea; dry mouth; stomatitis; insomnia; weakness; vertigo; tinnitus; paresthesias; rash; dark urine; urethral burning; disulfiram-like reaction with alcohol; candidiasis **Rare**: leukopenia; pancreatitis; seizures; peripheral neuropathy; encephalopathy; cerebellar syndrome with ataxia, dysarthria and MRI abnormalities
Podofilox (*Condylox*)	**Frequent**: local reactions with topical use **Occasional**: pain with intercourse; insomnia; tingling; bleeding; tenderness; chafing; malodor; dizziness; scarring; vesicle formation; crusting edema; dryness/peeling; foreskin irretraction; hematuria; vomiting and ulceration
Podophyllin resin (*Podofin 5%*, and others)	**Frequent**: burning, redness, pain, pruritus and swelling at application site

Continued on next page.

Drug	Adverse Effects
Probenecid (*Benemid*, and others)	**Frequent**: loss of appetite; headache; nausea; vomiting **Occasional**: dizziness **Rare**: nephrotic syndrome; pruritus; rash; drug-induced fever; allergic reaction; hemolytic anemia; leukopenia
Sinecatechins 15% ointment (*Veregen*)	**Frequent**: erythema, pruritus, burning, pain/discomfort, erosion/ulceration, edema and rash vesicular at application site **Occasional**: urethritis; perianal infection; pigmentation changes; dryness; eczema; hyperesthesia; necrosis; papules; discoloration; cervical dysplasia
Tinidazole (*Tindamax*)	**Occasional**: metallic taste; GI symptoms; rash **Rare**: weakness
Trichloroacetic acid	**Frequent**: local irritation at infusion site
Valacyclovir (*Valtrex*)	**Rare**: thrombotic thrombocytopenic purpura/hemolytic uremic syndrome in severely immunocompromised patients treated with high doses

of choice is topical 1% permethrin (*Nix*, and others) for pubic lice, and 5% permethrin (*Elimite*, and others) for scabies; both of these can be used in pregnancy. Oral ivermectin *(Stromectol),* 200 or 400 mcg/kg, is also effective as a single dose for treatment of lice or scabies, and can be repeated 8 days later for resistant infections with scabies. Crusted scabies, a serious complication usually seen in patients with AIDS or other immunodeficiencies, should be treated with both permethrin and ivermectin. Ivermectin is contraindicated for use in pregnant women.

GENITAL WARTS AND HUMAN PAPILLOMAVIRUS INFEC-TION — External genital warts are caused by human papillomavirus (HPV), usually type 6 or 11; other types (16, 18 and others) cause dysplasia and neoplasia of the cervix, anus and genital skin. No form of HPV-specific treatment has been shown to eradicate the virus or to modify the risk of cervical dysplasia or cancer, and no single treatment is uniformly effective in removing warts or preventing recurrence. Trichloroacetic acid, podophyllin, and cryotherapy (with liquid nitrogen or a cryoprobe) remain the most widely used provider-applied treatments for external genital warts. Imiquimod 5% cream *(Aldara)*, an immune modulator, and pod-ofilox 0.5% solution or gel *(Condylox)* offer the advantage of self-applica-tion by patients at home. Sinecatechins 15% ointment *(Veregen)* is another recently developed patient-applied option.[21] For all available treatments except surgical removal, the initial response rate is 60-70% and 20-30% will have a recurrence. The HPV vaccines *(Gardasil, Cervarix)* are highly effective in preventing HPV infection. *Cervarix* is recommended for rou-tine use in all females age 10-25 years old, and *Gardasil* is recommended for both males and females 9-26 years old.[22,23] The vaccines do not influ-ence the course of established infection and have no therapeutic role.

No treatment is recommended for subclinical HPV infection in the absence of dysplasia or neoplasia. The transient nature of most HPV infections in young women suggests that these infections and the low-grade cervical dysplasia often associated with them should both be treated conservatively because they usually regress spontaneously.

In Pregnancy – Imiquimod, podofilox, podophyllin and sinecatechins are not recommended for use during pregnancy. Topical trichloroacetic acid, cryotherapy, electrodesiccation or electrocauterization are options that can be used in pregnancy. Scissor excision or laser therapy is effec-tive and well-tolerated if the clinician is properly trained.

GENITAL HERPES — Acyclovir (*Zovirax,* and others), famciclovir (*Famvir*) or valacyclovir (*Valtrex*) taken orally for 7-10 days can shorten the duration of pain, systemic symptoms and viral shedding in initial herpes simplex virus (HSV) genital infection. Episodic treatment of symptomatic recurrent lesions with the same drugs can speed healing if treatment is started early. Continuous suppressive therapy substantially reduces symptomatic recurrences and subclinical shedding. Valacyclovir may be more effective than famciclovir in suppressing symptomatic recurrences and asymptomatic shedding of HSV-2.[24] Suppressive therapy with valacyclovir 500 mg daily reduces the frequency of HSV transmission to sex partners.[25]

Antiviral-resistant strains of HSV are uncommon; they occur mainly in immunodeficient patients treated with antiviral drugs. Long-term suppressive therapy has prevented emergence of drug-resistant HSV in stem-cell transplant recipients.

In Pregnancy – Although acyclovir is not approved for treatment of pregnant women, its use during pregnancy has not been associated with an increased risk of congenital abnormalities, and treatment is recommended for first episodes of genital herpes during pregnancy. Suppressive therapy with acyclovir in the last month of pregnancy can prevent symptomatic recurrences and thereby reduces the frequency of caesarean section, but its efficacy in reducing the risk of neonatal herpes is unknown.

1. MR Golden et al. Effect of expedited treatment of sex partners on recurrent or persistent gonorrhea or chlamydial infection. N Engl J Med 2005; 352:676.
2. CDC. Recommendations for partner services programs for HIV infection, syphilis, gonorrhea, and chlamydial infection. MMWR Recomm Rep 2008; 57(RR-9):1.
3. L Rahangdale et al. An observational cohort study of *Chlamydia trachomatis* treatment in pregnancy. Sex Transm Dis 2006; 33:106.
4. HL Johnson et al. Sexually transmitted infections during pregnancy. Curr Infect Dis Rep 2007; 9:125.
5. E Pitsouni et al. Single-dose azithromycin versus erythromycin or amoxicillin for *Chlamydia trachomatis* infection during pregnancy: a meta-analysis of randomised controlled trials. Int J Antimicrob Agents 2007; 30:213.
6. MR Hammerschlag et al. Treatment of neonatal chlamydial conjunctivitis with azithromycin. Pediatr Infect Dis J 1998; 17:1049.

7. D Richardson and D Goldmeier. Lymphogranuloma venereum: an emerging cause of proctitis in men who have sex with men. Int J STD AIDS 2007; 18:11.

8. CS Bradshaw et al. Etiologies of nongonococcal urethritis: bacteria, viruses, and the association with orogenital exposure. J Infect Dis 2006; 193:336.

9. HM Palmer et al. Emergence and spread of azithromycin-resistant *Neisseria gonorrhoeae* in Scotland. J Antimicrob Chemother 2008; 62:490.

10. TA Peterman et al. High incidence of new sexually transmitted infections in the year following a sexually transmitted infection: a case for rescreening. Ann Intern Med 2006; 145:564.

11. DN Fredricks et al. Molecular identification of bacteria associated with bacterial vaginosis. N Engl J Med 2005; 353:1899.

12. Tinidazole (*Tindamax*) – a new option for treatment of bacterial vaginosis. Med Lett Drugs Ther 2007; 49:73.

13. JD Sobel et al. Suppressive antibacterial therapy with 0.75% metronidazole vaginal gel to prevent recurrent bacterial vaginosis. Am J Obstet Gynecol 2006; 194:1283.

14. Drugs for vulvovaginal candidiasis. Med Lett Drugs Ther 2001; 43:3.

15. JD Sobel et al. Maintenance fluconazole therapy for recurrent vulvovaginal candidiasis. N Engl J Med 2004; 351:876.

16. D Soper. Trichomoniasis: under control or undercontrolled? Am J Obstet Gynecol 2004; 190:281.

17. G Riedner et al. Single-dose azithromycin versus penicillin G benzathine for the treatment of early syphilis. N Engl J Med 2005; 353:1236.

18. KK Holmes. Azithromycin versus penicillin G benzathine for early syphilis. N Engl J Med 2005; 353:1291.

19. NM Zetola and JD Klausner. Syphilis and HIV infection: an update. Clin Infect Dis 2007; 44:1222.

20. CM Marra et al. A pilot study evaluating ceftriaxone and penicillin G as treatment agents for neurosyphilis in human immunodeficiency virus-infected individuals. Clin Infect Dis 2000; 30:540.

21. Veregen: a botanical for treatment of genital warts. Med Lett Drugs Ther 2008; 50:15.

22. *Cervarix* – a second HPV vaccine. Med Lett Drugs Ther 2010; 52:37.

23. LR Baden et al. Human papillomavirus vaccine—opportunity and challenge. N Engl J Med 2007; 356:1990.

24. A Wald et al. Comparative efficacy of famciclovir and valacyclovir for suppression of recurrent genital herpes and viral shedding. Sex Tranm Dis 2006; 33:529.

25. L Corey and A Wald. Maternal and neonatal herpes simplex virus infections. N Engl J Med 2009; 361:1376.

Adult Immunization

Original publication date – April 2009

Although immunization programs have produced high vaccination rates in US infants and children, similar successes have not been achieved in adults.[1] Vaccines recommended for routine use in adults[2] are reviewed here. Vaccines for travel are reviewed separately.[3]

VACCINE PREPARATIONS

Live attenuated vaccines use a weakened form of the pathogen, which replicates after administration to induce an immune response. Their efficacy can be diminished by factors that damage the organism (e.g. heat or light) or interfere with replication (e.g. circulating antibodies). Compared to inactivated vaccines, live attenuated vaccines tend to have higher rates of adverse effects, particularly fever, but generally produce longer lasting immunity.

Inactivated vaccines are prepared from whole bacteria or virus, or a fractional antigenic component of one. Fractional vaccines are usually either protein- or polysaccharide-based. Protein-based vaccines typically include subunits of microbiologic protein or inactivated bacterial toxins (toxoids). Polysaccharide-based vaccines are generally less immunogenic than protein-based vaccines; they may be conjugated to a protein to increase the immune response.

VACCINE PREPARATIONS

Live Attenuated	Measles, Mumps, Rubella, Varicella, Zoster, Intranasal Influenza
Inactivated Whole organism	Hepatitis A
Fractional Pure polysaccharide	Pneumococcal *(Pneumovax)*, Meningococcal *(Menomune)*
Conjugate polysaccharide	Pneumococcal *(Prevnar)**, Meningococcal *(Menactra)*, *Haemophilus Influenzae* type b*
Protein	Acellular Pertussis, Tetanus, Diphtheria, Hepatitis B, Influenza, Human Papillomavirus

*Only FDA-approved for use in children.

VACCINES

Eight vaccines are currently recommended by the US Advisory Committee on Immunization Practices (ACIP) for routine use in adults: tetanus-diphtheria alone (Td) or combined with acellular pertussis (Tdap), pneumococcal, influenza, varicella, zoster, measles/mumps/rubella (MMR), and human papillomavirus (HPV). For some patients, hepatitis A and B and meningococcal vaccines are also recommended.

TETANUS, DIPHTHERIA AND PERTUSSIS — Tetanus toxoid and diphtheria toxoid were introduced into routine US childhood immunization programs in the late 1940s. Since then, rates of tetanus and diphtheria infection have substantially declined; sporadic cases occur in unvaccinated or incompletely vaccinated patients.[4]

Routine immunization has reduced the incidence of pertussis ("whooping cough") in children, but a substantial number of cases occur each year in adults in whom vaccine-induced immunity has waned over time.[5] In addition, susceptible adults may transmit the disease to unimmunized or partially immunized infants and children.

Inactivated adsorbed (aluminum-salt-precipitated) tetanus and diphtheria toxoid (Td) has been the standard booster vaccine for adults. Two vaccines containing protein components of acellular pertussis combined with diphtheria and tetanus toxoids (Tdap) are available for use as a one-time booster for adults ≤64 years of age.[6] Pediatric diphtheria, tetanus and acellular pertussis vaccine (DTaP) contains larger amounts of diphtheria and pertussis antigens than Tdap and is not licensed for use in adults.

Recommendations for Use – The ACIP recommends that adults with an uncertain history of primary vaccination receive 3 doses of a tetanus and diphtheria toxoid vaccine, one of which (preferably the first) should be Tdap. The first 2 doses should be administered at least 4 weeks apart and the third 6-12 months after the second. A booster dose of Td is recommended every 10 years. Adults who have completed a primary childhood series should be given a single dose of Tdap to replace a routine Td booster. For adults who have already received a Td booster, a single dose of Tdap should be given 10 years after the last Td. Healthcare workers and adults who will be exposed to infants can be immunized with a single dose of Tdap as soon as 2 years after their last Td to protect against pertussis. Adults ≤64 years old who require tetanus toxoid-containing vaccine as part of wound management should be given Tdap instead of Td if they have not previously received Tdap.[7]

Pregnant women who have not received Tdap should receive Tdap in the postpartum period if at least 2 years have elapsed since their last Td booster.[8] When protection against tetanus and diphtheria is indicated during pregnancy, Td is generally recommended. Tdap, although not well studied, has been used safely in pregnancy and could be given during the second or third trimester to protect against pertussis.[9]

Adverse Effects – Local reactions such as erythema and induration around the injection site are common with the Td vaccine, but are usually self-limited. Arthus-type reactions with extensive painful swelling can occur in adults with a history of repeated vaccination. Fever and injection site pain have been more frequent with Tdap. Most of the patients who received Tdap in clinical trials were previously immunized with whole-cell pertussis antigen; the incidence of reactions might be higher in coming years among patients who have already received multiple doses of a childhood vaccine containing acellular pertussis.

HUMAN PAPILLOMAVIRUS (HPV) — HPV is a sexually transmitted infection acquired by young women soon after initiation of sexual activity. In one study, the cumulative probability of infection was about 40% within 24 months of first sexual intercourse.[10] Although most HPV infections are cleared without clinical sequelae, persistent infection with an oncogenic HPV type can cause abnormalities in the cervical epithelium that may progress to cancer.

More than 30 types of HPV can infect the genital tract. Types 16 and 18 are responsible for more than 70% of cervical cancers and high-grade cervical intraepithelial neoplasia (CIN), a precursor of cervical cancer. Types 6 and 11 cause about 90% of genital warts.[11]

A recombinant quadrivalent human-papillomavirus-like particle vaccine (*Gardasil*) has been approved by the FDA to prevent diseases associated with infection with human papillomavirus (HPV) types 6, 11, 16 and 18, including genital warts, precancerous cervical, vaginal or vulvar lesions, and cervical cancer.[12] Two studies have shown that the quadrivalent vaccine may provide cross-protection against other HPV types as well.[13,14]

Recommendations for Use – HPV vaccination is recommended for women ≤26 years old and is administered in 3 separate 0.5-mL intramuscular injections into the deltoid or anterolateral thigh at 0, 2 and 6 months. Although HPV vaccine should ideally be administered before the onset of sexual activity,[15] women who have already been exposed to HPV or diagnosed with HPV (based on an abnormal Pap smear or presence of genital warts) should also be vaccinated. The duration of immunity is not known; booster doses are not currently recommended.

HPV vaccine has not been recommended for pregnant women due to limited data, but no adverse outcomes have been reported among women who became pregnant after receiving the vaccine.[16]

Adverse Effects – In clinical trials, adverse reactions at the injection site included pain, swelling, erythema and pruritus; discontinuation of the vaccine series was uncommon. Fever occurred 1-15 days post-vaccination in 10.3% of women who received the vaccine and in 8.6% who received placebo.

VARICELLA — Although universal childhood vaccination against varicella, introduced in the US in 1995, has resulted in a sharp decline in the incidence of varicella in both children and adults, susceptible adults should be vaccinated because those who develop primary varicella infection are at much higher risk than children of experiencing severe symptoms of the disease as well as complications.[17]

Each 0.5-mL dose of varicella vaccine *(Varivax)* contains at least 1350 plaque-forming units of a live attenuated Oka strain of varicella zoster virus (VZV).

Recommendations for Use – Persons born in the US before 1980 are considered immune to varicella, except for healthcare workers and pregnant women, who should be tested if they do not have other evidence of immunity. Two doses of vaccine separated by at least 4 weeks are recommended

VACCINES FOR ADULTS

Vaccines	Dose
TETANUS, DIPHTHERIA (TD)	
Tetanus and Diphtheria	0.5 mL IM
Adsorbed for Adult Use	(5 Lf T/2 Lf d)
(sanofi pasteur)	
TETANUS, DIPHTHERIA, ACELLULAR PERTUSSIS (TDAP)	
Adacel (sanofi pasteur)	0.5 mL IM[1]
Boostrix (GlaxoSmithKline)	0.5 mL IM[2]
HUMAN PAPILLOMAVIRUS (HPV)	
Gardasil (Merck)	0.5 mL IM
VARICELLA	
Varivax (Merck)	0.5 mL SC (1350 PFU)
ZOSTER	
Zostavax (Merck)	0.65 mL SC (19,400 PFU)
MEASLES, MUMPS, RUBELLA (MMR)	
MMR II (Merck)	0.5 mL SC[4]
INFLUENZA	
Inactivated	0.5 mL IM
Afluria (CSL Biotherapies)	(15 mcg of each antigen)
Fluarix (GSK)	
Fluvirin (Novartis)	
Fluzone (sanofi pasteur)	
Live attenuated	0.1 mL x2 intranasal
Flumist (MedImmune)	($10^{6.5-7.5}$ FFU)

* Approved age ranges for use of these vaccines in children and adolescents are not included here.
** **A:** vaccine recommended by the ACIP for adults in the age category who lack evidence of immunity (i.e. lack evidence of immunization or have no prior evidence of infection); **B:** vaccine recommended if another risk factor is present on the basis of medical, occupational, lifestyle, or other indications.
1. Each dose of *Adacel* contains 2.5 mcg of detoxified pertussis toxin, 5 mcg of filamentous hemagglutinin, 3 mcg of pertactin, 5 mcg of fimbriaetypes 2 and 3 in addition to 5 Lf of tetanus toxoid and 2 Lf of diphtheria toxoid.
2. Each dose of *Boostrix* contains 5 Lf of tetanus toxoid, 2.5 Lf of diptheria toxoid, 8 mcg of inactivated PT (pertussis toxin), 8 mcg of filamentous hemagglutinin, and 2.5 mcg of pertactin.

FDA-Approved Adult Age Range*	Recommendation**	Schedule
≥19 yrs	A	1 booster dose q10yrs
19-64 yrs	A	1 lifetime booster dose
19-26 yrs	A	3 doses (0, 2 and 6 mos)[3]
≥19 yrs	A	2 doses (0, 4-8 wks)
≥60 yrs	A	1 dose
≥19 yrs	A (19-51 yrs) B (≥52 yrs)	1-2 doses[5] 1-2 doses[5]
≥18 yrs	B (18-49 years) A (≥50 yrs)	1 dose/yr 1 dose/yr
18-49 yrs	B	1 dose/yr

3. Minimum interval between 1st and 2nd dose is 4 weeks, between 2nd and 3rd dose is 12 weeks, and between 1st and 3rd dose is 24 weeks.
4. Each dose contains approximately 1,000 $TCID_{50}$ (50% tissue culture infectious dose) of measles virus; 20,000 $TCID_{50}$ of mumps virus; and 1,000 $TCID_{50}$ of rubella virus.
5. Second dose must be administered at least 28 days after the first. 1-2 doses for measles and mumps and 1 dose for rubella.

Continued on next page.

VACCINES FOR ADULTS (continued)

Vaccines	Dose
PNEUMOCOCCAL	
Pneumovax 23 (Merck)	0.5 mL IM or SC
	(25 mcg of each antigen)
HEPATITIS A	
Havrix (GSK)	1 mL IM (1440 EL.U.)
Vaqta (Merck)	1 mL IM (50 U)
HEPATITIS B	
Engerix-B (GSK)	1 mL IM (20 mcg)[8]
Recombivax-HB (Merck)	1 mL IM (10 mcg)[8]
HEPATITIS A/B	
Twinrix (GSK)	1 mL IM (720 EL.U./20 mcg)
	(1 mL)
MENINGOCOCCAL[12]	
Menactra (sanofi pasteur)	0.5 mL IM
	(4 mcg of each antigen)
Menomune (sanofi pasteur)	0.5 mL SC
	(50 mcg of each antigen)

7. One-time revaccination after 5 years at or after age 65 if vaccinated before age 65, and for high-risk patients.
8. Dose for hemodialysis is 40 mcg given at 0, 1 and 6 months *(Recombivax)* or 0, 1, 2, and 6 months *(Engerix-B)*.
9. A 4-dose schedule at 0, 1, 2 and 12 months is also FDA-approved.
10. Minimum interval between doses 1 and 2 is 4 weeks, between doses 2 and 3 is 8 weeks, and between doses 1 and 3 is 16 weeks.

for non-immune adults. Evidence of immunity to varicella is demonstrated by: a history of typical varicella, laboratory evidence of immunity or confirmation of disease, documentation of vaccination, or healthcare provider-diagnosed zoster. Adult vaccination programs should target those in close contact with persons at risk for severe disease (healthcare workers or family contacts of immunosuppressed persons), and those at

FDA-Approved Adult Age Range*	Recommendation**	Schedule
19-64 yrs	B	1-2 doses[7]
≥65 yrs	A	1 dose
≥19 yrs	B	2 doses (0 and 6-12 mos)
≥19 yrs	B	2 doses (0 and 6-18 mos)
>19 yrs	B	3 doses (0, 1 and 6 mos)[9,10]
>19 yrs	B	3 doses (0, 1 and 6 mos)[10]
≥18 yrs	B	3 doses (0, 1 and 6 mos)[11]
18-55 yrs	B	1 dose[13]
≥19 yrs	B	1 dose[13]

11. Minimum interval between doses 1 and 2 is 4 weeks and between doses 2 and 3 is 5 months. A 4-dose schedule at 0, 7, 21-30 days and 12 months   may also be used.
12. Meningococcal conjugate vaccine *(Menactra)* is preferred for adults ≤55 years.
13. Revaccination every 5 years if ongoing risk has been recommended for those previously vaccinated with *Menomune*, preferably with *Menactra* in those ≤55 years old. No data for *Menactra*, but likely lasts longer than *Menomune*.

high risk of being exposed to or transmitting the virus, such as college students, teachers, childcare workers, adults living with young children, residents and staff in institutional settings, international travelers and military personnel. Newly arrived adult immigrants from tropical countries may also be susceptible to varicella.[18] Immunity is probably permanent in most vaccinees.

Non-immune pregnant women should receive the first dose of varicella vaccine postpartum before hospital discharge.

Adverse Effects – Local injection-site reactions are common in vaccinated adults. Other adverse effects include fever and injection-site or rarely generalized varicella-like rash. Spread of vaccine virus from healthy vaccinees who develop a varicella-like rash to susceptible contacts has been reported, but is rare. Recipients who have a vaccine-related rash should avoid, if possible, contact with susceptible individuals who are at high risk of complications of varicella, such as immunocompromised persons, pregnant women, and neonates of non-immune mothers.[19]

Contraindications – Because it is a live vaccine, *Varivax* is contraindicated in pregnant women and patients who are immunosuppressed as a result of disease (e.g. lymphoproliferative malignancies) or treatment (cytotoxic chemotherapy, systemic corticosteroids). However, HIV-infected patients without evidence of immunity to varicella who do not have evidence of severe underlying immunosuppression (CD4 count <200 cells/mcL, $\leq$14% of total) should be considered for this vaccination if it is indicated. It should not be given to patients with a history of anaphylaxis to neomycin.

ZOSTER — Following primary infection, varicella-zoster virus (VZV) persists in a latent form in sensory ganglia; VZV-specific cell-mediated immunity (CMI) prevents latent virus from reactivating and multiplying to cause herpes zoster (zoster; "shingles"). When CMI falls below a critical threshold, as it can in older persons and immunosuppressed patients, latent VZV can reactivate.

Currently more than 90% of adults in the US have had varicella and are at risk for zoster.[20] A live attenuated vaccine (*Zostavax*) is available to prevent zoster in persons $\geq$60 years old.[21] Each 0.65-mL dose of *Zostavax* contains about 14 times as much VZV as *Varivax*.

Recommendations for Use – A single dose of *Zostavax* is recommended for all immunocompetent persons ≥60 years old, including those who have had a previous episode of zoster. The amount of time that should elapse between the last episode of zoster and vaccination is not clear. An interval of at least 12 months has been suggested,[22] but some Medical Letter consultants would recommend even longer intervals (3-4 years).

Adverse Effects – Reactions to the vaccine at the injection site (erythema, pain, tenderness, swelling and pruritus) are generally mild. Varicella-like rash at the injection site has occurred but is less common than with varicella vaccination. Transmission of the vaccine virus from vaccine recipients to other susceptible persons has not been reported with *Zostavax*, but has occurred very rarely in contacts of *Varivax* recipients who developed a varicella-like rash after vaccination.

Contraindications – *Zostavax* is contraindicated in pregnant women and persons who are immunosuppressed as a result of disease (e.g. lymphoproliferative malignancies) or treatment (cytotoxic chemotherapy, systemic corticosteroids) and in those with a history of an anaphylactic reaction to neomycin.

MEASLES, MUMPS, RUBELLA (MMR) — Routine vaccination of children with MMR vaccine has decreased rates of measles, mumps and rubella by 99% in the US.[23] Sporadic outbreaks continue to occur and often originate with a traveler from another country.[24-26] Congenital rubella syndrome is no longer considered a public health threat, largely due to high rates of immunity in women of childbearing age.

The components of MMR are not currently available as separate monovalent formulations and their future availability is uncertain. An adult who has received one dose of a monovalent vaccine and requires another dose should receive MMR as the second dose. The trivalent MMR vaccine is recommended for routine adult immunization.

Each 0.5-mL subcutaneous dose of MMR vaccine contains live attenuated measles and mumps virus, both derived from chick embryo cell culture, and rubella virus derived from human diploid cell culture.

Recommendations for Use – In most adults, one dose of MMR is sufficient. A second dose, given at least 28 days after the first, may be required in some situations to ensure protection against measles or mumps.

Adults born before 1957 (1970 in Canada) can be considered immune to **measles**. All other adults should receive at least 1 dose of MMR vaccine unless they have a physician-documented history of measles or laboratory evidence of immunity. Two doses of vaccine, separated by at least 28 days, are recommended for adults who were previously vaccinated with the killed (or an unknown) measles vaccine used in the 1960s, and for students in postsecondary educational institutions, healthcare workers, travelers to countries where measles is endemic, and adults with a recent measles exposure.

Adults born before 1957 can also be considered immune to **mumps**. Adults born during or after 1957 should receive MMR vaccine if they do not have a history of physician-diagnosed mumps, laboratory evidence of immunity, or immunity through vaccination. According to the ACIP, 1 dose of vaccine is sufficient for adults who are not at high risk of mumps exposure. A second dose of vaccine given at least 28 days after the first dose is recommended for adults who live in communities experiencing a mumps outbreak and are in an affected age group, and for students in postsecondary educational institutions, healthcare workers, and those who are traveling to a country where mumps is endemic.

Adults born before 1957 can be considered immune to **rubella**. One dose of MMR vaccine should be administered to all adults born during or after 1957 whose rubella vaccination history is unreliable or who lack serologic evidence of immunity to rubella, particularly nonpregnant women of childbearing age. Women who are pregnant and who do not have evidence of immunity to rubella should receive MMR vaccine upon completion of pregnancy, ideally before discharge from the healthcare facility.

Vaccination should be considered for healthcare workers born before 1957 who do not have other evidence of immunity to the 3 diseases.[4]

Adverse Effects – Adverse events associated with MMR vaccination include pain and erythema at the injection site (7-29%), fever and rash (5%, most commonly associated with the measles component), and transient arthralgias (up to 25% of postpubertal women receiving rubella vaccine). Systemic anaphylactic reactions and thrombocytopenia occur very rarely. There is no convincing evidence to support a causal link between MMR vaccination and autism or Guillain-Barré Syndrome.[23, 27]

Contraindications – Because the MMR vaccine is a live attenuated virus vaccine, it is contraindicated in pregnant women and in patients with moderate to severe immunodeficiency. HIV-infected patients who do not have evidence of severe underlying immunosuppression (CD4 count < 200 cells/mcL, ≤14% of total) are an exception and should be vaccinated if it is indicated.[28] Patients with a history of anaphylaxis to neomycin should not receive the vaccine. Patients with a history of egg allergy without anaphylaxis can be vaccinated.

INFLUENZA — Influenza vaccine is about 70% effective (lower in the elderly) in preventing infection; effectiveness varies annually depending on the match between the vaccine and circulating strains.[29] A prospective cohort study in healthy working adults aged 50-64 years found that administration of influenza vaccine (well matched to circulating strains) reduced the occurrence of influenza-like illness by about 45% and morbidity associated with influenza-like illness by >60%.[30]

All influenza vaccines contain two influenza A strains and one influenza B strain selected annually based on surveillance data from the CDC. Two types of influenza vaccine are available in the US: an inactivated intramuscular vaccine and a live attenuated intranasal vaccine *(FluMist)*.

No commercial vaccine is available for pathogenic strains of avian influenza (H5N1, H7N2, H9N2, H7N3, H7N7), but an inactivated vaccine against avian H5N1 influenza is FDA-approved and is being included in the US Strategic National Stockpile.

Recommendations for Use – Based on the duration of protective antibodies and the timing of influenza circulation, the optimal time for annual vaccination in the US is in October or November, but the vaccine should be offered until the end of the influenza season in the late spring. Routine vaccination should be targeted to adults at high risk of influenza infection or complications, including those ≥50 years old, adults of any age with chronic medical conditions, and women in any trimester of pregnancy during the influenza season. One study found that vaccinating women during the third trimester reduced proven influenza illness in infants <6 months of age by 63%.[31] Healthcare workers and close contacts of high-risk persons should also be vaccinated. International travelers should consider vaccination.

The live attenuated intranasal vaccine *(Flumist)* is approved only for healthy, non-pregnant adults <50 years old. It should not be used in patients who are immunosuppressed and is not recommended for those with asthma, reactive airways disease or chronic cardiovascular, pulmonary, renal or metabolic disease.[32]

In comparative clinical trials in children, the live attenuated vaccine was more efficacious than inactivated vaccine, even against antigenically drifted strains of influenza A and B,[33-35] but the inactivated vaccine appears to be more effective than the live attenuated vaccine in previously immunized adults.[36]

Adverse Effects – Except for soreness at the injection site, adverse reactions to inactivated influenza vaccine are uncommon. Fever, myalgia and malaise can occur. In some years, vaccination has been associated rarely with Guillain-Barré syndrome.[37] The live attenuated intranasal vaccine is also generally well tolerated, but can cause rhinorrhea, nasal congestion and sore throat. After receiving the live-virus vaccine, healthcare workers, family members and other close contacts of severely immunosuppressed patients (in special care units) should avoid contact with the immunosuppressed person for 7 days because of the theoretical risk of transmission of vaccine-strain virus.

Contraindications – Both types of vaccine are grown in eggs and should not be given to persons with a history of anaphylactic reactions to egg proteins.

PNEUMOCOCCAL — A 23-valent pneumococcal polysaccharide vaccine (PPSV23; *Pneumovax* – Merck) has been available for many years for use in adults. PPSV23 contains 25 mcg of purified capsular polysaccharide antigen from each of 23 serotypes of *Streptococcus pneumoniae*. The serotypes contained in the vaccine account for 85-90% of the strains that cause invasive disease. In addition, cross-reactivity occurs with capsular antigens from other strain types that account for an additional 8% of bacteremic disease.[38]

Observational studies have suggested that vaccination against *pneumoniae* with PPSV can reduce the incidence of pneumococcal bacteremia and decrease pneumonia-related morbidity and mortality in adults,[39] but randomized controlled trials and cohort studies have not consistently shown a decrease in pneumonia, either all-cause or pneumococcal.[40,41]

A conjugate vaccine containing 7 serotypes of pneumococcus (PCV7; *Prevnar* – Wyeth) is FDA-approved only for use in infants and toddlers and has substantially decreased rates of invasive pneumococcal disease in young children.[42,43] It has also been shown to decrease pneumococcal carriage of vaccine serotypes in household contacts of vaccine recipients and rates of invasive pneumococcal disease have declined in adults since the vaccine was approved.[44,45] Compared to PPSV23, PCV7 has induced superior immune responses to vaccine serotypes in elderly adults; an investigational 13-valent conjugate vaccine is currently being studied for the prevention of pneumococcal pneumonia in adults.[46]

Recommendations for Use – A one-time dose of pneumococcal poly-saccharide vaccine has been recommended by the ACIP for all adults ≥65 years of age. Now the ACIP has broadened the recommendation to include adults <65 years of age who have asthma or who smoke.[47] The vaccine continues to be recommended for persons of any age with chronic illnesses that place them at moderate or high risk for invasive pneumococcal disease, such as those with diabetes, heart disease, pulmonary disease, liver disease, kidney disease, asplenia or immunocompromising conditions, recipients of organ or bone marrow transplants or cochlear implants, or residents of long-term care facilities.

Persons who receive an initial dose of pneumococcal vaccine before 65 years of age should be revaccinated once at or after age 65, at least 5 years after initial vaccination. A second dose may also be given after 5 years to persons with chronic renal failure or nephrotic syndrome, asplenia or other underlying immunosuppression regardless of age.

Adverse Effects – Mild to moderate soreness and erythema at the injection site are common. One retrospective study found no increase in adverse effects among persons who received ≥3 doses.[48]

HEPATITIS A — Hepatitis A virus (HAV) infection is frequently reported in the US and is endemic in certain communities in the western and southwestern states and in Alaska. In the US, the prevalence of anti-HAV antibodies increases from about 10% in preadolescent children to about 75% in elderly adults.[49] Vaccination is now part of routine pediatric immunization in the US.

Two inactivated hepatitis A whole-virus vaccines *(Vaqta, Havrix)* are available in the US. *Twinrix*, the combination hepatitis A and B vaccine, contains the same hepatitis A component as in *Havrix* at half the dose. All 3 vaccines are equally effective.

Recommendations for Use – Hepatitis A vaccine is recommended for adults with a medical, occupational or behavioral risk of hepatitis A infection. Medical indications include clotting factor disorders or chronic liver disease, such as chronic active hepatitis C and/or B virus infection. Occupational indications include work with HAV in a laboratory setting. Behavioral indications include illicit (injection and non-injection) drug users and men who have sex with men. Hepatitis A vaccine is also recommended for close contacts of adopted children from countries with high rates of hepatitis A and for susceptible travelers going anywhere other than Canada, Australia, New Zealand, Japan or western Europe.[50] Hepatitis A vaccination in adults usually consists of 2 doses separated by at least 6 months. After a single dose, *Havrix* provides protection for at least 12 months, and *Vaqta* for at least 18 months. Patients who receive *Twinrix* need 3 doses at 0, 1 and 6 months. An accelerated 4-dose schedule is also licensed for *Twinrix* with doses at 0, 7 and 21-30 days and a fourth dose at 12 months.[51] Patients who have received a first dose of one vaccine will respond to a second dose of the other.

Booster doses are not recommended for immunocompetent adults who have completed a primary vaccination series.[52,53]

Adverse Effects – Local injection site reactions such as pain, swelling or erythema occur in 20-50% of vaccine recipients. Mild systemic complaints such as malaise, low-grade fever or fatigue occur in less than 10%.

HEPATITIS B — Transmission of hepatitis B virus occurs through sexual contact, contact with infected blood or other body fluids, and through

ADULT VACCINES ACCORDING TO RISK GROUP*

Risk Groups	HPV	Td/ Tdap	Influenza
Pregnancy	NR	✓[1]	✓[2]
Immunocompromising conditions (except HIV)[6,7]	✓	✓	✓[2]
Diabetes; chronic cardiac or pulmonary[8] disease, or chronic alcoholism	✓	✓	✓[2]
Asplenia[9,10] (including terminal complement component deficiency)	✓	✓	✓[11]
Kidney failure; End-stage renal disease (including hemodialysis)	✓	✓	✓[2]
Chronic liver disease	✓	✓	✓
HIV[7]			
CD4 count <200 cells/mcL	✓	✓	✓[2]
CD4 count >200 cells/mcL	✓	✓	✓[2]
Healthcare workers	✓	✓	✓

* See table that begins on page 306 for age restrictions
✓: Recommended; RF: Recommended if another risk factor is present; C: Contraindicated; NR: No recommendation

1. Women who are pregnant and have not had a Td booster in ≥10 years could receive Td during pregnancy or Tdap postpartum if sufficient tetanus/diptheria protection is likely until delivery. If they have received Td between 2 and 10 years prior, they should receive Tdap in the postpartum period (TV Murphy et al. MMWR Recomm Rep 2008; 57(RR-4):1). Tdap, although not well studied, has been used safely in pregnancy (SA Gall. Clin Obstet Gynecol 2008; 51:486).
2. Only inactivated influenza vaccine is recommended.
3. Pregnant women who are not immune to rubella and/or varicella should receive one dose of MMR vaccine and/or varicella vaccine after delivery and before discharge from the hospital. Dose 2 of varicella should be given 4-8 weeks after dose 1.
4. Patients with leukemia, lymphoma or other malignancies in remission with no recent history (≥3 months) of chemotherapy are not considered severely immunosuppressed for the purpose of receiving live-virus vaccines.
5. Wait at least 1 month after discontinuing long-term administration of high-dose corticosteroids before giving a live-virus vaccine. The definition of high-dose or long-term corticosteroids is considered by most clinicians to be equivalent to ≥2 mg/kg/d or ≥20 mg/d of prednisone or its equivalent for ≥14 days. Short-term (<2 weeks treatment), low to moderate doses, long-term alternate day treatment with short-acting preparations, maintenance physiologic doses (replacement therapy), or steroids administered topically, by aerosol or by intra-articular, bursal or tendon injection are not considered contraindications to live-virus vaccines.

Pneumo-coccal	MMR	Vari-cella	Zoster	Hep B	Hep A	Meningo-coccal
RF	C[3]	C[3]	C	RF	RF	RF
✓	C[4,5]	C[4,5]	C[4,5]	RF	RF	RF
✓	✓	✓	✓	RF	RF	RF
✓	✓	✓	✓	RF	RF	✓
✓	✓	✓	✓	✓[12]	RF	RF
✓	✓	✓	✓	✓	✓	RF
✓	C	C	C	✓	RF	RF
✓	✓	✓	NR	✓	RF	RF
RF	✓	✓	✓	✓	RF	RF

6. See also recommendations for hematopoietic stem cell transplant recipients (MMWR Recomm Rep 2006; 55 [RR-15]:28).
7. If possible, indicated vaccines should be given before starting chemotherapy, treatment with other immunosuppressive drugs or radiation.
8. Chronic pulmonary disease: chronic pneumonitis, chronic obstructive pulmonary disease, chronic bronchitis or asthma.
9. Includes functional or anatomic asplenia, including elective splenectomy. When possible, persons undergoing elective splenectomy should receive the indicated vaccines >2 weeks prior to surgery.
10. *Haemophilus influenzae* type B (Hib) vaccine should also be considered.
11. No data exist on the risk for severe or complicated influenza in persons with asplenia. However, influenza is a risk factor for secondary bacterial infections that can be life-threatening in asplenic patients.
12. Hemodialysis patients should receive a 40 mcg/ml or two 20 mcg/mL doses of Hepatitis B vaccine.

perinatal exposure. Universal vaccination of infants has been standard in the US since 1991.

Available formulations of hepatitis B vaccine contain hepatitis B surface antigen (HBsAg) protein grown in baker's yeast using recombinant DNA technology, which is then purified and adsorbed to aluminum hydroxide. Each 1.0 mL dose of *Engerix-B* contains 20 mcg of HBsAg, while each 1.0 mL dose of *Recombivax HB* contains 10 mcg of HBsAg. The hepatitis B component in the combined hepatitis A and B vaccine *(Twinrix)* is the same antigenic component as in *Engerix-B*. All available vaccines are equally effective.

Recommendations for Use – Hepatitis B immunization is recommended for adults with a medical, occupational or behavioral risk of infection. Medical indications include hemodialysis or treatment with clotting-factor concentrates. Occupational indications include health care or public safety work with potential exposure to blood or body fluids. Behavioral indications include injection drug use, sex with more than one partner in the previous 6 months, recently acquired sexually transmitted infection, and men who have sex with men.

Other populations who should receive hepatitis B vaccination include clients of facilities that treat sexually transmitted infections (STIs), HIV or drug abuse, residents and staff members of institutions for the developmentally disabled, inmates of correctional facilities, household contacts and sex partners of those with chronic hepatitis B infection, and travelers who will be in countries with intermediate or high prevalence of hepatitis B infection for more than 6 months, or who may undergo medical or dental procedures in such countries.[54]

Primary immunization with hepatitis B vaccine usually consists of 3 doses given at 0, 1, and 6 months. An alternate schedule of 3 doses given at 0, 1 and 2 months, followed by a fourth dose at 12 months, is approved only for *Engerix-B* in the US and is intended for use in certain special populations, including those who have been recently exposed to the virus and travelers to high-risk areas. An interrupted hepatitis B vaccination series does not have to be restarted. A 3-dose series started with one vaccine may be completed with the other. Patients who receive *Twinrix* need 3 doses at 0, 1 and 6 months. An accelerated 4-dose schedule is also licensed for *Twinrix* with doses at 0, 7 and 21-30 days and a fourth dose at 12 months.[51]

Booster doses are not recommended for most adults who have completed a primary immunization series.[52]

Adverse Effects – The most common adverse effects of hepatitis B vaccination are pain at the injection site. Fever occurs in <10% of recipients.

MENINGOCOCCAL — About 2000-3000 cases of meningococcal disease occur in the US each year. The case fatality rate is 10% for meningitis and up to 40% for meningococcemia. Rates of meningococcal disease are highest in infancy, but a second peak occurs in adolescence and young adulthood, and about 3% of cases occur in college students, especially freshmen living in dormitories. Five major serogroups of *Neisseria meningitidis*—A, B, C, Y and W-135—cause most human infection.[55]

Two quadrivalent vaccines are available against *N. meningitidis* serogroups A, C, Y, and W135. *Menomune* contains meningococcal capsular polysaccharides. *Menactra* contains the same capsular polysaccharides conjugated to diphtheria toxoid.[56] Neither vaccine provides protection against serogroup B, which does not have an immunogenic polysaccharide capsule.

Each 0.5 mL dose of *Menactra* contains 4 mcg of meningococcal polysaccharide from each of the four serogroups conjugated to 48 mcg of diphtheria toxoid protein. Each dose of *Menomune* contains 50 mcg of meningococcal polysaccharide from each of the four serogroups. In adults, both vaccines are effective and induce serotype-specific antibody responses in over 90% of recipients.[55]

Recommendations for Use – Vaccination is recommended for adults with anatomic or functional asplenia or terminal complement component deficiencies, first-year college students living in dormitories, laboratory personnel routinely exposed to isolates of *N. meningitidis*, military recruits, and persons who travel to or reside in countries in which meningococcal disease is hyperendemic or epidemic, particularly those in the "meningitis belt" of sub-Saharan Africa. The government of Saudi Arabia also requires vaccination for pilgrims during the annual Hajj.

A single dose of vaccine is recommended. The conjugate vaccine is preferred for adults $\leq$55 years old, although the polysaccharide vaccine is an acceptable alternative.

For adults previously vaccinated with the polysaccharide vaccine, revaccination after 5 years (preferably with the conjugate vaccine for adults $\leq$55 years old) is recommended for those who remain at high risk. The duration of protection with conjugate vaccine is likely to be longer, but data are not yet available.

Adverse Effects – The most common adverse reactions to *Menactra* have been headache, fatigue and malaise, in addition to pain, redness and induration at the site of injection. The rates of these reactions are higher than with *Menomune*, but similar to those with tetanus toxoid. Guillian-Barré syndrome has been reported rarely in adolescents who received *Menactra*, but cause and effect have not been established.[57]

OTHER VACCINES

***Haemophilus Influenzae* Type b (Hib)** – Most adults do not require routine immunization with Hib conjugate vaccine, which is FDA-approved for use only in children. Adults with chronic medical conditions such as sickle cell disease, HIV infection, leukemia, lymphoma or other immunodeficiencies, or those with anatomic or functional asplenia or a history of bone marrow or organ transplant are at increased risk for invasive disease due to Hib. Vaccination of these patients could be considered, but its efficacy is unknown.

1. GA Poland et al. Standards for adult immunization practices. Am J Prev Med 2003; 25:144.
2. Centers for Disease Control and Prevention (CDC). Recommended Adult Immunization Schedule—United States, 2009. MMWR 2008; 57:Q1.
3. Advice for travelers. Treat Guidel Med Lett 2006; 4:25.
4. Centers for Disease Control and Prevention (CDC). Epidemiology and Prevention of Vaccine-Preventable Diseases (The Pink Book). W Atkinson et al, eds. 10th Edition. Washington, DC: Public Health Foundation, 2008. Available at www.cdc.gov/vaccines/pubs/pinkbook/default.htm. Accessed March 11, 2009.
5. SE Raguckas et al. Pertussis resurgence: diagnosis, treatment, prevention, and beyond. Pharmacotherapy 2007; 27:41.
6. Adacel and Boostrix: Tdap vaccines for adolescents and adults. Med Lett Drugs Ther 2006; 48:5.
7. K Kretsinger et al. Preventing tetanus, diphtheria, and pertussis among adults: use of tetanus toxoid, reduced diphtheria toxoid and acellular pertussis vaccine: recommendations of the Advisory Committee on Immunization Practices (ACIP) and recommendation of ACIP, supported by the Healthcare Infection Control Practices Advisory Committee (HICPAC) for use of Tdap among health-care personnel. MMWR Recomm Rep 2006; 55 (RR-17):1.
8. TV Murphy et al. Prevention of pertussis, tetanus and diphtheria among pregnant and postpartum women and their infants: recommendations of the Advisory Committee on Immunization Practices (ACIP). MMWR Recomm Rep 2008; 57 (RR-4):1.
9. SA Gall. Vaccines for pertussis and influenza: recommendations for use in pregnancy. Clin Obstet Gynecol 2008; 51:486.
10. RL Winer et al. Genital human papillomavirus infection: incidence and risk factors in a cohort of female university students. Am J Epidemiol 2003; 157:218.
11. KA Ault. Human papillomavirus vaccines: an update for gynecologists. Clin Obstet Gynecol 2008; 51:527.
12. A human papillomavirus vaccine. Med Lett Drugs Ther 2006; 48:65.
13. DR Brown et al. The impact of quadrivalent human papillomavirus (HPV; Types 6, 11, 16, and 18) L1 virus-like particle vaccine on infection and disease due to oncogenic non-vaccine HPV types in generally HPV-naïve women aged 16-26 years. J Infect Dis 2009; 199:926.
14. CM Wheeler et al. The impact of quadrivalent human papillomavirus (HPV; Types 6, 11, 16, and 18) L1 virus-like particle vaccine on infection and disease due to oncogenic non-vaccine HPV types in sexually active women aged 16-26 years. J Infect Dis 2009; 199:936.
15. A Hildesheim and R Herrero. Human papillomavirus vaccine should be given before sexual debut for maximum benefit. J Infect Dis 2007; 196:1431.
16. FUTURE II Study Group. Quadrivalent vaccine against human papillomavirus to prevent high-grade cervical lesions. N Engl J Med 2007; 356:1915.

17. M Marin et al. Varicella among adults: data from an active surveillance project, 1995-2005. J Infect Dis 2008; 197 (suppl 2):S94.

18. P Merrett et al. Strategies to prevent varicella among newly arrived adult immigrants and refugees: a cost-effectiveness analysis. Clin Infect Dis 2007; 44:1040.

19. M Marin et al. Prevention of varicella: recommendations of the Advisory Committee on Immunization Practices (ACIP). MMWR Recomm Rep 2007; 56 (RR-4):1.

20. R Harpaz et al. Prevention of herpes zoster: recommendations of the Advisory Committee on Immunization Practices (ACIP). MMWR Recomm Rep 2008; 57 (RR-5):1.

21. Herpes zoster vaccine (Zostavax). Med Lett Drugs Ther 2006; 48:73.

22. GA Poland and W Schaffner. Immunization guidelines for adult patients: an annual update and a challenge. Ann Intern Med 2009; 150:53.

23. JC Watson et al. Measles, Mumps, and Rubella — Vaccine use and strategies for elimination of measles, rubella, and congenital rubella syndrome and control of mumps: recommendations of the Advisory Committee on Immunization Practices (ACIP). MMWR Recomm Rep 1998; 47(RR-8);1.

24. A Hviid et al. Mumps. Lancet 2008; 371:932.

25. AA Parker et al. Implications of a 2005 measles outbreak in Indiana for sustained elimination of measles in the United States. N Engl J Med 2006; 355:447.

26. Measles outbreak. Med Lett Drugs Ther 2008; 50:41.

27. JS Gerber and PA Offit. Vaccines and autism: a tale of shifting hypotheses. Clin Infect Dis 2009; Jan 7 [Epub ahead of print].

28. AT Kroger et al. General recommendations on immunization. Recommendations of the Advisory Committee on Immunization Practices (ACIP). MMWR Recomm Rep 2006; 55 (RR-15):1.

29. AE Fiore et al. Prevention and control of influenza: recommendations of the Advisory Committee on Immunization Practices (ACIP), 2008. MMWR Recomm Rep 2008; 57 (RR-7):1.

30. KL Nichol et al. Burden of influenza-like illness and effectiveness of influenza vaccination among working adults aged 50-64 years. Clin Infect Dis 2009; 48:292.

31. K Zaman et al. Effectiveness of maternal influenza immunization in mothers and infants. N Engl J Med 2008; 359:1555.

32. Influenza vaccine 2008-2009. Med Lett Drugs Ther 2008; 50:77.

33. S Ashkenazi et al. Superior relative efficacy of live attenuated influenza vaccine compared with inactivated influenza vaccine in young children with recurrent respiratory tract infections. Pediatr Infect Dis J 2006; 25:870.

34. DM Fleming et al. Comparison of the efficacy and safety of live attenuated cold-adapted influenza vaccine, trivalent, with trivalent inactivated influenza virus vaccine in children and adolescents with asthma. Pediatr Infect Dis J 2006; 25:860.

35. RB Belshe et al. Live attenuated versus inactivated influenza vaccine in infants and young children. N Engl J Med 2007; 356:685.

36. Z Wang et al. Live attenuated or inactivated influenza vaccines and medical encounters for respiratory illnesses among US military personnel. JAMA 2009; 301:945.

37. DN Juurlink et al. Guillain-Barré syndrome after influenza vaccination in adults: a population-based study. Arch Intern Med 2006; 166:2217.

38. Prevention of pneumococcal disease: recommendations of the Advisory Committee on Immunization Practices (ACIP). MMWR Recomm Rep 1997; 46 (RR-8):1.

39. DN Fisman et al. Prior pneumococcal vaccination is associated with reduced death, complications, and length of stay among hospitalized adults with community-acquired pneumonia. Clin Infect Dis 2006; 42:1093.

40. LA Jackson and EN Janoff. Pneumococcal vaccination of elderly adults: new paradigms for protection. Clin Infect Dis 2008; 47:1328.

41. A Huss et al. Efficacy of pneumococcal vaccination in adults: a meta-analysis. CMAJ 2009; 180:48.

42. Centers for Disease Control and Prevention (CDC). Pneumonia hospitalizations among young children before and after introduction of pneumococcal conjugate vaccine—United States, 1997-2006. Centers for Disease Control and Prevention. MMWR Morb Mortal Wkly Rep 2009; 58:1.

43. Centers for Disease Control and Prevention (CDC). Invasive pneumococcal disease in children 5 years after conjugate vaccine introduction – eight states, 1998-2005. MMWR Morb Mortal Wkly Rep 2008; 57:144.

44. HE Hsu et al. Effect of pneumococcal conjugate vaccine on pneumococcal meningitis. N Engl J Med 2009; 360:244.

45. EV Millar et al. Indirect effect of 7-valent pneumococcal conjugate vaccine on pneumococcal colonization among unvaccinated household members. Clin Infect Dis 2008; 47:989.

46. E Hak et al. Rationale and design of CAPITA: a RCT of 13-valent conjugated pneumococcal vaccine efficacy among older adults. Neth J Med 2008; 66:378.

47. GA Poland and W Schaffner. Immunization guidelines for adult patients: an annual update and a challenge. Ann Intern Med 2009; 150:53.

48. FJ Walker et al. Reactions after 3 or more doses of pneumococcal polysaccharide vaccine in adults in Alaska. Clin Infect Dis 2005; 40:1730.

49. Advisory Committee on Immunization Practices (ACIP). AE Fiore et al. Prevention of hepatitis A through active or passive immunization: recommendations of the Advisory Committee on Immunization Practices (ACIP). MMWR Recomm Rep 2006; 55 (RR-7):1.

50. Advisory Committee on Immunization Practices (ACIP). Centers for Disease Control and Prevention (CDC). Update: Prevention of hepatitis A after exposure to hepatitis A virus and in international travelers. Updated recommendations of the Advisory Committee on Immunization Practices (ACIP). MMWR Morb Mortal Wkly Rep 2007; 56:1080.

51. JS Keystone and JH Hershey. The underestimated risk of hepatitis A and hepatitis B: benefits of an accelerated vaccination schedule. Int J Infect Dis 2008; 12:3.

52. P Van Damme and K Van Herck. A review of the long-term protection after hepatitis A and B vaccination. Travel Med Infect Dis 2007; 5:79.

53. LL Hammitt et al. Persistence of antibody to hepatitis A virus 10 years after vaccination among children and adults. J Infect Dis 2008; 198:1776.

54. EE Mast et al. A comprehensive immunization strategy to eliminate transmission of hepatitis B virus infection in the United States: recommendations of the Advisory Committee on Immunization Practices (ACIP) part II: immunization of adults. MMWR Recomm Rep 2006; 55 (RR-16):1.
55. P Gardner. Clinical practice. Prevention of meningococcal disease. N Engl J Med 2006; 355:1466.
56. Menactra: a meningococcal conjugate vaccine. Med Lett Drugs Ther 2005; 47:29.
57. Center for Disease Control and Prevention (CDC). Update: Guillain-Barré syndrome among recipients of Menactra meningococcal conju-gate vaccine—United States, June 2005-September 2006. MMWR Morb Mortal Wkly Rep 2006; 55:1120.

Cervarix — A Second HPV Vaccine
Originally published in The Medical Letter – May 2010; 52:37

The FDA has approved a recombinant human papillomavirus (HPV) vaccine (*Cervarix* – GlaxoSmithKline) for use in girls and women 10-25 years old to prevent infection with HPV types 16 and 18, which have been associated with cervical cancer. A recombinant quadrivalent HPV vaccine (*Gardasil* – Merck) already on the market in the US prevents infection with HPV types 6, 11, 16 and 18.[1]

BACKGROUND — HPV is commonly acquired by young women soon after initiation of sexual activity, with a cumulative incidence of 40% within 16 months.[2] Although most HPV infections clear spontaneously without clinical sequelae, persistent infection can cause abnormalities in the cervical epithelium that may progress to cancer. HPV types 16 and 18 are responsible for more than 70% of cervical cancers and high-grade cervical intraepithelial neoplasia (CIN), a precursor of cervical cancer. Types 6 and 11 cause about 90% of genital warts.

THE NEW VACCINE — *Cervarix* is a non-infectious vaccine prepared from highly purified virus-like particles (VLPs) of the major capsid L1 protein of HPV types 16 and 18. It includes AS04, a toll-like receptor agonist, as an adjuvant.

CLINICAL STUDIES — Among 18,644 women 15-25 years old randomly assigned to receive either the bivalent HPV vaccine or hepatitis A vaccine, the HPV vaccine's efficacy against grade 2+ cervical intraepithelial neoplasia (CIN2+) containing HPV 16 or 18 DNA was 93% during a mean follow-up period of 34.9 months. In addition, it provided cross-protection against persistent infections with HPV 45 and other non-vaccine HPV types (but not types 6 and 11).[3] Follow-up data available for up to 6.4 years have demonstrated sustained immunogenicity and long-term efficacy[4]; similar data are available for up to 5 years with *Gardasil*.

HPV VACCINES

	Gardasil	*Cervarix*
FDA-approved indications	Females 9-26 yrs old • Prevention of cervical cancer caused by HPV 16 and 18 • Prevention of genital warts caused by HPV 6 and 11 Males 9-26 yrs old • Prevention of genital warts caused by HPV types 6 and 11	Females 10-25 yrs old • Prevention of cervical cancer caused by HPV 16 and 18
Formulations	0.5 mL single dose vial; 0.5 mL pre-filled syringe	0.5 mL single dose vial; 0.5 mL pre-filled syringe
Administration	0.5 mL intramuscular injection at 0, 2, and 6 months	0.5 mL intramuscular injection at 0, 1, and 6 months
Cost[1] (series)	$469.50	$463.05

1. Cost according to AWP listings in *Red Book Update* April 2010.

A randomized prospective trial (sponsored by GlaxoSmithKline) comparing the two HPV vaccines found higher serum neutralizing antibody titers and a higher incidence of adverse reactions, mostly injection site reactions, after vaccination with *Cervarix*.[5] Whether the higher immune response offers any clinical benefits remains to be determined.

ADVERSE EFFECTS — Local pain, redness and swelling at the injection site are common with *Cervarix*.

RECOMMENDATIONS — Vaccination is recommended routinely for girls 11-12 years old and also for girls 13-25 years old who have not been vaccinated previously. Vaccination is not a substitute for cervical cancer screening (Pap smears). HPV vaccine is not recommended for use in pregnant women.

CONCLUSION — *Cervarix* can prevent disease associated with HPV types 16 and 18, which cause >70% of cervical cancer, and can induce higher serum antibody levels than those achieved with *Gardasil*. Whether these high levels lead to greater long-term protection is unknown. *Gardasil* does, and *Cervarix* does not, protect against HPV types 6 and 11, which cause about 90% of genital warts in both sexes.

1. A human papillomavirus vaccine. Med Lett Drugs Ther 2006; 48:65.
2. RL Winer et al. Genital human papillomavirus infection: incidence and risk factors in a cohort of female university students. Am J Epidemol 2003; 157:218.
3. J Paavonen et al for the HPV PATRICIA study group. Efficacy of human papillomavirus (HPV)-16/18 AS04-adjuvanted vaccine against cervical infection and precancer caused by oncogenic HPV types (PATRICIA): final analysis of a double-blind, randomised study in young women. Lancet 2009; 374:301.
4. B Romanowski et al for the GlaxoSmithKline Vaccine HPV-007 study group. Sustained efficacy and immunogenicity of the human papillomavirus (HPV)-16/18 AS04-adjuvanted vaccine: analysis of a randomized placebo-controlled trial up to 6.4 years. Lancet 2009; 374:1975.
5. MH Einstein et al. Comparison of the immunogenicity and safety of *Cervarix* and *Gardasil* human papillomavirus (HPV) cervical cancer vaccines in healthy women aged 18-45 years. Hum Vaccin 2009; 5:705.

Pneumococcal Vaccination of Adults: Polysaccharide or Conjugate?

Originally published in The Medical Letter – June 2009; 51:1314

A 23-valent polysaccharide vaccine (PPSV23; *Pneumovax 23* – Merck) is the only pneumococcal vaccine approved for use in adults. A more immunogenic conjugate vaccine containing 7 pneumococcal serotypes (PCV7; *Prevnar* – Wyeth) is generally used only in children <5 years old, but apparently has reduced the incidence of pneumococcal disease due to these serotypes in adults as well, presumably as a result of herd immunity. Some authors have suggested that perhaps PPSV23 should be withdrawn.[1]

POLYSACCHARIDE VACCINE — PPSV23 contains the capsular polysaccharide antigens of 23 pneumococcal serotypes. It has reduced the risk of invasive pneumococcal disease (meningitis or bacteremic pneumonia), but not mortality, in immunocompetent older adults.[2] PPSV23 has not been shown to reduce the risk of invasive pneumococcal disease (IPD) in immunocompromised patients.[3]

The US Advisory Committee on Immunization Practices (ACIP) recommends a one-time dose of PPSV23 for all adults ≥65 years old.[4] Persons who received an initial dose before age 65 should be revaccinated once at or after age 65, at least 5 years following the initial vaccination. PPSV23 is also recommended for adults who smoke or have asthma and for patients ≥2 years old with chronic illnesses or immunosuppression.

CONJUGATE VACCINE — PCV7 contains the capsular polysaccharide antigens of 7 pneumococcal serotypes conjugated to a protein carrier, mutant diphtheria toxin, which increases immunogenicity. Annual rates of IPD in children <5 years declined by 77% between 1999, the year before PCV7 became part of routine infant immunizations, and 2005.[5] PCV7 does not contain the 19A serotype, which is currently the most prevalent in invasive pneumococcal disease in children and the second most common in older adults.[6] All of the PCV7 serotypes and 19A are present in PPSV23. A 13-valent conjugate vaccine (PCV13) that includes the PCV7 serotypes and 19A is under investigation in adults and children.[7]

PCV7 in Adults – Clinical trials of PCV7 in adults have used immunogenicity rather than pneumococcal disease as their endpoint. A clinical trial comparing vaccination with PPSV23 to vaccination with PCV7 in pneumococcal vaccine-naïve adults ≥70 years old found higher immune responses in patients who received PCV7 vaccine.[8] In another study, the immune response to twice the standard pediatric dose of PCV7 in adults 70-79 years old vaccinated with PPSV23 at least 5 years earlier, was greater than it was with PPSV23 revaccination.[9]

CONCLUSION — Compared to the pneumococcal polysaccharide vaccine (PPSV23; *Pneumovax 23)*, the currently available pneumococcal conjugate vaccine (PCV7, *Prevnar*) has the advantage of greater immunogenicity, but the disadvantages of a narrower spectrum of pneumococcal serotypes and, in adults, the absence of clinical efficacy data. Until the results of studies with a conjugate vaccine for adults containing additional pneumococcal serotypes, including 19A, become available, there is no good reason to stop using PPSV23.

1. A Huss et al. Efficacy of pneumococcal vaccination in adults: a meta-analysis. CMAJ 2009; 180:48.
2. SA Moberley et al. Vaccine for preventing pneumococcal infection in adults. Cochrane Database Syst Rev 2008; (1): CD000422.
3. CG Whitney et al. Rethinking recommendations for use of pneumococcal vaccines in adults. Clin Infect Dis 2001; 33:662.
4. Adult immunization. Treat Guidel Med Lett 2009; 7:27.
5. CDC. Invasive pneumococcal disease in children 5 years after conjugate vaccine introduction–eight states, 1998–2005. MMWR Morb Mortal Wkly Rep 2008; 57:144.
6. LA Hicks et al. Incidence of pneumococcal disease due to non-pneumococcal conjugate vaccine (PCV7) serotypes in the United States during the era of widespread PCV7 vaccination, 1998-2004. J Infect Dis 2007; 196:1346.
7. EC Dinleyici and ZA Yargic. Pneumococcal conjugated vaccines: impact of PCV-7 and new achievements in the postvaccine era. Expert Rev Vaccines 2008; 7:1367.

8. A de Roux et al. Comparison of pneumococcal conjugate polysaccharide and free poly-saccharide vaccines in elderly adults: conjugate vaccine elicits improved antibacterial immune responses and immunological memory. Clin Infect Dis 2008; 46:1015.
9. LA Jackson et al. Immunogenicity of varying dosages of 7-valent pneumococcal polysac-charide-protein conjugate vaccine in seniors previously vaccinated with 23-valent pneu-mococcal polysaccharide vaccine. Vaccine 2007; 25:4029.

ADVICE FOR
Travelers

Original publication date – November 2009

Patients planning to travel to other countries often ask physicians for information about appropriate vaccines and prevention of diarrhea and malaria. More detailed advice for travelers is available from the Centers for Disease Control and Prevention (CDC) at www.cdc.gov/travel. Guidelines are also available from the Infectious Diseases Society of America (IDSA).[1]

VACCINES

Common travel vaccines are listed in the table on the next page. In addition to travel-specific vaccines, all travelers (including children) should be up to date on routine vaccines. Guidelines for routine adult immunization have been published in a separate issue.[2] Immunocompromised or pregnant patients generally should not receive live virus vaccines, such as those for measles and yellow fever, although in some situations the benefit might outweigh the risk.

CHOLERA — The risk of cholera in tourists is very low. The parenteral vaccine previously licensed in the US is no longer available. An oral, whole-cell recombinant vaccine called *Dukoral* is available in some European countries (Crucell/SBL Vaccines) and in Canada (Sanofi Pasteur). It is not currently recommended for routine use in travelers, but

SOME VACCINES FOR TRAVEL

Vaccines	Adult Dose (Volume)	Pediatric Age
HEPATITIS A		
Havrix (GSK)	1440 EU IM (1 mL)	1-18 yrs
Vaqta (Merck)	50 U IM (1 mL)	1-18 yrs
HEPATITIS B		
Engerix-B (GSK)	20 mcg IM (1 mL)	Birth-19 yrs
Recombivax-HB (Merck)	10 mcg IM (1 mL)	Birth-19 yrs
HEPATITIS A/B		
Twinrix (GSK)	720 EU/20 mcg IM (1 mL)	Not approved for <18 yrs
JAPANESE ENCEPHALITIS		
Ixiaro (Novartis)	0.5 mL IM	Not approved for <17 yrs
JE-Vax (Sanofi Pasteur)	1 mL SC	1-3 yrs / >3 yrs
MENINGOCOCCAL		
Menomune (Sanofi Pasteur)	50 mcg of each antigen SC (0.5 mL)	≥2 yrs[2]
Menactra (Sanofi Pasteur)	4 mcg of each antigen IM (0.5 mL) (18-55 yrs)	≥2 yrs

1. Protection likely lasts at least 12 months after a single dose.
2. According to the CDC it is safe for children < 2 years old who require vaccination for the Hajj.

might be considered for those who plan to work in refugee camps or as healthcare providers in endemic areas.

HEPATITIS A — Hepatitis A vaccine, which is now part of routine childhood immunization in the US, is recommended for all unvaccinated

Pediatric Dose (Volume)	Standard Primary Schedule	Duration of Protection
720 EU IM (0.5 mL) 25 U IM (0.5 mL)	0 and 6-12 mos 0 and 6-18 mos	Probably lifelong after completion of primary series[1]
10 mcg IM (0.5 mL) 5 mcg IM (0.5 mL)	0, 1 and 6 mos 0, 1 and 6 mos	Probably lifelong after completion of primary series
—	0, 1 and 6 mos	Probably lifelong after completion of primary series
—	0, 28 days	No data
0.5 mL SC 1 mL SC	0, 7 and 14 or (preferably) 30 days	Not established; a single booster is usually given after 24 months if ongoing risk
50 mcg of each antigen SC (0.5 mL) 4 mcg of each antigen IM (0.5 mL)	Single dose Single dose	Repeat every 5 yrs[3] with *Menactra* if ongoing risk Repeat every 5 yrs[3] if ongoing risk

3. Repeat after three years for children vaccinated at 2-6 years of age.

Continued on next page.

travelers going anywhere other than Australia, Canada, western Europe, Japan or New Zealand.[3]

Vaccination of adults and children usually consists of two IM doses separated by 6-18 months. Additional booster doses are not needed.[4,5] Two

SOME VACCINES FOR TRAVEL (continued)

Vaccines	Adult Dose (Volume)	Pediatric Age
RABIES		
Imovax (Sanofi Pasteur)	≥2.5 IU of rabies antigen IM (1 mL)	Birth
RabAvert (Novartis)	≥2.5 IU of rabies antigen IM (1 mL)	Birth
TYPHOID		
Vivotif (Crucell/Berna)	1 cap PO (contains 2-6x10^9 viable CFU of *S. typhi* Ty21a)	≥6 yrs
Typhim Vi (Sanofi Pasteur)	25 mcg IM (0.5 mL)	≥2 yrs
YELLOW FEVER		
YF-Vax (Sanofi Pasteur)	4.74 log$_{10}$ plaque forming units of 17D204 attenuated YF virus SC (0.5 mL)	≥9 mos

4. Regimen for pre-exposure prophylaxis. If a previously vaccinated traveler is exposed to a potentially rabid animal, post-exposure prophylaxis with 2 additional vaccine doses separated by 3 days should be initiated as soon as possible.

hepatitis A vaccines are available in the US: *Havrix* and *Vaqta*. Patients who received a first dose of one vaccine will respond to a second dose of the other. Second doses given up to 8 years after the first dose have produced protective antibody levels.[6]

Antibodies reach protective levels 2-4 weeks after the first dose. Even when exposure to the disease occurs sooner than 4 weeks after vaccina-

Pediatric Dose (Volume)	Standard Primary Schedule	Duration of Protection
≥2.5 IU of rabies antigen IM (1 mL)	0, 7 and 21 or 28 days[4]	Routine boosters not necessary; for those engaging in frequent high-risk activities (cavers, veterinarians, laboratory workers), serologic testing is recommended every 2 yrs with booster doses if low levels[5]
≥2.5 IU of rabies antigen IM (1 mL)	0, 7 and 21 or 28 days[4]	
1 cap PO (contains 2-6x10⁹ viable CFU of *S. typhi* Ty21a)	1 cap every other day x 4 doses	Repeat every 5 yrs if ongoing risk
25 mcg IM (0.5 mL)	Single dose	Repeat every 2 yrs if ongoing risk
4.74 log₁₀ plaque forming units of 17D204 attenuated YF virus SC (0.5 mL)	Single dose	Booster dose every 10 yrs if ongoing risk

5. Minimal acceptable antibody level is complete virus neutralization at a 1:5 serum dilution by the rapid fluorescent focus inhibition test.

tion, the traveler is usually protected because of the relatively long incubation period of hepatitis A (average 28 days). For immunosuppressed patients and those with chronic liver disease who will be traveling to an endemic area in ≤2 weeks, immune globulin (0.02 mL/kg IM) should be given in addition to the initial dose of vaccine. The same dose should be given to children under 1 year of age and other travelers who cannot receive the vaccine if traveling for ≤3 months; a dose of 0.06 mL/kg IM

LOW-RISK AREAS FOR HEPATITIS A & B*

Hepatitis A	Hepatitis B
Australia	Argentina
Canada	Australia
Japan	Canada[1]
New Zealand	Chile
United States	Costa Rica
Western Europe (all countries)	Cuba
	Hungary
	Mexico
	New Zealand
	Nicaragua
	Panama
	Paraguay
	United States[1]
	Uruguay
	Western Europe[2]

* All other areas are intermediate to high risk; vaccine is indicated.
1. Risk is intermediate in Alaska natives and is high in indigenous populations of northern Canada.
2. Risk is intermediate in Greece, Portugal and Spain.

should be given if traveling for >3 months. For travel durations of >5 months, the dose should be repeated.[7]

HEPATITIS B — Vaccination against hepatitis B is recommended for travelers going to intermediate- or high-risk areas (see table above for low-risk areas). Travelers going anywhere who engage in behaviors that may increase the risk of transmission, such as unprotected sexual contact with new partners, dental treatment, skin perforation practices (tattoos, acupuncture, ear piercing) or invasive medical treatment (injections, stitching), should be immunized against hepatitis B.

Two hepatitis B vaccines are available in the US: *Engerix-B* and *Recombivax-HB*. Primary immunization usually consists of 3 doses given IM at 0, 1 and 6 months. An alternate schedule of 3 doses given at 0, 1 and 2 months, followed by a fourth dose at 12 months, is approved for *Engerix-B* in the US. A 2-dose schedule of adult *Recombivax-HB* at 0 and 4-6 months is approved in the US for adolescents 11-15 years old. An accelerated schedule of 0, 7 and 14 days, followed by a booster dose at 6 months, can also be used with either vaccine, but is not FDA-approved.

An interrupted hepatitis B vaccination series can be completed without being restarted. A 3-dose series started with one vaccine may be completed with the other. Post-vaccination serologic testing is recommended for healthcare workers, infants born to HBsAg-positive mothers, hemodialysis patients, HIV-infected and other immunocompromised patients, and sex- and needle-sharing partners of HBsAg-positive patients.

HEPATITIS A/B — A combination vaccine *(Twinrix)* containing the same antigenic components as pediatric *Havrix* and *Engerix-B* is available for patients ≥18 years old. It is given in 3 doses at 0, 1 and 6 months. An accelerated schedule of 0, 7 and 21-30 days with a booster dose at 12 months is also approved.[8]

The combination vaccine can be used to complete an immunization series started with monovalent hepatitis A and B vaccines. *Twinrix Junior* is available outside the US for children 1-15 years old.

INFLUENZA — Influenza may be a risk in the tropics year-round and in temperate areas of the Southern Hemisphere from April to September. Outbreaks have occurred on cruise ships and on organized group tours in any latitude or season.[9]

Seasonal influenza vaccine directed against strains in the Northern Hemisphere is sometimes available in the US until the end of June and the US Advisory Committee on Immunization Practices (ACIP) recommends that persons for whom seasonal influenza vaccine is indicated[10] consider being vaccinated before travel to the Southern Hemisphere during influenza season or to the tropics at any season, or when traveling in a group with persons from the Southern Hemisphere during their influenza season (April-September).[11] In some years, the vaccine strains are the same in both hemispheres. If the vaccine strains are different, high-risk patients from the Northern Hemisphere who travel to the Southern Hemisphere during that region's influenza season could also consider being immunized on arrival because the vaccine active against strains in the Southern Hemisphere is rarely available in the Northern Hemisphere.

A monovalent vaccine is available to protect against the currently (2009) circulating pandemic influenza A (H1N1) virus.[12] It can be given at the same time as the seasonal vaccine, except not the 2 live attenuated formulations together. Both the seasonal and monovalent influenza vaccines are prepared in eggs. Hypersensitivity reactions could occur.

There is no commercial influenza vaccine available for pathogenic strains of avian influenza (H5N1, H7N2, H9N2, H7N3, H7N7), but an inactivated vaccine against avian H5N1 is FDA-approved and is being included in the US Strategic National Stockpile.

JAPANESE ENCEPHALITIS — Japanese encephalitis is an uncommon but potentially fatal mosquito-borne viral disease that occurs in rural Asia, especially near pig farms and rice paddies. It is usually seasonal (May-October), but may occur year-round in equatorial regions. The attack rate in travelers has been very low.[13]

Vaccination is recommended for travelers >1 year old who expect a long stay ($\geq$1 month) in endemic areas or heavy exposure to mosquitoes (such as adventure travelers) during the transmission season. Vaccination also should be considered for travelers spending less than a month in endemic areas during the transmission season if they will be sleeping without air conditioning, screens or bed nets, or spending considerable time outside in rural or agricultural areas, especially in the evening or at night.[14] Some Medical Letter consultants suggest that, given the rarity of the disease in US residents, compulsive use of insect repellents and judicious avoidance of exposure to mosquitoes might be reasonable alternatives to vaccination for short-term travelers.

Two formulations are FDA-approved in the United States: *JE-Vax*, which is a mouse-brain preparation, and the recently approved *Ixiaro*, a non-mouse-brain vaccine, which is preferred for use in adults, but has not been approved for use in children in the US.[15] In clinical trials, 2 doses of *Ixiaro* (one is not enough) appeared to be as effective as *JE-Vax*, and considerably safer.[16]

MEASLES — The measles vaccine is no longer available in a monovalent formulation. It is available as an attenuated live-virus vaccine in combination with mumps and rubella (MMR). Adults born in or after 1957 (1970 in Canada) and healthcare workers of any age who have not received 2 doses of live measles vaccine (not the killed vaccine that was commonly used in the 1960s) after their first birthday and do not have a physician-documented history of infection or laboratory evidence of immunity should receive two doses of MMR vaccine, separated by at least 28 days.[17]

Previously unvaccinated children ≥12 months old should receive 2 doses of MMR vaccine at least 28 days apart before traveling outside the US. Children 6-11 months old should receive 1 dose before traveling, but will still need two subsequent doses for routine immunization, one at 12-15 months and one at 4-6 years.

MENINGOCOCCAL — A single dose of meningococcal vaccine is recommended for adults and children ≥2 years old who are traveling to areas where epidemics are occurring, or to anywhere in the "meningitis belt" (semi-arid areas of sub-Saharan Africa extending from Senegal and

Guinea eastward to Ethiopia) from December to June. Saudi Arabia requires a certificate of immunization for pilgrims during the Hajj. Immunization should also be considered for travelers to other areas where *Neisseria meningitidis* is hyperendemic or epidemic, particularly for those who will have prolonged contact with the local population, such as those living in a dormitory or refugee camp, or working in a healthcare setting.[18-20]

Two quadrivalent vaccines are available against *N. meningitidis* serogroups A, C, Y and W135. *Menomune* contains meningococcal capsular polysaccharides. *Menactra,* which contains capsular polysaccharides conjugated to diphtheria toxoid, is preferred, but *Menomune* is an acceptable alternative. Neither vaccine provides protection against serogroup B, which does not have an immunogenic polysaccharide capsule. Group B infections are rare in sub-Saharan Africa.

The most common adverse reactions to *Menactra* have been headache, fatigue and malaise in addition to pain, redness and induration at the site of injection. The rates of these reactions are higher than with *Menomune*, but similar to those with tetanus toxoid. Guillain-Barré syndrome has been reported rarely in adolescents who received *Menactra*, but cause and effect have not been established.[21]

POLIO — Adults who have not previously been immunized against polio should receive a primary series of inactivated polio vaccine (IPV) if traveling to areas where polio is still endemic (Nigeria, India, Pakistan, Afghanistan) or to areas with documented outbreaks or circulating vaccine-derived strains (see table on next page).[22] Previously unimmunized children should also receive a primary series of IPV.

If protection is needed within 4 weeks, a single dose of IPV is recommended, but provides only partial protection. Adult travelers to risk areas who have previously completed a primary series and have never had a booster should receive a single booster dose of IPV.

COUNTRIES WITH A RISK OF POLIO[1]

Afghanistan	Djibouti	Nepal
Angola	Equatorial Guinea	Niger
Bangladesh	Eritrea	Nigeria
Benin	Ethiopia	Pakistan
Bhutan	Gabon	Rwanda
Burkina Faso	Gambia	Senegal
Burundi	Ghana	Sierra Leone
Cameroon	Guinea	Somalia
Central African	Guinea-Bissau	Sudan
Republic	India	Tanzania
Chad	Kenya	Togo
Congo	Liberia	Uganda
Côte d'Ivoire	Mali	Zambia
Democratic Republic	Mauritania	
of the Congo	Namibia	

1. Centers for Disease Control and Prevention. Update on the Global Status of Polio. October 1, 2009. Available at: http://wwwnc.cdc.gov/travel/content/in-thenews/polio-outbreaks.aspx.

RABIES — Rabies is highly endemic in parts of Africa, Asia (particularly India) and Central and South America, but the risk to travelers is generally low. Pre-exposure immunization against rabies is recommended for travelers with an occupational risk of exposure, for those (especially children) visiting endemic areas where immediate access to medical treatment, particularly rabies immune globulin, tends to be limited, and for outdoor-adventure travelers.[23,24] The 2 vaccines available in the US *(Imovax, RabAvert)* are similar; both are given in the deltoid (not gluteal) muscle at 0, 7 and 21 or 28 days.

After a bite or scratch from a potentially rabid animal, patients who received pre-exposure prophylaxis should promptly receive 2 additional doses of vaccine at days 0 and 3. Without pre-exposure immunization, the ACIP recommends rabies immune globulin (RIG) and is now recommending 4 doses (over 14 days) of vaccine instead of 5 doses (over 28 days). Patients with immunosuppression should still receive 5 doses of vaccine.[25] The reduced vaccine dosing schedule may not be included in the prescribing information from the manufacturers of the approved vaccines. According to the CDC, cell culture rabies vaccines available outside the US are acceptable alternatives to FDA-approved vaccines; neural tissue vaccines have high rates of serious adverse effects.[26] RIG is a blood product, and its purity and potency may be less reliable, if it is available at all, in developing countries.

TETANUS, DIPHTHERIA AND PERTUSSIS — Previously unimmunized children should receive 3 or (preferably) 4 doses of pediatric diphtheria, tetanus and acellular pertussis vaccine (DTaP) before travel. An accelerated schedule can be used beginning at age 6 weeks, with the second and third doses given 4 weeks after the previous dose, and the fourth dose 6 months after the third.

Adults with an uncertain history of primary vaccination should receive 3 doses of a tetanus and diphtheria toxoid vaccine. Two vaccines (*Adacel*; *Boostrix*) containing protein components of acellular pertussis combined with diphtheria and tetanus toxoids (Tdap) are available for adults $\leq$64 years of age.[27] One of the 3 doses (preferably the first) should be Tdap. The first 2 doses should be administered at least 4 weeks apart and the third 6-12 months after the second. DTaP contains larger amounts of diphtheria and pertussis antigens than Tdap and is not licensed for use in adults.

Inactivated adsorbed (aluminum-salt-precipitated) tetanus and diphtheria toxoid (Td) has been the standard booster vaccine for adults. A booster dose of Td is recommended every 10 years. Persons 11-64 years old who have completed a primary childhood series and have not yet received Tdap should receive a single dose of Tdap at the time of their next scheduled routine Td booster. Tdap can be given less than 10 years after the last Td to provide pertussis protection before travel.

TICK-BORNE ENCEPHALITIS (TBE) — TBE occurs in temperate areas of Europe and Asia, from eastern France to northern Japan, and from northern Russia to Albania.[28,29] The risk is greatest from April to November. Humans acquire the disease through the bite of a tick or, rarely, from eating unpasteurized dairy (mostly goat) products. Immunization is recommended only for travelers who will spend extensive time outdoors in rural areas. The vaccine, which is not approved in the US but is available in Canada and Europe (*Encepur* – Novartis; *FSME-Immun* – Baxter AG), is usually given in 3 doses over 9-12 months, but can be given (*Encepur*) over 3 weeks (0, 7 and 21 days). *FSME-Immun* can be obtained in Canada by contacting the Special Access Programme, Health Canada (613-941-2108).

The usual duration of protection after the primary series is 3 years; with the accelerated schedule of *Encepur*, it may be only 12-18 months. Boosters give 5 years of protection for patients <50 years old and 3 years for those ≥50 years old.

TYPHOID — Typhoid vaccine is recommended for travelers to South Asia and other developing countries in East and Southeast Asia, Central and South America, the Caribbean and Africa, especially if they will be visiting friends or relatives or traveling outside routine tourist destinations.[30,31]

A live attenuated oral vaccine *(Vivotif)* is available for adults and children ≥6 years old. It is taken every other day as a single capsule (at least 1 hour before eating) for a total of 4 capsules, beginning no later than 2 weeks before departure; it protects for about 5 years. The capsules must be refrigerated. Antibiotics should be avoided for at least 72 hours before the first capsule. A purified capsular polysaccharide parenteral vaccine *(Typhim Vi)* for adults and children ≥2 years old is given as a single IM dose at least 2 weeks before departure. Re-vaccination is recommended every 2 years (3 years in Canada).

A combined hepatitis A/typhoid vaccine (*Vivaxim* – Sanofi Pasteur) is available in Canada.

YELLOW FEVER — Yellow fever vaccine *(YF-Vax)*, a single-dose attenuated live virus vaccine prepared in eggs, should be given at least 10 days before travel to endemic areas, which include much of tropical South America and sub-Saharan Africa between 15°N and 15°S.[32] Some countries in Africa require an International Certificate of Vaccination against yellow fever, or a physician's waiver letter, from all entering travelers; other countries in Africa, South America and Asia require evidence of vaccination from travelers coming from or traveling through endemic or infected areas. The vaccine is available in the US only from providers certified by state health departments.[33] Boosters are given every 10 years, but immunity probably lasts much longer. If other injectable or intranasal live vaccines are not administered simultaneously with yellow fever vaccine, administration should be separated by one month to avoid a diminished immune response to the vaccines.

Yellow fever vaccine is contraindicated in travelers who have symptomatic HIV infection (and possibly in those with CD4 counts <200 cells/mm^3), are immunocompromised or have egg allergy. Yellow fever vaccine-associated viscerotropic disease, a severe systemic illness that can cause fatal organ failure, has been reported rarely. It has occurred only in first-time recipients, especially those with thymus disorders. Vaccine-associated neurologic disease (encephalitis, Guillain-Barré, Bell's palsy) has also occurred. The vaccine should be avoided if possible in infants <9 months old and it is contraindicated in infants <6 months old.[34] Travelers >60 years of age also have a relatively high risk of systemic adverse effects.[35]

TRAVELERS' DIARRHEA

The most common cause of travelers' diarrhea, usually a self-limited illness lasting several days, is infection with noninvasive enterotoxigenic

(ETEC) or enteroaggregative (EAEC) strains of *Escherichia coli*. Infections with *Campylobacter*, *Shigella*, *Salmonella*, *Aeromonas*, viruses and parasites are less common. Children tend to have more severe illness and are particularly susceptible to dehydration. Travelers to areas where hygiene is poor should avoid raw vegetables, fruit they have not peeled themselves, unpasteurized dairy products, cooked food not served steaming hot, and tap water, including ice.

Treatment – For mild diarrhea, loperamide (*Imodium*, and others), an over-the-counter synthetic opioid (4-mg loading dose, then 2 mg orally after each loose stool to a maximum of 16 mg/d for adults), often relieves symptoms in <24 hours. It should not be used if fever or bloody diarrhea are present, and some patients complain of constipation after use. Loperamide is approved for use in children >2 years old.

If diarrhea is moderate to severe, persists >3 days or is associated with high fever or bloody stools, self-treatment for 1-3 days with ciprofloxacin, levofloxacin, norfloxacin or ofloxacin is usually recommended.[36] Azithromycin, taken as a single 1000-mg dose or 500 mg daily for 1-3 days, is an alternative[37,38] and is the drug of choice for travelers to areas with a high prevalence of fluoroquinolone-resistant *Campylobacter*, such as Thailand and India.[39,40] Azithromycin can be used in pregnant women and children (10 mg/kg/d x 3d), and in patients who do not respond to a fluoroquinolone in 48 hours.

A non-absorbed oral antibiotic derived from rifampin, rifaximin is approved for treatment of travelers' diarrhea caused by noninvasive strains of *E. coli* in travelers ≥12 years of age. In clinical trials in patients with diarrhea mostly caused by *E. coli*, it has been similar in efficacy to ciprofloxacin, with fewer adverse effects.[41] It should not be used in infections associated with fever or blood in the stool or those caused by *C. jejuni, Salmonella, Shigella* or other invasive pathogens, or during pregnancy.

ANTIMICROBIAL DRUGS FOR TREATMENT OF TRAVELERS' DIARRHEA

Drug	Dosage	Cost[1]
Azithromycin	1000 mg once	
generic	or 500 mg once/d	$42.54
Zithromax (Pfizer)	x 3d	64.29
Ciprofloxacin		
generic	500 mg bid x 1-3d	31.44[2]
Cipro (Bayer)		36.30
sustained release		
generic	1000 mg once/d x 1-3d	32.64
Cipro XR		33.78
Levofloxacin	500 mg once/d x 1-3d	
Levaquin (Ortho-McNeil)		44.37
Norfloxacin – *Noroxin* (Merck)	400 mg bid x 1-3d	24.84
Ofloxacin – generic	300 mg bid x 1-3d	32.88
Rifaximin – *Xifaxan* (Salix)	200 mg tid x 3d	49.23

1. Cost of 3 days' treatment based on August 2009 data from retail pharmacies nationwide available from Wolters Kluwer Health.
2. 20 500-mg tablets cost $4 at some discount pharmacies.

One meta-analysis found that combinations of an antibacterial plus loperamide were more effective than an antibacterial alone in decreasing the duration of illness.[42]

Packets of oral rehydration salts (*Ceralyte*, *ORS*, and others) mixed in potable water can prevent and treat dehydration, particularly in children and the elderly. They are available from suppliers of travel-related products and some pharmacies in the US, and from pharmacies overseas.

Prophylaxis – Medical Letter consultants generally do not prescribe antibiotic prophylaxis for travelers' diarrhea, but rather instruct the patient to begin self-treatment when symptoms are distressing or persistent. Some travelers, however, such as immunocompromised patients or those with time-dependent activities who cannot risk the temporary incapacitation associated with diarrhea, might benefit from prophylaxis.[43] In such patients, ciprofloxacin 500 mg, levofloxacin 500 mg, ofloxacin 300 mg or norfloxacin 400 mg can be given once daily during travel and for 2 days after return and are generally well tolerated. In one 2-week study among travelers to Mexico, rifaximin (200 mg 1-3x/d) was effective in preventing travelers' diarrhea.[44] Bismuth subsalicylate (*Pepto-Bismol*, and others) can prevent diarrhea in travelers who take 2 tablets 4 times a day for the duration of travel, but it is less effective than antibiotics. It is not recommended for children <3 years old.

MALARIA

No drug is 100% effective for prevention of malaria; travelers should be told to take protective measures against mosquito bites in addition to medication.[45] Countries with a risk of malaria are listed in the table on the next page. Some countries with endemic malaria transmission may not have malaria in the most frequently visited major cities and rural tourist resorts. Travelers to malarious areas should be reminded to seek medical attention if they have fever either during their trip or up to a year (especially during the first 2 months) after they return. Travelers to developing countries, where counterfeit and poor quality drugs are common, should consider buying antimalarials before travel.

CHLOROQUINE-SENSITIVE MALARIA — Chloroquine is the drug of choice for prevention of malaria in the few areas that still have chloroquine-sensitive malaria (see table on the next page, footnotes 4, 6 and 7). Patients who cannot tolerate chloroquine should take atovaquone/proguanil, doxycycline, mefloquine or, in some circumstances, primaquine in the same doses used for chloroquine-resistant malaria (see table on page 348).

COUNTRIES WITH A RISK OF MALARIA[1]

AFRICA

Angola	Democratic	Kenya[3]	São Tomé and
Benin	Republic of the	Liberia	Príncipe
Botswana[3]	Congo	Madagascar	Senegal
Burkina Faso	Djibouti	Malawi	Sierra Leone
Burundi	Equatorial	Mali	Somalia
Cameroon	Guinea	Mauritania	South Africa[3]
Cape Verde[2]	Eritrea[3]	Mayotte	Sudan
Central African	Ethiopia[3]	Mozambique	Swaziland
Republic	Gabon	Namibia	Tanzania
Chad	Gambia, The	Niger	Togo
Comoros	Ghana	Nigeria	Uganda
Congo	Guinea	Rwanda	Zambia
Côte d'Ivoire	Guinea-Bissau		Zimbabwe

AMERICAS

Argentina[3,4]	Costa Rica[3,4]	Guatemala[3,4]	Panama[3,6]
Bahamas, The[3,4,5]	Dominican	Guyana[3]	Paraguay[3,4]
Belize[3,4]	Republic[3,4]	Haiti[4]	Peru[3]
Bolivia[3]	Ecuador[3]	Honduras[3,4]	Suriname[3]
Brazil	El Salvador[3,4]	Mexico[3,4]	Venezuela[3]
Colombia[3]	French Guiana[3]	Nicaragua[3,4]	

ASIA

Afghanistan	India	Myanmar[3]	Timor-Leste
Armenia[3,4]	Indonesia[3]	Nepal[3]	(East Timor)
Azerbaijan[3,4]	Iran[3]	Pakistan	Turkey[3,4]
Bangladesh[3]	Iraq[3,4]	Philippines[3]	Uzbekistan[4]
Bhutan[3]	Korea, North[4]	Saudi Arabia[3]	Vietnam[3]
Cambodia[3]	Korea, South[3,4]	Sri Lanka	Yemen
China[7]	Laos[3]	Tajikistan	
Georgia[3,4]	Malaysia[3]	Thailand[3]	

OCEANIA

Papua New	Solomon Islands	Vanuatu
Guinea		

1. Only includes countries for which prophylaxis is recommended. Regional variation in risk may exist within a country. More detailed information is available at www.cdc.gov/malaria and by phone for medical personnel from the Malaria Branch of the CDC at 770-488-7788.
2. Limited to Island of Saõ Tiago.
3. No malaria in major urban areas.
4. Chloroquine is the drug of choice for prophylaxis.
5. Only Great Exuma Island.
6. Chloroquine is recommended in Bocas del Toro province.
7. Chloroquine is recommended except in Hainan and Yunnan provinces.

CHLOROQUINE-RESISTANT MALARIA — Three drugs of choice with similar efficacy, listed with their dosages in the table on the next page, are available in the US for prevention of chloroquine-resistant malaria.

A fixed-dose combination of **atovaquone and proguanil** *(Malarone)* taken once daily is generally the best tolerated prophylactic,[46] but it can cause headache, insomnia, GI disturbances and mouth ulcers. Single case reports of Stevens-Johnson syndrome and hepatitis have been published. Atovaquone/proguanil should not be given to patients with severe renal impairment (CrCl <30 mL/min). There have been isolated case reports of treatment-related resistance to atovaquone/proguanil in *Plasmodium falciparum* in Africa, but Medical Letter consultants do not believe there is a high risk for acquisition of resistant disease.[47-50] In one study of malaria prophylaxis, atovaquone/proguanil was as effective and better tolerated than mefloquine in nonimmune travelers.[51] The protective efficacy of atovaquone/proguanil against *P. vivax* is variable ranging from 84% in Indonesian New Guinea[52] to 100% in Colombia.[53] Some Medical Letter consultants prefer other drugs if traveling to areas where *P. vivax* predominates.

Mefloquine has the advantage of once-a-week dosing, but is contraindicated in patients with a history of any psychiatric disorder (including severe anxiety and depression), and also in those with a history of seizures or cardiac conduction abnormalities.[54] Dizziness, headache, insomnia and disturbing dreams are the most common CNS adverse effects. The drug's adverse effects in children are similar to those in adults. If a patient develops psychological or behavioral abnormalities such as depression, restlessness or confusion while taking mefloquine, another drug should be substituted. Mefloquine should not be given together with quinine, quinidine or halofantrine due to potential prolongation of the QT interval; caution is required when using these drugs to treat patients who have taken mefloquine prophylaxis.

DRUGS OF CHOICE FOR PREVENTION OF MALARIA[1]

Drug	Adult dosage
All *Plasmodium* species in chloroquine-sensitive areas[2]	
Drug of Choice[3,4]:	
Chloroquine phosphate[5]	500 mg (300 mg base)
(*Aralen*, and others)	PO once/wk
All *Plasmodium* species in chloroquine-resistant areas[2]	
Drug of Choice[3]:	
Atovaquone/proguanil[6]	1 adult tablet daily
(*Malarone, Malarone Pediatric*)	
OR Doxycycline[7]	100 mg PO daily
(*Vibramycin*, and others)	
OR Mefloquine[8]	250 mg PO once/wk[9]
Alternative:	
Primaquine phosphate[11,12]	30 mg base PO daily

1. No drug guarantees protection against malaria. Travelers should be advised to seek medical attention if fever develops after they return. Insect repellents, insec-ticide-impregnated bed nets and proper clothing are important adjuncts for malaria prophylaxis.
2. Chloroquine-resistant *P. falciparum* occurs in all malarious areas except Central America (including Panama north and west of the Canal Zone), Mexico, Haiti, the Dominican Republic, Paraguay, northern Argentina, North and South Korea, Georgia, Armenia, most of rural China and some countries in the Middle East (chloroquine resistance has been reported in Yemen, Saudi Arabia and Iran). *P. vivax* with decreased susceptibility to chloroquine is a significant problem in Papua New Guinea and Indonesia. There are also a few reports of resistance from Myanmar, India, the Solomon Islands, Vanuatu, Guyana, Brazil, Colombia and Peru (JK Baird et al, Curr Infect Dis Rep 2007; 9:39). Chloroquine-resistant *P. malariae* has been reported from Sumatra (JD Maguire et al, Lancet 2002; 360:58).
3. Primaquine is given for prevention of relapse after infection with *P. vivax* or *P. ovale*. Some experts also prescribe primaquine phosphate 30 mg base/d (0.6 mg base/kg/d for children) for 14d after departure from areas where these species are endemic (Presumptive Anti-Relapse Therapy [PART], "terminal prophylaxis"). Since this is not always effective as prophylaxis (E Schwartz et al, N Engl J Med 2003; 349:1510), others prefer to rely on surveillance to detect cases when they occur, particularly when exposure was limited or doubtful. See also footnote 11.
4. Alternatives for patients who are unable to take chloroquine include atovaquone/proguanil, mefloquine, doxycycline or primaquine dosed as for chloroquine-resistant areas.
5. Chloroquine should be taken with food to decrease gastrointestinal adverse effects. If chloroquine phosphate is not available, hydroxychloroquine sulfate is as effective; 400 mg of hydroxychloroquine sulfate is equivalent to 500 mg of chloroquine phosphate.

Pediatric dosage	Duration
5 mg/kg base (300 mg max) PO once/wk	Start: 1-2 wks before travel Stop: 4 wks after leaving malarious zone
5-8 kg: ½ peds tab/d 9-10 kg: ¾ peds tab/d 11-20 kg: 1 peds tab/d 21-30 kg: 2 peds tabs/d 31-40 kg: 3 peds tabs/d >40 kg: 1 adult tab/d	Start: 1-2d before travel Stop: 1 wk after leaving malarious zone
2 mg/kg/d PO, up to 100 mg/d	Start: 1-2d before travel Stop: 4 wks after leaving malarious zone
5-10 kg: $^1/_8$ tab once/wk[9,10] 11-20 kg: ¼ tabs once/wk[9,10] 21-30 kg: ½ tab once/wk[9] 31-45 kg: ¾ tab once/wk[9] >45 kg: 1 tab once/wk[9]	Start: 1-2 wks before travel Stop: 4 wks after leaving malarious zone
0.6 mg/kg base PO daily	Start: 1d before travel Stop: 1 wk after leaving malarious zone

6. Atovaquone/proguanil is available as a fixed-dose combination tablet: adult tablets (*Malarone*; 250 mg atovaquone/100 mg proguanil) and pediatric tablets (*Malarone Pediatric*; 62.5 mg atovaquone/25 mg proguanil). To enhance absorption and reduce nausea and vomiting, it should be taken with food or a milky drink. The drug should not be given to patients with severe renal impairment (creatinine clearance <30 mL/min).

7. Doxycycline should be taken with adequate water to avoid esophageal irritation. It can be taken with food to minimize gastrointestinal adverse effects. It is contraindicated in children <8 years old.

8. In the US, a 250-mg tablet of mefloquine contains 228 mg mefloquine base. Outside the US, each 275-mg tablet contains 250 mg base. Mefloquine can be given to patients taking ß-blockers if they do not have an underlying arrhythmia; it should not be used in patients with conduction abnormalities. Mefloquine should not be taken on an empty stomach; it should be taken with at least 8 oz. of water.

9. Most adverse events occur within 3 doses. Some Medical Letter consultants favor starting mefloquine 3 weeks prior to travel and monitoring the patient for adverse events; this allows time to change to an alternative regimen if mefloquine is not tolerated.

10. For pediatric doses <½ tablet, it is advisable to have a pharmacist crush the tablet, estimate doses by weighing, and package them in gelatin capsules. There is no data for use in children <5 kg, but based on dosages in other weight groups, a dose of 5 mg/kg can be used.

11. Patients should be screened for G-6-PD deficiency before treatment with primaquine. It should be taken with food to minimize nausea and abdominal pain.

12. Not FDA-approved for this indication.

Doxycycline (*Vibramycin*, and others), which frequently causes GI disturbances and can cause photosensitivity and vaginitis, offers an inexpensive once-daily alternative. Doxycycline should not be taken concurrently with antacids, oral iron or bismuth salts

A fourth drug, **primaquine phosphate,** can also be used for prophylaxis, especially in areas where *P. vivax* is the predominant species, but in other areas should be reserved for travelers unable to take any other drug; it is somewhat less effective than the alternatives against *P. falciparum.* However, several studies have shown that daily primaquine can provide effective prophylaxis against chloroquine-resistant *P. falciparum* and *P. vivax.*[55] Some experts also prescribe primaquine for prophylaxis after departure from areas where *P. vivax* and *P. ovale* are endemic (see table on previous page, footnote 3).

Primaquine can cause hemolytic anemia in patients with glucose-6-phosphate dehydrogenase (G-6-PD) deficiency, which is most common in African, Asian, and Mediterranean peoples. Travelers should be screened for G-6-PD deficiency before treatment with the drug. Primaquine should be taken with food to reduce GI effects.

MEFLOQUINE-RESISTANT MALARIA — Doxycycline or atovaquone/proguanil is recommended for prophylaxis against mefloquine-resistant malaria, which occurs in the malarious areas of Thailand and in the areas of Myanmar and Cambodia that border on Thailand. It has also been reported on the borders between Myanmar and China, and Laos and Myanmar, and in southern Vietnam.

PREGNANCY — Malaria in pregnancy is particularly serious for both mother and fetus; prophylaxis is indicated if travel cannot be avoided. Chloroquine has been used extensively and safely for prophylaxis of chloroquine-sensitive malaria during pregnancy. Mefloquine is not approved for use during pregnancy. It has, however, been reported to be safe for prophylactic use during the second or third trimester of pregnancy and possibly during early pregnancy as well.[56,57] The safety of atovaquone/proguanil in pregnancy has not been established, and its use is not recommended. However, outcomes were normal in 24 women treated with the combination in the second and third trimester,[58] and proguanil alone has been used in pregnancy without evidence of toxicity. Doxycycline and primaquine are contraindicated in pregnancy.

PREVENTION OF INSECT BITES

To minimize insect bites, travelers should wear light-colored, long-sleeved shirts, pants, socks and covered shoes. They should sleep in air conditioned or screened areas and use insecticide-impregnated bed nets. Mosquitoes that transmit malaria are most active between dusk and dawn; those that transmit dengue fever bite during the day, particularly during early morning and late afternoon.[59]

DEET — The most effective topical insect repellent is N, N-diethyl-m-toluamide (DEET).[60] Applied on exposed skin, DEET repels mosquitoes, as well as ticks, chiggers, fleas, gnats and some flies. DEET is available in formulations of 5-100% even though increasing the concentration above 50% does not seem to improve efficacy. Medical Letter consultants prefer concentrations of 30-35%. A long-acting DEET formulation originally developed for the US Armed Forces (US Army Extended Duration Topical Insect and Arthropod Repellent – EDTIAR) containing 25-33% DEET *(Ultrathon)* protects for 6-12 hours. A microencapsulated sustained-release formulation containing 20% DEET *(Sawyer Controlled Release)* is also available and can provide longer protection than similar concentrations of other DEET formulations.

According to the CDC, DEET is probably safe in children and infants >2 months old; the American Academy of Pediatrics recommends use of concentrations containing no more than 30%. One study found that applying DEET regularly during the second and third trimesters of pregnancy did not result in any adverse effects on the fetus.[61] DEET has been shown to decrease the effectiveness of sunscreens when it is applied after the sunscreen; nevertheless, sunscreen should be applied first because it may increase the absorption of DEET when DEET is applied first.[62]

PICARIDIN — Picaridin has been available in Europe and Australia for many years. Data on the 7% and 15% formulations *(Cutter Advanced)* currently sold in the US are limited. The 20% formulation (*Natrapel 8 Hour*; *GoReady*) has been shown to protect for up to 8 hours; in clinical trials it has been about as effective as 20% DEET.[63-65]

PERMETHRIN — An insecticide available in liquid and spray form, permethrin (*Duranon*, *Permanone*, and others) can be used on clothing, mosquito nets, tents and sleeping bags for protection against mosquitoes and ticks. After application to clothing, it remains active for several weeks through multiple launderings. Using permethrin-impregnated mosquito nets while sleeping is helpful when rooms are not screened or air-conditioned. If bednets or tents are immersed in the liquid, the effect can last for about 6 months. The combination of DEET on exposed skin and permethrin on clothing provides increased protection.

SOME OTHER INFECTIONS

DENGUE — Dengue fever is a viral disease transmitted by mosquito bites that occurs worldwide in tropical and subtropical areas, including cities. Epidemics have occurred in recent years in Southeast Asia (especially Thailand), South Central Asia, sub-Saharan Africa, the South Pacific and Australia, Central and South America and the Caribbean. It has also been reported in travelers from the US vacationing at popular tourist destinations in Puerto Rico, the US Virgin Islands and Mexico.[66] Prevention of mosquito bites during the day, particularly in early morning and late afternoon, is the primary way to protect against dengue fever; no vaccine is currently available.

LEPTOSPIROSIS — Leptospirosis, a bacterial disease that occurs in many domestic and wild animals, is endemic worldwide, but the highest incidence is in tropical and subtropical areas. Transmission to humans usually occurs through contact with fresh water or damp soil contaminated by the urine of infected animals.[67] Travelers at increased risk, such as adventure travelers and those who engage in recreational water activities, should consider prophylaxis with doxycycline 200 mg orally once a week, beginning 1-2 days before and continuing throughout the period of exposure. No human vaccine is available in the US.

NON-INFECTIOUS RISKS OF TRAVEL

Many non-infectious risks are associated with travel. Injuries, particularly **traffic accidents** and **drowning**, which account for the majority of travel-related deaths, and **sunburn** occur in many travelers.

HIGH ALTITUDE ILLNESS — Rapid exposure to altitudes >8,000 feet (2500 meters) may cause acute mountain sickness (headache, fatigue, nausea, anorexia, insomnia, dizziness); pulmonary and cerebral edema can occur.[68] Sleeping altitude appears to be especially important in determining whether symptoms develop. The most effective preventive measure is pre-acclimatization by a 2- to 4-day stay at intermediate altitude (6000-8000 feet) and gradual ascent to higher elevations.

Acetazolamide, a carbonic anhydrase inhibitor taken in a dosage of 125-250 mg twice daily (or 500 mg daily with the slow-release formulation *Diamox Sequels*) beginning 1-2 days before ascent and continuing at high altitude for 48 hours or longer, decreases the incidence and severity of acute mountain sickness.[69] The recommended dose for children is 5 mg/kg/d in 2 or 3 divided doses. Although acetazolamide, a sulfone, has little cross-reactivity with sulfa drugs, hypersensitivity reactions to acetazolamide are more likely to occur in those who have had severe (life-threatening) allergic reactions to sulfa drugs.[70]

Symptoms can be treated after they occur by descent to a lower altitude or by giving supplemental oxygen, especially during sleep. When descent is impossible, dexamethasone (*Decadron*, and others) 4 mg q6h, acetazolamide 250-500 mg q12h, or the two together, may help. Nifedipine (*Procardia*, and others), 20-30 mg twice daily may also be helpful.

VENOUS THROMBOEMBOLISM — Prolonged immobilization, particularly during air travel, increases the risk of lower extremity deep vein thrombosis (DVT). Travelers with risk factors for thrombosis (past history of thrombosis, obesity, malignancy, increased platelets) are at even higher risk. Nevertheless, flight-related symptomatic pulmonary embolism is rare.[71]

To minimize the risk, travelers should be advised to walk around or, if necessary, exercise while sitting by flexing/extending ankles and knees, to drink extra fluids, and to avoid alcohol and caffeine. Compression stockings can decrease the risk of asymptomatic DVT.[72] Giving a single dose of a low-molecular-weight heparin as prophylaxis to travelers at high risk reduced the incidence of DVT in a clinical trial.[73]

JET LAG — Disturbance of body and environmental rhythms resulting from a rapid change in time zones gives rise to jet lag, which is characterized by insomnia, decreased quality of sleep, loss of concentration, irritability and GI disturbances. It is usually more severe after eastward travel.[74]

A variety of interventions have been tried, but none is proven to be effective. Shifting daily activities to correspond to the time zone of the destination country before arrival along with taking short naps, remaining well hydrated, avoiding alcohol and pursuing activities in sunlight on arrival may help. The dietary supplement melatonin (0.5-5 mg started on the first night of travel and continued for 1-5 days after arrival) has been reported to facilitate the shift of the sleep-wake cycle and decrease symptoms in some patients. A program of appropriately timed light exposure and avoidance in the new time zone may adjust the "body clock" and reduce jet lag.[75] In one study, zolpidem (*Ambien*, and others) started the first night after travel and taken for 3 nights was helpful.[76]

MOTION SICKNESS — Therapeutic options for motion sickness remain limited.[77] A transdermal patch or oral formulation of the prescription cholinergic blocker scopolamine can decrease symptoms. *Transderm Scop* is applied to the skin behind the ear at least 4 hours before exposure and changed, alternating ears, every 3 days. The oral 8-hour tablet *(Scopace)* is taken 1 hour before exposure. Oral promethazine (*Phenergan*, and others) is a highly sedating alternative. Over-the-counter drugs such as dimenhydrinate (*Dramamine*, and others) or meclizine (*Bonine*, and others) are less effective, but may be helpful for milder symptoms.

1. DR Hill et al. The practice of travel medicine: guidelines by the Infectious Diseases Society of America. Clin Infect Dis 2006; 43:1499.
2. Adult immunization. Treat Guidel Med Lett 2009; 7:27.
3. D Daniels et al. Surveillance for acute viral hepatitis-United States, 2007. MMWR Surveill Summ 2009; 58(SS03):1.
4. P Van Damme et al. Hepatitis A booster vaccination: is there a need? Lancet 2003; 362:1065.
5. JN Zuckerman et al. Hepatitis A and B booster recommendations: implications for travelers. Clin Infect Dis 2005; 41:1020.
6. S Iwarson et al. Excellent booster response 4 to 8 years after a single primary dose of an inactivated hepatitis A vaccine. J Travel Med 2004; 11:120.
7. Advisory Committee on Immunization Practices (ACIP) Centers for Disease Control and Prevention (CDC). Update: prevention of hepatitis A after exposure to hepatitis A virus and in international travelers. Updated recommendations of the Advisory Committee on Immunization Practices (ACIP). MMWR Morb Mortal Wkly Rep 2007; 56:1080.
8. BA Connor and DJ Patron. Use of an accelerated immunization schedule for combined hepatitis A and B protection in the corporate traveler. J Occup Environ Med 2008; 50:945.
9. DO Freedman and K Leder. Influenza: changing approaches to prevention and treatment in travelers. J Travel Med 2005; 12:36.
10. Seasonal trivalent influenza vaccine for 2009-2010. Med Lett Drugs Ther 2009; 51:73.
11. Centers for Disease Control and Prevention (CDC). Use of northern hemisphere influenza vaccines by travelers to the southern hemisphere. MMWR Morb Mortal Weekly Rep 2009; 58:312.
12. H1N1 Vaccine for prevention of pandemic influenza. Med Lett Drugs Ther 2009; 51:77.

13. MR Buhl and L Lindquist. Japanese encephalitis in travelers: review of cases and seasonal risk. J Travel Med 2009; 16:217.

14. ACIP provisional recommendations for the use of Japanese encephalitis virus vaccines, June 24, 2009. Available at www.cdc.gov/vaccines/recs/provisional/downloads/je-july2009-508.pdf. Accessed October 5, 2009.

15. A new Japanese encephalitis vaccine (*Ixiaro*). Med Lett Drugs Ther 2009; 51:66.

16. ST Duggan and GL Plosker. Japanese enecphalitis vaccine (inactivated, adsorbed) [IXIARO]. Drugs 2009; 69:115.

17. ACIP Provisional Recommendations for measles-mumps-rubella (MMR) 'evidence of immunity' requirements for healthcare personnel. Available at: www.cdc.gov/vaccines/recs/provisional/default.htm. Accessed October 5, 2009.

18. A Wilder-Smith. Meningococcal disease: risk for international travellers and vaccine strategies. Travel Med Infect Dis 2008; 6:182.

19. OO Bilukha and N Rosenstein; National Center for Infectious Diseases, Centers for Disease Control and Prevention (CDC). Prevention and control of meningococcal disease. recommendations of the Advisory Committee on Immunization Practices (ACIP). MMWR Recomm Rep 2005; 54 (RR-7):1.

20. Committee to Advise on Tropical Medicine and Travel (CATMAT). Statement on meningococcal vaccination for travellers. An Advisory Committee Statement (ACS). Can Commun Dis Rep 2009; 35(ACS-4):1.

21. CDC Vaccine safety updates. GBS and Menactra meningococcal vaccine. Available at: www.cdc.gov/vaccinesafety/updates/gbsfact sheet.htm. Accessed October 5, 2009.

22. Centers for Disease Control and Prevention (CDC). Update on vaccine-derived polioviruses—worldwide, January 2008-June 2009. MMWR Morb Mortal Wkly Rep 2009; 58:1002.

23. CE Rupprecht and RV Gibbons. Clinical practice. Prophylaxis against rabies. N Engl J Med 2004; 351:2626.

24. FX Meslin. Rabies as a traveler's risk, especially in high-endemicity areas. J Travel Med 2005; 12 Suppl 1:S30.

25. ACIP provisional recommendations for the prevention of human rabies. July 10, 2009. Available at www.cdc.gov/vaccines/recs/provisional/downloads/rabies-July 2009-508.pdf. Accessed October 5, 2009.

26. SE Manning et al. Human rabies prevention—United States, 2008: recommendations of the Advisory Committee on Immunization Practices (ACIP). MMWR Recomm Rep 2008; 57 (RR-3):1.

27. Adacel and Boostrix: Tdap vaccines for adolescents and adults. Med Lett Drugs Ther 2006; 48:5.

28. A Banzhoff et al. Protection against tick-borne encephalitis (TBE) for people living in and traveling to TBE-endemic areas. Travel Med Infect Dis 2008; 6:331.

29. U Kunze. Is there a need for a travel vaccination against tick-borne encephalitis? Travel Med Infect Dis 2008; 6:380.

30. MF Lynch et al. Typhoid fever in The United States, 1999-2006. JAMA 2009; 302:859.

31. JA Whitaker et al. Rethinking typhoid fever vaccines: implications for travelers and people living in highly endemic areas. J Travel Med 2009; 16:46.

32. ED Barnett. Yellow fever: epidemiology and prevention. Clin Infect Dis 2007; 44:850.

33. Search for yellow fever vaccination clinics. Updated Jan 28, 2008. Available at: wwwn.cdc.gov/travel/yellow-fever-vaccination-clinics-search.aspx. Accessed Oct 5, 2009.

34. AW McMahon et al. Neurologic disease associated with 17D-204 yellow fever vaccination: a report of 15 cases. Vaccine 2007; 25:1727.

35. ED Barnett et al. Yellow fever vaccines and international travelers. Expert Rev Vaccines 2008; 7:579.

36. HL DuPont et al. Expert review of the evidence base for self-therapy of travelers' diarrhea. J Travel Med 2009; 16:161.

37. JA Adachi et al. Azithromycin found to be comparable to levofloxacin for the treatment of US travelers with acute diarrhea acquired in Mexico. Clin Infect Dis 2003; 37:1165.

38. CD Ericsson et al. Loperamide plus azithromycin more effectively treats travelers' diarrhea in Mexico than azithromycin alone. J Travel Med 2007; 14:312.

39. D Jain et al. *Campylobacter* species and drug resistance in a north Indian rural community. Trans R Soc Trop Med Hyg 2005; 99:207.

40. DR Tribble et al. Traveler's diarrhea in Thailand: randomized, double-blind trial comparing single-dose and 3-day azithromycin-based regimens with a 3-day levofloxacin regimen. Clin Infect Dis 2007; 44:338.

41. AL Pakyz. Rifaximin: a new treatment for travelers' diarrhea. Ann Pharmacother 2005; 39:284.

42. MS Riddle et al. Effect of adjunctive loperamide in combination with antibiotics on treatment outcomes in traveler's diarrhea: a systematic review and meta-analysis. Clin Infect Dis 2008; 47:1007.

43. HL DuPont et al. Expert review of the evidence base for prevention of travelers' diarrhea. J Travel Med 2009; 16:149.

44. HL DuPont et al. A randomized, double-blind, placebo-controlled trial of rifaximin to prevent travelers' diarrhea. Ann Intern Med 2005; 142:805.

45. DO Freedman. Clinical practice. Malaria prevention in short-term travelers. N Engl J Med 2008; 359:603.

46. PJ van Genderen et al. The safety and tolerance of atovaquone/proguanil for the long-term prophylaxis of plasmodium falciparum malaria in non-immune travelers and expatriates [corrected]. J Travel Med 2007; 14:92.

47. E Schwartz et al. Genetic confirmation of atovaquone-proguanil-resistant Plasmodium falciparum malaria acquired by a nonimmune traveler to East Africa. Clin Infect Dis 2003; 37:450.

48. A Färnert et al. Evidence of *Plasmodium falciparum* malaria resistant to atovaquone and proguanil hydrochloride: case reports. BMJ 2003; 326:628.

49. S Kuhn et al. Emergence of atovaquone-proguanil resistance during treatment of *Plasmodium falciparum* malaria acquired by a non-immune North American traveller to west Africa. Am J Trop Med Hyg 2005; 72:407.

50. CT Happi et al. Confirmation of emergence of mutations associated with atovaquone-proguanil resistance in unexposed *Plasmodium falciparum* isolates from Africa. Malaria J 2006; 5:82.

51. D Overbosch et al. Atovaquone-proguanil versus mefloquine for malaria prophylaxis in nonimmune travelers: results from a randomized, double-blind study. Clin Infect Dis 2001; 33:1015.
52. J Ling et al. Randomized, placebo-controlled trial of atovaquone/proguanil for the prevention of *Plasmodium falciparum* or *Plasmodium vivax* malaria among migrants to Papua, Indonesia. Clin Infect Dis 2002; 35:825.
53. J Soto et al. Randomized, double-blind, placebo-controlled study of Malarone for malaria prophylaxis in non-immune Colombian soldiers. Am J Trop Med Hyg 2006; 75:430.
54. LH Chen et al. Controversies and misconceptions in malaria chemoprophylaxis for travelers. JAMA 2007; 297:2251.
55. DR Hill et al. Primaquine: report from CDC expert meeting on malaria chemoprophylaxis I. Am J Trop Med Hyg 2006; 75:402.
56. Centers for Disease Control and Prevention. CDC Health Information for International Travel 2010. Atlanta: U.S. Department of Health and Human Services, Public Health Service, 2009, p 469.
57. BL Smoak et al. The effects of inadvertent exposure of mefloquine chemoprophylaxis on pregnancy outcomes and infants of US Army servicewomen. J Infect Dis 1997; 176:831.
58. R McGready et al. The pharmacokinetics of atovaquone and proguanil in pregnant women with acute falciparum malaria. Eur J Clin Pharmacol 2003; 59:545.
59. Committee to Advise on Tropical Medicine and Travel (CATMAT). Statement on personal protective measures to prevent arthropod bites. Can Commun Dis Rep 2005; 31 (ACS-4):1.
60. TM Katz et al. Insect repellents: historical perspectives and new developments. J Am Acad Dermatol 2008; 58:865.
61. R McGready et al. Safety of the insect repellent N,N-diethyl-M-toluamide (DEET) in pregnancy. Am J Trop Med Hyg 2001; 65:285.
62. Sunscreens: an update. Med Lett Drugs Ther 2008; 50:70.
63. A Badolo et al. Evaluation of the sensitivity of *Aedes aegypti* and *Anopheles gambiae* complex mosquitoes to two insect repellents: DEET and KBR 3023. Trop Med Int Health 2004; 9:330.
64. SP Frances et al. Laboratory and field evaluation of commercial repel-lent formulations against mosquitoes (diptera: culcidae) in Queensland, Australia. Aust J Entomol 2005; 44:431.
65. C Constantini et al. Field evaluation of the efficacy and persistence of insect repellents DEET, IR3535, and KBR 3023 against *Anopheles gambiae* complex and other Afrotropical vector mosquitoes. Trans R Soc Trop Med Hyg 2004; 98:644.
66. A Wilder-Smith and DJ Gubler. Geographic expansion of dengue: the impact of international travel. Med Clin North Am 2008; 92:1377.
67. A Pavli and HC Maltezou. Travel-acquired leptospirosis. J Travel Med 2008; 15:447.
68. SA Gallagher and PH Hackett. High-altitude illness. Emerg Med Clin North Am 2004; 22:329.
69. B Basnyat et al. Acetazolamide 125 mg BD is not significantly different from 375 mg BD in the prevention of acute mountain sickness: the prophylactic acetazolamide dosage comparison for efficacy (PACE) trial. High Alt Med Biol 2006; 7:17.

70. BL Strom et al. Absence of cross-reactivity between sulfonamide antibiotics and sulfonamide nonantibiotics. N Engl J Med 2003; 349:1628.
71. D Chandra et al. Meta-analysis: travel and risk for venous thromboembolism. Ann Intern Med 2009; 151:180.
72. M Clarke et al. Compression stockings for preventing deep vein thrombosis in airline passengers. Cochrane Database Syst Rev 2006; (2):CD004002.
73. MR Cesarone et al. Venous thrombosis from air travel: the LON-FLIT3 study–prevention with aspirin vs low-molecular-weight heparin (LMWH) in high-risk subjects: a randomized trial. Angiology 2002; 53:1.
74. RL Sack. The pathophysiology of jet lag. Travel Med Infect Dis 2009; 7:102.
75. J Waterhouse et al. Jet lag: trends and coping strategies. Lancet 2007; 369:1117.
76. AO Jamieson et al. Zolpidem reduces the sleep disturbance of jet lag. Sleep Med 2001; 2:423.
77. JF Golding and MA Gresty. Motion sickness. Curr Opin Neurol 2005; 18:29.

PRINCIPAL ADVERSE EFFECTS OF ANTIMICROBIAL DRUGS

Adverse effects of antimicrobial drugs vary with dosage, duration of administration, concomitant therapy, renal and hepatic function, immune competence, and the age of the patient. The principal adverse effects of antimicrobial agents are listed in the following table. The designation of adverse effects as "frequent," "occasional" or "rare" is based on published reports and on the experience of Medical Letter consultants. Information about adverse interactions between drugs, including probable mechanisms and recommendations for clinical management, are available in The Medical Letter Adverse Drug Interactions Program.

ABACAVIR (*Ziagen*)
Frequent: hypersensitivity reaction with fever, GI or respiratory symptoms and rash
Occasional: arthralgias; anemia; syndrome of lactic acidosis with hepatomegaly and steatosis
Rare: anaphylaxis; pancreatitis; hyperglycemia

ABACAVIR-LAMIVUDINE (*Epzicom*) — See individual drugs

ACYCLOVIR (*Zovirax*, others)
Frequent: local irritation at infusion site
Occasional: local reactions with topical use; rash, nausea, diarrhea, headache, vertigo and arthralgias with oral use; decreased renal function sometimes progressing to renal failure; metabolic encephalopathy; bone marrow depression; abnormal hepatic function in immunocompromised patients
Rare: lethargy or agitation; tremor, disorientation; hallucinations; transient hemiparesthesia

ADEFOVIR (*Hepsera*)
Frequent: asthenia; headache; abdominal pain
Occasional: exacerbation of hepatitis B with drug discontinuation
Rare: increased serum creatinine; azotemia and renal tubular dysfunction

with high doses (30-60 mg/d) and/or pre-existing renal impairment

ALBENDAZOLE (*Albenza*)
Occasional: abdominal pain; increased aminotransferases; reversible alopecia
Rare: leukopenia; rash; renal toxicity

AMANTADINE (*Symmetrel*, others)
Frequent: livedo reticularis and ankle edema; insomnia; dizziness; lethargy
Occasional: depression; psychosis; confusion; slurred speech; visual disturbance; sudden loss of vision; increased seizures in epilepsy; congestive heart failure; orthostatic hypotension; urinary retention; GI disturbance; rash
Rare: seizures; leukopenia; neutropenia; eczematoid dermatitis; photosensitivity; oculogyric episodes

AMIKACIN (*Amikin*)
Occasional: vestibular damage; renal damage; fever; rash
Rare: auditory damage; CNS reactions; blurred vision; neuromuscular blockade and apnea, may be reversible with calcium salts; paresthesias; hypotension; nausea; vomiting

AMINOSALICYLIC ACID (*Paser*)
Frequent: GI disturbance

Occasional: allergic reactions; liver damage; renal irritation; hematologic abnormalities; thyroid enlargement; malabsorption syndrome
Rare: acidosis; hypokalemia; encephalopathy; vasculitis; hypoglycemia in diabetics

AMOXICILLIN — See Penicillins

AMOXICILLIN/CLAVULANIC ACID — See Penicillins

AMPHOTERICIN B DEOXYCHOLATE (*Fungizone*, others)
Frequent: renal damage; hypokalemia; thrombophlebitis at site of peripheral vein infusion; anorexia; nausea; weight loss; bone marrow suppression with reversible decline in hematocrit; headache; chills, fever, vomiting during infusion, possibly with delirium, hypotension or hypertension, wheezing, and hypoxemia
Occasional: hypomagnesemia; normocytic, normochromic anemia
Rare: hemorrhagic gastroenteritis; rash; blurred vision; peripheral neuropathy; seizures; anaphylaxis; arrhythmias; acute liver failure; reversible nephrogenic diabetes insipidus; hearing loss; acute pulmonary edema; spinal cord damage with intrathecal use

AMPHOTERICIN B LIPID FORMULATIONS (*Ambisone, Abelcet, Amphotec*) — See page 152.

AMPICILLIN — See Penicillins

AMPICILLIN/SULBACTAM — See Penicillins

AMPRENAVIR (*Agenerase*)
Frequent: GI disturbance; oral and perioral paresthesias; rash; hypersensitivity with fever
Occasional: hyperglycemia; increased aminotransferases; hyperlipidemia; abnormal fat distribution

Rare: severe rash including Stevens-Johnson syndrome; hemolytic anemia

ANIDULAFUNGIN (*Eraxis*)
Occasional: Infusion-related rash; urticaria; flushing; pruritus; dyspnea and hypotension; fever; nausea; vomiting; hypokalemia
Rare: hepatitis

ARTEMETHER (*Artenam*)
Occasional: neurological toxicity; possible increase in length of coma in cerebral malaria; seizures; QTc prolongation

ARTEMETHER/LUMEFANTRINE (*Coartem/Riamet*)
Frequent: abdominal pain; anorexia; headache; dizziness; diarrhea; vomiting; nausea; palpitations; arthralgia; myalgia; asthenia; fatigue; pruritus; rash; sleep disorder; cough
Occasional: somnolence; involuntary muscle contractions; paresthesia; hypoesthesia; abnormal gait; ataxia
Rare: hypersensitivity

ARTESUNATE
Occasional: neurological toxicity; ataxia; slurred speech; possible increase in length of coma in cerebral malaria; seizures; QTc prolongation
Rare: neutropenia with high doses (6 mg/kg/d)

ATAZANAVIR (*Reyataz*)
Frequent: hyperbilirubinemia; nausea; rash
Occasional: increased cholesterol and triglycerides; depression; headache; dizziness; fatigue; fever
Rare: insomnia; peripheral neuropathy; PR prolongation; heart block; angioedema; alopecia; Stevens-Johnson syndrome; gout; kidney stones; myasthenia; hepatitis; pancreatitis; diabetes

ATOVAQUONE (*Mepron, Malarone* [with *proguanil*])
Frequent: headache; rash; nausea

Occasional: diarrhea; increased amino-transferases; cholestasis; insomnia; mouth ulcers
Rare: Stevens-Johnson syndrome; hepatitis

AZITHROMYCIN (*Zithromax*, others)
Occasional: GI disturbance; headache; dizziness; vaginitis
Rare: angioedema; cholestatic jaundice; photosensitivity; reversible dose-related hearing loss; QTc prolongation; CDAD

AZT — See Zidovudine

AZTREONAM (*Azactam*)
Occasional: local reaction at injection site; rash; diarrhea; nausea; vomiting; increased aminotransferases
Rare: thrombocytopenia

BACITRACIN — many manufacturers
Frequent: nephrotoxicity; GI disturbance
Occasional: rash; hematologic abnormalities
Rare: anaphylaxis

BENZNIDAZOLE (*Rochagan*)
Frequent: rash; dose-dependent polyneuropathy; GI disturbance; psychic disturbances

BITHIONOL (*Bitin*)
Frequent: photosensitivity reactions; nausea; vomiting; diarrhea; abdominal pain; urticaria
Rare: leukopenia; hepatitis

CAPREOMYCIN (*Capastat*)
Occasional: renal damage; eighth nerve damage; hypokalemia and other electrolyte abnormalities; pain, induration, excessive bleeding, and sterile abscess at injection site
Rare: allergic reactions; leukocytosis, leukopenia; neuromuscular blockade and apnea with large IV doses, reversed by neostigmine

CARBENICILLIN — See Penicillins

CASPOFUNGIN (*Cancidas*)
Occasional: fever; rash; increased aminotransferases; GI disturbance; facial flushing; hypokalemia
Rare: anaphylaxis; Stevens-Johnson syndrome; exfoliative dermatitis

CEPHALOSPORINS
(cefaclor - *Ceclor*; cefadroxil - *Duricef*, others; cefazolin - *Ancef*, others; cefdinir - *Omnicef*; cefditoren pivoxil - *Spectracef*; cefepime - *Maxipime*; cefixime - *Suprax*; cefoperazone - *Cefobid*; cefotaxime - *Claforan*; cefotetan; cefoxitin - *Mefoxin*; cefpodoxime - *Vantin*; cefprozil - *Cefzil*; ceftaroline - *Teflaro*; ceftazidime - *Fortaz, Tazidime, Tazicef, Ceptaz*; ceftibuten - *Cedax*; ceftizoxime - *Cefizox*; ceftriaxone - *Rocephin*; cefuroxime - *Kefurox, Zinacef*; cefuroxime axetil - *Ceftin*; cephalexin - *Keflex*, others; cephapirin - *Cefadyl*, others; cephradine - *Velosef*, others; loracarbef - *Lorabid*
Frequent: thrombophlebitis with IV use; serum-sickness-like reaction with prolonged parenteral administration; moderate to severe diarrhea, especially with cefoperazone and cefixime
Occasional: hypersensitivity reactions, rarely anaphylactic; pain at injection site; GI disturbance; hypoprothrombinemia, hemorrhage with cefamandole, cefoperazone or cefotetan; rash and arthritis ("serum-sickness") with cefaclor or cefprozil, especially in children; cholelithiasis with ceftriaxone; vaginal candidiasis (especially with cefdinir); carnitine deficiency with prolonged use of cefditoren
Rare: hemolytic anemia; hematologic abnormalities; hepatic dysfunction; renal damage; acute interstitial nephritis; CDAD; seizures; encephalopathy; toxic epidermal necrolysis

CHLORAMPHENICOL (*Chloromycetin*, others)
Occasional: hematologic abnormalities; gray syndrome (cardiovascular collapse); GI disturbance

Rare: fatal aplastic anemia, even with eye drops or ointment; allergic and febrile reactions; peripheral neuropathy; optic neuritis and other CNS injury; CDAD

CHLOROQUINE HCL and **CHLORO-QUINE PHOSPHATE** (*Aralen*, others)
Occasional: pruritus; vomiting; headache; confusion; depigmentation of hair; partial alopecia; skin eruptions; corneal opacity; weight loss; extraocular muscle palsies; exacerbation of psoriasis, eczema, and other exfoliative dermatoses; myalgias; photophobia; QTc prolongation
Rare: irreversible retinal injury (especially when total dosage exceeds 100 grams); discoloration of nails and mucus membranes; nerve-type deafness; peripheral neuropathy and myopathy; heart block; torsades de pointes; hematologic abnormalities; hematemesis; seizures; neuropsychiatric changes

CIDOFOVIR (*Vistide*)
Frequent: nephrotoxicity; ocular hypotony; neutropenia
Occasional: metabolic acidosis; uveitis; Fanconi syndrome

CIPROFLOXACIN (*Cipro*, others) — See Fluoroquinolones

CLARITHROMYCIN (*Biaxin*, others)
Occasional: nausea; diarrhea; abdominal pain; abnormal taste; headache; dizziness; QTc prolongation
Rare: reversible dose-related hearing loss; pancreatitis; torsades de pointes; psychic disturbance (mania); CDAD

CLINDAMYCIN (*Cleocin*, others)
Frequent: diarrhea; hypersensitivity reactions
Occasional: CDAD can occur even with topical use
Rare: hematologic abnormalities; esophageal ulceration; hepatotoxicity; polyarthritis

CLOFAZIMINE (*Lamprene*)
Frequent: ichthyosis; pigmentation of skin, cornea and retina; urine discoloration; dryness and irritation of eyes; GI disturbance
Occasional: headache; retinal degeneration
Rare: splenic infarction, bowel obstruction, and GI bleeding with high doses

COLISTIMETHATE — See Polymyxins

CROTAMITON (*Eurax*)
Occasional: rash

CYCLOSERINE (*Seromycin*, others)
Frequent: anxiety; depression; confusion; disorientation; paranoia; hallucinations; somnolence; headache
Occasional: peripheral neuropathy; liver damage; malabsorption syndrome; folate deficiency
Rare: suicide; seizures; coma

DAPSONE
Frequent: rash; headache; GI disturbance; anorexia; infectious mononucleosis-like syndrome
Occasional: cyanosis due to methemoglobinemia and sulfhemoglobinemia; other hematologic abnormalities, including hemolytic anemia; nephrotic syndrome; liver damage; peripheral neuropathy; hypersensitivity reactions; increased risk of lepra reactions; insomnia; irritability; uncoordinated speech; agitation; acute psychosis
Rare: renal papillary necrosis; severe hypoalbuminemia; epidermal necrolysis; optic atrophy; agranulocytosis; neonatal hyperbilirubinemia after use in pregnancy

DAPTOMYCIN (*Cubicin*)
Occasional: GI disturbance; rash, injection site reaction; fever; headache; insomnia; dizziness
Rare: increased CPK and rhabdomyolysis; eosinophilic pneumonia; peripheral neuropathy; hypersensitivity reactions; CDAD

DARUNAVIR (*Prezista*)/**RITONAVIR** — See also Ritonavir

Frequent: GI disturbance
Occasional: headache; increased aminotransferases; increased cholesterol and triglycerides; rash
Rare: Stevens-Johnson syndrome; erythema multiforme; hepatitis

DELAVIRDINE *(Rescriptor)* — Similar to nevirapine, but rash may be less severe and hepatotoxicity is less common

DEMECLOCYCLINE — See Tetracyclines

DICLOXACILLIN — See Penicillins

DIDANOSINE (ddI; *Videx*)
    Frequent: peripheral neuropathy; GI disturbance
    Occasional: pancreatitis; hyperuricemia; increased aminotransferases; constipation; loss of taste; hypokalemia; headache; fever; rash; syndrome of lactic acidosis with hepatomegaly and steatosis; retinal depigmentation
    Rare: non-cirrhotic portal hypertension hepatic failure; retinal atrophy in children

DIETHYLCARBAMAZINE CITRATE *(Hetrazan)*
    Frequent: severe allergic or febrile reactions in patients with microfilaria in the blood or the skin; GI disturbance
    Rare: encephalopathy

DILOXANIDE FUROATE *(Furamide)*
    Frequent: flatulence
    Occasional: nausea; vomiting; diarrhea
    Rare: diplopia; dizziness; urticaria; pruritus

DORIPENEM *(Doribax)* — Similar to imipenem, but less likely to cause seizures

DOXYCYCLINE — See Tetracyclines

EFAVIRENZ *(Sustiva)*
    Frequent: dizziness; headache; inability to concentrate; insomnia and somno-

lence; rash
    Occasional: vivid dreams; nightmares; depression; hallucinations; hypersensitivity reaction with fever, GI or respiratory symptoms and rash; Stevens-Johnson syndrome; increased cholesterol and triglycerides
    Rare: pancreatitis; peripheral neuropathy; psychosis; photosensitivity reactions; gynecomastia

EFAVIRENZ-EMTRICITABINE-TENOFOVIR *(Atripla)* — See individual drugs.

EFLORNITHINE
(Difluoromethylornithine, DFMO, *Ornidyl*)
    Frequent: anemia; leukopenia
    Occasional: diarrhea; thrombocytopenia; seizures
    Rare: hearing loss

EMTRICITABINE (FTC, *Emtriva*)
    Frequent: headache; dizziness; insomnia; weakness; rash; GI disturbance; increased CPK
    Occasional: dream disturbances; increased triglycerides; hyperpigmentation of palms and soles; syndrome of lactic acidosis with hepatomegaly and steatosis; exacerbation of hepatitis B with drug discontinuation

EMTRICITABINE-TENOFOVIR *(Truvada)* — See individual drugs.

ENFUVIRTIDE *(Fuzeon)*
    Frequent: injection site reactions; insomnia; depression; increased triglycerides; neuropathy
    Occasional: rash; eosinophilia
    Rare: hypersensitivity reactions; increased bacterial pneumonias

ENTECAVIR *(Baraclude)*
    Occasional: headache; fatigue; nausea; dizziness; syndrome of lactic acidosis with hepatomegaly and steatosis; exacerbation of hepatitis B with drug discontinuation

Principal Adverse Effects of Antimicrobial Drugs

ERTAPENEM (*Invanz*)
Occasional: phlebitis; nausea; vomiting; diarrhea
Rare: seizures; CDAD

ERYTHROMYCIN (*Ery-Tab*, others)
Frequent: GI disturbance
Occasional: stomatitis; cholestatic hepatitis especially with erythromycin estolate in adults; QTc prolongation
Rare: allergic reactions, including severe respiratory distress; CDAD; hemolytic anemia; pancreatitis; transient hearing loss with high doses, prolonged use, or in patients with renal insufficiency; ventricular arrhythmias and torsades de pointes; aggravation of myasthenia gravis; hypothermia; hypertrophic pyloric stenosis following treatment of infants

ETHAMBUTOL (*Myambutol*)
Occasional: optic neuritis; allergic reactions; GI disturbance; mental confusion; precipitation of acute gout
Rare: peripheral neuritis; possible renal damage; thrombocytopenia; toxic epidermal necrolysis; lichenoid skin eruption

ETHIONAMIDE (*Trecator-SC*)
Frequent: GI disturbance
Occasional: liver damage; CNS disturbance; peripheral neuropathy; allergic reactions; gynecomastia; depres-sion; myalgias; hypotension
Rare: hypothyroidism; optic neuritis; arthritis; impotence

ETRAVIRINE (*Intelence*)
Occasional: rash; nausea; peripherial neuropathy; hypertension
Rare: Stevens-Johnson syndrome; erythema multiforme; increased aminotransferases; increased cholesterol and triglycerides

FAMCICLOVIR (*Famvir*)
Occasional: headache; nausea; diarrhea

FLUCONAZOLE (*Diflucan*, others)
Occasional: GI disturbance; increased aminotransferases; headache; rash; QTc prolongation
Rare: severe hepatic toxicity; exfoliative dermatitis; anaphylaxis; Stevens-Johnson syndrome; toxic epidermal necrolysis; hair loss; leukopenia

FLUCYTOSINE (*Ancobon*)
Frequent: hematologic abnormalities, including pancytopenia and fatal agranulo-cytosis; GI disturbance, including severe diarrhea and ulcerative colitis; hepatic dysfunction; rash
Occasional: confusion; hallucinations
Rare: anaphylaxis

FLUOROQUINOLONES
(ciprofloxacin – *Cipro*, others; gemifloxacin (*Factive)*; levofloxacin – *Levaquin*; moxi-floxacin – *Avelox*; norfloxacin – *Noroxin*; ofloxacin – *Floxin*)
Occasional: GI disturbance; dizziness; headache; tremors; restlessness; confu-sion; rash; Candida infections of the phar-ynx and vagina; eosinophilia; neutropenia; leukopenia; increased aminotransferases; hyper- and hypoglycemia; increased serum creatinine concentration; insomnia; photosensitivity reactions, especially with lomefloxacin; QTc prolongation
Rare: hallucinations; delirium; psychosis; vertigo; seizures; paresthesias; blurred vision and photophobia; severe hepatitis; hyper- and hypoglycemia; CDAD; interstitial nephritis; vasculitis; possible exacer-bation of myasthenia gravis; serum-sick-ness-like reaction; anaphylaxis; toxic epi-dermal necrolysis; anemia; tendinitis or tendon rupture; ventricular tachycardia and torsades de pointes; rhabdomyolysis with ofloxacin

FOSAMPRENAVIR (*Lexiva*)
Frequent: headache; fatigue; rash; GI disturbance
Occasional: depression; increased cho-lesterol and triglycerides; increased lipase and aminotransferases; perioral numbness or tingling

Rare: neutropenia; Stevens-Johnson syndrome

FOSCARNET (*Foscavir*)
Frequent: renal dysfunction; anemia; nausea; electrolyte disturbances
Occasional: headache; vomiting; fatigue; genital ulceration; seizures; neuropathy; hematologic abnormalities
Rare: Nephrogenic diabetes insipidus; cardiac arrhythmias; hypertension

FOSFOMYCIN (*Monurol*)
Frequent: diarrhea
Occasional: vaginitis

FURAZOLIDONE (*Furoxone*)
Frequent: nausea; vomiting
Occasional: allergic reactions, including pulmonary infiltrates; hypotension; urticaria; fever; vesicular rash; hypoglycemia; headache
Rare: hemolytic anemia in G6PD deficiency and neonates; disulfiram-like reaction with alcohol; polyneuritis

GANCICLOVIR (*Cytovene*)
Frequent: neutropenia; thrombocytopenia
Occasional: headache; anemia; fever; rash; abnormal liver function; neurological toxicity; phlebitis
Rare: hypertension; cardiac arrhythmias; GI disturbance; eosinophilia; hypoglycemia; alopecia; pruritus; urticaria; renal toxicity; psychiatric disturbances; seizures

GEMIFLOXACIN — See Fluoroquinolones

GENTAMICIN (*Garamycin*)
Occasional: vestibular damage; renal damage; rash
Rare: auditory damage; neuromuscular blockade and apnea, reversible with calcium or neostigmine; neurotoxicity; polyneuropathy; anaphylaxis

GRISEOFULVIN (*Fulvicin-U/F*, others)
Occasional: GI disturbance; allergic and photosensitivity reactions

Rare: proteinuria; hematologic abnormalities; confusion; paresthesias; exacerbation of lupus; fixed-drug eruption; reversible liver damage; lymphadenopathy; exacerbation of leprosy

HALOFANTRINE (*Halfan*)
Occasional: diarrhea; abdominal pain; pruritus; QTc and PR prolongation
Rare: cardiac arrhythmias and torsades de pointes

IMIPENEM-CILASTATIN (*Primaxin*)
Occasional: phlebitis; pain at injection-site; fever; urticaria; rash; pruritus; diarrhea; nausea, vomiting and transient hypotension during intravenous infusion
Rare: seizures; CDAD

INDINAVIR (*Crixivan*)
Frequent: hyperbilirubinemia; dysuria; flank pain; hematuria; crystalluria; kidney stones
Occasional: pyuria; interstitial nephritis; hemolytic anemia; increased aminotransferases; GI disturbance; reflux esophagitis; glucose intolerance; hyperlipidemia; abnormal fat distribution; increased bleeding in hemophiliacs; paronychia; alopecia; dry skin and mucous membranes
Rare: rash; hyperprolactinemia; cholelithiasis

INTERFERON ALFA (*Alferon N, Infergen, Intron A, Roferon-A, Rebetron* with ribavirin; Pegylated interferon alfa 2b-*Peg-Intron*)
Frequent: Transient flu-like syndrome; fatigue; myalgia; anorexia; GI disturbance; increased aminotransferases; rash; dry skin or pruritus; alopecia; bone marrow suppression; depression; anxiety; insomnia
Occasional: Paresthesias; alopecia; diaphoresis; reactivation of herpes labialis; hypo- and hyperthyroidism; tinnitus; activation of autoimmune diseases, including diabetes; mania; hallucinations; psychosis
Rare: Visual disturbance and retinopathy; hypertension; cardiac arrhythmias; pneu-

monitis; stroke; renal failure; nephrotic
syndrome; hearing loss; capillary leak
syndrome with monoclonal gammopathy;
hypersensitivity reactions

IODOQUINOL (*Yodoxin*, others)
Occasional: rash; acne; enlargement of the
thyroid gland; GI disturbance; anal pruritus
Rare: optic neuritis, atrophy and loss of
vision; peripheral neuropathy after prolonged use in high dosage (months);
hypersensitivity reactions in patients with
iodine sensitivity

ISONIAZID (*Nydrazid*, others)
Occasional: peripheral neuropathy; liver
damage, may be chronic, progressive or
fatal, risk increases with age; glossitis
and GI disturbance; hypersensitivity reactions; fever
Rare: hematologic abnormalities; red cell
aplasia; depression; agitation; auditory and
visual hallucinations; paranoia; optic neuritis; hyperglycemia; folate and vitamin B_6
deficiency; pellagra-like rash; keratitis;
lupus erythematosus-like syndrome;
Stevens-Johnson syndrome

ITRACONAZOLE (*Sporanox*, others)
Occasional: nausea; vomiting; epigastric
pain; hepatic toxicity; headache; dizziness;
edema; hypertension; hypokalemia; rash
Rare: congestive heart failure; anaphylaxis; Stevens-Johnson syndrome

IVERMECTIN (*Stromectol*)
Occasional: Mazzotti-type reaction seen
in onchocerciasis, including fever, pruritus, tender lymph nodes, headache, and
joint and bone pain
Rare: hypotension; hepatitis

KANAMYCIN (*Kantrex*, others)
Occasional: eighth-nerve damage affect-
ing mainly hearing that may be irreversible and may not be detected until
after therapy has been stopped (more likely with renal impairment); renal damage
Rare: rash; fever; peripheral neuritis; par-

enteral or intraperitoneal administration
may produce neuromuscular blockade and
apnea, not reversed by neostigmine or calcium gluconate

KETOCONAZOLE (*Nizoral*, others)
Frequent: nausea; vomiting
Occasional: decreased testosterone synthesis; gynecomastia; oligospermia and
impotence in men; rash; pruritus; dizziness; abdominal pain; hepatitis; constipation; diarrhea; fever and chills; photophobia; headache
Rare: hepatotoxicity and jaundice;
increased aminotransferases or fatal hepatic necrosis; severe epigastric burning and
pain; may interfere with adrenal function;
anaphylaxis

LAMIVUDINE (3TC; *Epivir*)
Occasional: exacerbation of hepatitis B
with drug discontinuation
Rare: headache; dizziness; nasal symptoms; rash; nausea; pancreatitis; neuropathy; syndrome of lactic acidosis with
hepatomegaly and steatosis

LEVOFLOXACIN — See Fluoroquinolones

LINCOMYCIN (*Lincocin*, others)
Frequent: diarrhea
Occasional: CDAD; hypersensitivity reac-
tions
Rare: hematologic abnormalities; hypoten-
sion with rapid IV injection; amphylaxis

LINEZOLID (*Zyvox*)
Frequent: GI disturbance; bone marrow
suppression particularly thrombocytopenia, risk greater with treatment >10 days;
increased aminotransferases
Rare: peripheral nerve and optic neuropathy; bradycardia; seizures

LOPINAVIR/RITONAVIR (*Kaletra*)
Similar to ritonavir, but adverse effects are
less common; nephrotoxicity has not been
reported

Rare: pancreatitis, may be fatal; bradyarrhythmia

LORACARBEF — See Cephalosporins

MARAVIROC *(Selzentry)*
  Occasional: cough; pyrexia; upper respiratory tract infection; rash; musculoskeletal symptoms; abdominal pain; postural dizziness
  Rare: hepatotoxicity; cardiac ischaemia or MI

MEBENDAZOLE *(Vermox)*
  Occasional: diarrhea; abdominal pain
  Rare: leukopenia; agranulocytosis; hypospermia

MEFLOQUINE *(Lariam)*
  Frequent: GI disturbance; vertigo; lightheadedness; nightmares; visual disturbances; headache; insomnia
  Occasional: confusion; depression; restlessness
  Rare: psychosis; hypotension; convulsions; coma; paresthesias; pneumonitis

MEGLUMINE ANTIMONIATE *(Glucantime)* — Similar to sodium stibogluconate

MELARSOPROL *(Mel B)*
  Frequent: myocardial damage; albuminuria; hypertension; colic; Herxheimer-type reaction; encephalopathy; vomiting; peripheral neuropathy
  Rare: shock

MEROPENEM *(Merrem)* — Similar to imipenem, but less likely to cause seizures

METHENAMINE MANDELATE *(Mandelamine*, others) and
METHENAMINE HIPPURATE *(Hiprex, Urex)*
  Occasional: GI disturbance; dysuria; hypersensitivity reactions

METHICILLIN — See Penicillins

METRONIDAZOLE *(Flagyl*, others)
  Frequent: nausea; headache; anorexia; metallic taste
  Occasional: vomiting; diarrhea; dry mouth; stomatitis; insomnia; weakness; vertigo; tinnitus; paresthesias; rash; dark urine; urethral burning; disulfiram-like reaction with alcohol; candidiasis
  Rare: leukopenia; pancreatitis; seizures; peripheral neuropathy; encephalopathy; cerebellar syndrome with ataxia, dysarthria and MRI abnormalities

MICAFUNGIN *(Mycamine)*
  Occasional: fever; headache; GI disturbance; hypokalemia; leukopenia; thrombocytopenia; phlebitis at injection site; increased aminotransferases; renal dysfunction
  Rare: rash; pruritus; facial swelling; anaphylaxis; hemolysis

MICONAZOLE *(Monistat)*
  Occasional: intense, persistent pruritus; rash; local burning and irritation; abdominal cramps
  Rare: hypersensitivity reactions

MILTEFOSINE *(Impavido)*
  Frequent: GI disturbance; motion sickness; increased creatinine

MINOCYCLINE — See Tetracyclines

MOXIFLOXACIN — See Fluoroquinolones

NAFCILLIN — See Penicillins

NALIDIXIC ACID *(NegGram*, others)
  Frequent: GI disturbance; rash; visual disturbance
  Occasional: CNS disturbance; acute intracranial hypertension in young children and rarely in adults; photosensitivity reactions, sometimes persistent; seizures; hyperglycemia
  Rare: cholestatic jaundice; blood dyscrasias; fatal immune hemolytic anemia; arthralgia or arthritis; lupus-like syn-

drome; confusion; depression; excitement; visual hallucinations

NELFINAVIR *(Viracept)*
  Frequent: mild to moderate diarrhea
  Occasional: increased aminotransferases; rash; nausea; glucose intolerance; increased bleeding in hemophiliacs; hyperlipidemia; abnormal fat distribution

NEOMYCIN
  Occasional: eighth-nerve and renal damage, same as with kanamycin but hearing loss may be more frequent and severe and may occur with oral, intraarticular, irrigant, or topical use; GI disturbance; malabsorption with oral use; contact dermatitis with topical use
  Rare: neuromuscular blockade and apnea that may be reversed by intravenous neostigmine or calcium gluconate

NEVIRAPINE *(Viramune)*
  Frequent: rash, can progress to Stevens-Johnson syndrome
  Occasional: fever; nausea; headache; hepatotoxicity, which can be fatal; vivid dreams

NICLOSAMIDE *(Niclocide)*
  Occasional: nausea; abdominal pain

NIFURTIMOX *(Lampit)*
  Frequent: anorexia; vomiting; weight loss; loss of memory; sleep disorders; tremor; paresthesias; weakness; polyneuritis
  Rare: convulsions; fever; pulmonary infiltrates and pleural effusion

NITAZOXANIDE *(Alinia)*
  Occasional: GI disturbance; headache
  Rare: yellow discoloration of sclera; hypersensitivity reactions; increased creatinine; dizziness; flatulence; malaise; salivary gland enlargement; discolored urine; anemia; leukocytosis

NITROFURANTOIN *(Macrodantin, others)*
  Frequent: GI disturbance; allergic reactions, including pulmonary infiltrates
  Occasional: lupus-like syndrome; hematologic abnormalities; hemolytic anemia; peripheral neuropathy, sometimes severe; interstitial pneumonitis and pulmonary fibrosis
  Rare: cholestatic jaundice; chronic active hepatitis, sometimes fatal; focal nodular hyperplasia of liver; pancreatitis; lactic acidosis; parotitis; trigeminal neuralgia; crystalluria; increased intracranial pressure; severe hemolytic anemia in G6PD deficiency

NORFLOXACIN — See Fluoroquinolones

NYSTATIN *(Mycostatin, others)*
  Occasional: hypersensitivity reactions; fixed drug eruption; GI disturbance

OFLOXACIN — See Fluoroquinolones

ORNIDAZOLE *(Tiberal)*
  Occasional: dizziness; headache; GI disturbance
  Rare: reversible peripheral neuropathy

OSELTAMIVIR PHOSPHATE *(TamiFlu)*
  Occasional: nausea; vomiting; headache
  Rare: neuropsychiatric events, including suicide and delirium, particularly in children and adolescents

OXACILLIN — See Penicillins

OXAMNIQUINE *(Vansil)*
  Occasional: fever; headache; dizziness; somnolence and insomnia; rash; nausea; diarrhea; increased aminotransferases; ECG changes; EEG changes; orange-red discoloration of urine
  Rare: seizures; neuropsychiatric disturbances

OXYTETRACYCLINE — See Tetracyclines

PARA-AMINOSALICYLIC ACID — See Aminosalicylic acid

PAROMOMYCIN (aminosidine; *Humatin*)
 Frequent: GI disturbance with oral use
 Rare: eighth-nerve damage (mainly auditory) and renal damage when given IV; vertigo; pancreatitis

PENICILLINS
(amoxicillin – *Amoxil*, others; amoxicillin/clavulanic acid – *Augmentin*; ampicillin – *Principen*, others; ampicillin/sulbactam – *Unasyn*; carbenicillin indanyl – *Geocillin*; dicloxacillin – *Dycill*, others; methicillin; mezlocillin – *Mezlin*; nafcillin – *Nafcil*, others; oxacillin; penicillin G; penicillin V; piperacillin – *Pipracil*; piperacillin/tazobactam – *Zosyn*; ticarcillin – *Ticar*; ticarcillin/clavulanic acid – *Timentin*)
 Frequent: allergic reactions, rarely anaphylaxis, erythema multiforme or Stevens Johnson syndrome; rash (more common with ampicillin and amoxicillin than with other penicillins); diarrhea (most common with ampicillin and amoxicillin/clavulanic acid); nausea and vomiting with amoxicillin/clavulanic acid
 Occasional: hemolytic anemia; neutropenia; platelet dysfunction with high doses of piperacillin, ticarcillin, nafcillin, or methicillin; cholestatic hepatitis with amoxicillin/clavulanic acid; CDAD
 Rare: hepatic damage with semisynthetic penicillins; granulocytopenia or agranulocytosis with semisynthetic penicillins; renal damage with semisynthetic peni-cillins and penicillin G; muscle irritability and seizures, usually after high doses in patients with impaired renal function; hyperkalemia and arrhythmias with IV potassium penicillin G given rapidly; bleeding diathesis; Henoch-Schönlein purpura with ampicillin; thrombocytopenia with methicillin and mezlocillin; terror, hallucinations, disorientation, agitation, bizarre behavior and neurological reactions with high doses of procaine penicillin G, oxacillin, or ticarcillin; hypokalemic alkalosis and/or sodium overload with high doses of ticarcillin or nafcillin; hemorrhagic cystitis with methicillin;

GI bleeding with dicloxacillin; tissue damage with extravasation of nafcillin

PENTAMIDINE ISETHIONATE (*Pentam 300, NebuPent*, others)
 Frequent: hypotension; hypoglycemia often followed by diabetes mellitus; vomiting; hematologic abnormalities; renal damage; pain at injection site; GI disturbance
 Occasional: may aggravate diabetes; shock; hypocalcemia; liver damage; cardiotoxicity; delirium; rash; QTc prolongation
 Rare: Herxheimer-type reaction; anaphylaxis; acute pancreatitis; hyperkalemia; torsades de pointes

PERMETHRIN (*Nix*, others)
 Occasional: burning; stinging; numbness; increased pruritus; pain; edema; erythema; rash

PIPERACILLIN — See Penicillins

PIPERACILLIN/TAZOBACTAM — See Penicillins

POLYMYXINS
(colistimethate – *Coly-Mycin*, polymyxin B – generic)
 Occasional: renal damage; peripheral neuropathy; thrombophlebitis at IV injection site with polymyxin B
 Rare: hypersensitivity reactions; neuromuscular blockade and apnea with parenteral administration, not reversed by neostig-mine but may be by IV calcium chloride

POSACONAZOLE (*Noxafil*)
 Frequent: GI disturbance; headache; fatigue
 Occasional: rash; dry skin; taste disturbance; dizziness; paresthesias; flushing; QTc prolongation; increased aminotransferases
 Rare: angioedema; anaphylaxis; toxic epidermal necrolysis; hemolytic uremic syn-

drome/thrombotic thrombocytopenic purpura; arrhythmias

PRAZIQUANTEL *(Biltricide)*
Frequent: abdominal pain; diarrhea; malaise; headache; dizziness
Occasional: sedation; fever; sweating; nausea; eosinophilia
Rare: pruritus; rash; edema; hiccups

PRIMAQUINE PHOSPHATE
Frequent: hemolytic anemia in G6PD deficiency
Occasional: neutropenia; GI disturbance; methemoglobinemia
Rare: CNS symptoms; hypertension; arrhythmias

PROGUANIL *(Paludrine; Malarone* [with atovaquone])
Occasional: oral ulceration; hair loss; scaling of palms and soles; urticaria
Rare: hematuria (with large doses); vomiting; abdominal pain; diarrhea (with large doses); thrombocytopenia

PYRANTEL PAMOATE *(Antiminth,* others)
Occasional: GI disturbance; headache; dizziness; rash; fever

PYRAZINAMIDE
Frequent: arthralgia; hyperuricemia
Occasional: liver damage; GI disturbance; acute gout; rash
Rare: photosensitivity reactions; acute hypertension

PYRIMETHAMINE *(Daraprim)*
Occasional: hematologic abnormalities; folic acid deficiency
Rare: rash; vomiting; seizures; shock; possibly pulmonary eosinophilia; fatal cutaneous reactions with pyrimethamine-sulfadoxine *(Fansidar)*

QUINACRINE
Frequent: disulfiram-like reaction with alcohol; nausea; vomiting; colors skin and

urine yellow
Occasional: headache; dizziness
Rare: rash; fever; psychosis; extensive exfoliative dermatitis in patients with psoriasis

QUININE DIHYDROCHLORIDE and QUININE SULFATE
Frequent: cinchonism (tinnitus, head-ache, nausea, abdominal pain, visual disturbance)
Occasional: deafness; hemolytic anemia and other hematologic abnormalities; photosensitivity reactions; hypoglycemia; arrhythmias; hypotension; fever
Rare: blindness; sudden death if injected too rapidly; hypersensitivity reaction with TTP-HUS

QUINUPRISTIN/DALFOPRISTIN *(Synercid)*
Frequent: local irritation and thrombophlebitis with peripheral IV administration; arthralgias; myalgias; increase in conjugated bilirubin
Occasional: nausea; rash; increased aminotransferases

RALTEGRAVIR *(Isentress)*
Occasional: diarrhea; nausea; headache
Rare: increases in serum creatine kinase; myopathy; rhabdomyolysis

RIBAVIRIN *(Copegus, Rebetol, Virazole, Rebetron* [with interferon alfa])
Occasional: hemolytic anemia; headache; depression; fatigue; abdominal cramps; nausea; elevation of bilirubin; teratogenic and embryo-lethal in animals and mutagenic in mammalian cells; rash; conjunctivitis; bronchospasm with aerosol use; hyperuricemia

RIFABUTIN *(Mycobutin)* — Similar to rifampin; also iritis, uveitis, leukopenia, arthralgia

RIFAMPIN *(Rifadin, Rimactane)*
Frequent: colors urine, tears, saliva, CSF, contact lenses, and lens implants

red-orange
Occasional: liver damage; GI disturbance; hypersensitivity reactions
Rare: flu-like syndrome, sometimes with thrombocytopenia, hemolytic anemia, shock, and renal failure, particularly with intermittent therapy; acute organic brain syndrome; acute adrenal crisis in patients with adrenal insufficiency; renal damage; severe proximal myopathy

RIFAMPIN-ISONIAZID *(Rifamate)* — See individual drugs

RIFAMPIN-ISONIAZID-PYRAZI-NAMIDE *(Rifater)* — See individual drugs

RIFAPENTINE *(Priftin)* — Similar to rifampin; higher rate of hyperuricemia

RIFAXIMIN *(Xifaxan)*
Occasional: headache
Rare: abnormal dreams; allergic dermatitis; hypersensitivity reactions; photosensitivity; motion sickness

RIMANTADINE *(Flumadine)* — Similar to amantadine, but lower risk of CNS effects

RITONAVIR *(Norvir)*
Frequent: GI disturbance; asthenia; elevated serum triglycerides and cholesterol
Occasional: anorexia; altered taste; increased aminotransferases; cholestasis; glucose intolerance; abnormal fat distribution; circumoral and peripheral paresthesias; rash; increased bleeding in hemophiliacs; PR prolongation
Rare: nephrotoxicity; hyperprolactinemia

SAQUINAVIR *(Invirase)*/ **RITONAVIR** — See also Ritonavir
Occasional: GI disturbance; glucose intolerance; hyperlipidemia; abnormal fat distribution; increased aminotransferases; increased bleeding in hemophiliacs; PR and QTc prolongation
Rare: rash; hyperprolactinemia; torsades de pointes

SODIUM STIBOGLUCONATE *(Pentostam)*
Frequent: myalgia and arthralgia (typically large joint, may or may not be symmetric); malaise; fatigue and weakness; headache; anorexia; nausea; increased aminotransferases; increased amylase and lipase; T-wave flattening or inversion;
Occasional: vomiting; abdominal pain; liver damage; bradycardia; leukopenia; thrombocytopenia; rash
Rare: diarrhea; pruritus; myocardial damage; hemolytic anemia; renal damage; shock; sudden death

SPECTINOMYCIN *(Trobicin)*
Occasional: soreness at injection site; urticaria; dizziness; insomnia; nausea; chills; fever; decreased urine output; hypersensitivity reactions

SPIRAMYCIN *(Rovamycine)*
Occasional: GI disturbance
Rare: hypersensitivity reactions

STAVUDINE (D4T; *Zerit*)
Frequent: peripheral neuropathy
Occasional: increased aminotransferases; syndrome of lactic acidosis with hepatomegaly and steatosis; abnormal fat distribution; hyperlipidemia
Rare: rash; pancreatitis

STREPTOMYCIN
Frequent: eighth-nerve damage (mainly vestibular), sometimes permanent; paresthesias; rash; fever; eosinophilia
Occasional: pruritus; anaphylaxis; renal damage
Rare: hematologic abnormalities; neuromuscular blockade and apnea with parenteral administration, usually reversed by neostigmine; optic neuritis; hepatic necrosis; myocarditis; hemolytic anemia; renal failure; toxic erythema; Stevens-Johnson syndrome

SULFONAMIDES
Frequent: hypersensitivity reactions

(rash, photosensitivity, fever)

Occasional: kernicterus in newborn; renal damage; liver damage; Stevens-Johnson syndrome (particularly with long-acting sulfonamides); hemolytic anemia; other hematologic abnormalities; vasculitis

Rare: transient acute myopia; CDAD; reversible infertility in men with sulfasalazine; CNS toxicity with trimethoprim/sulfamethoxazole in patients with AIDS

SURAMIN SODIUM

Frequent: vomiting; pruritus; urticaria; paresthesias; hyperesthesia of hands and feet; peripheral neuropathy; photophobia

Occasional: kidney damage; hematologic abnormalities; shock; optic atrophy

TELAVANCIN *(Vibativ)*

Frequent: taste disturbance; nausea; vomiting; foamy urine

Occasional: renal failure

Rare: QTc prolongation

TELBIVUDINE *(Tyzeka)*

Frequent: headache; fatigue

Occasional: nausea; vomiting; syndrome of lactic acidosis with hepatomegaly and steatosis; exacerbation of hepatitis B with drug discontinuation

Rare: myopathy

TELITHROMYCIN *(Ketek)*

Frequent: GI disturbance; headache; dizziness

Occasional: visual disturbances including blurred vision, diplopia; difficulty focusing; rash

Rare: serious hepatotoxicity; anaphylaxis; edema; muscle cramps; QTc prolongation; exacerbation of myasthenia gravis

TENOFOVIR *(Viread)*

Occasional: GI disturbance; rash; headache; renal toxicity; syndrome of lactic acidosis with hepatomegaly and steatosis; exacerbation of hepatitis B with drug discontinuation

TERBINAFINE *(Lamisil)*

Frequent: headache; GI disturbance

Occasional: taste disturbance; increased aminotransferases; rash; pruritus; urticaria; toxic epidermal necrolysis; erythema multiforme

Rare: hepatitis; anaphylaxis; pancytopenia; agranulocytosis; severe neutropenia; changes in ocular lens and retina; parotid swelling; congestive heart failure

TETRACYCLINES

(demeclocycline – *Declomycin*; doxycycline – *Vibramycin*, others; minocycline – *Minocin*, others; oxytetracycline – *Terramycin*, others; tetracycline hydrochloride – *Sumycin*, others)

Frequent: GI disturbance; bone lesions and staining and deformity of teeth in children up to 8 years old, and in the newborn when given to pregnant women after the fourth month of pregnancy

Occasional: malabsorption; enterocolitis; photosensitivity reactions (most frequent with demeclocycline); vestibular toxicity with minocycline; increased azotemia with renal insufficiency (except doxycycline, but exacerbation of renal failure with doxycycline has been reported); renal insufficiency with demeclocycline in cirrhotic patients; hepatitis; parenteral doses may cause serious liver damage, especially in pregnant women and patients with renal disease receiving ≥1 gram/day; esophageal ulcerations; cutaneous and mucosal hyperpigmentation; tooth discoloration in adults with minocycline

Rare: hypersensitivity reactions, including serum sickness and anaphylaxis; CDAD; hemolytic anemia and other hematologic abnormalities; drug-induced lupus with minocycline; autoimmune hepatitis; increased intracranial pressure; fixed-drug eruptions; diabetes insipidus with demeclocycline; transient acute myopia; blurred vision, diplopia; papilledema; photoonycholysis and onycholysis; acute interstitial nephritis with minocycline; aggravation of myasthenic symptoms with IV injection, reversed with calcium; possibly transient neuropathy

THIABENDAZOLE (*Mintezol*)
Frequent: nausea; vomiting; vertigo; headache; drowsiness; pruritus
Occasional: leukopenia; crystalluria; hallucinations and other psychiatric reactions; visual and olfactory disturbance; rash; erythema multiforme
Rare: shock; tinnitus; intrahepatic cholestasis; seizures; angioneurotic edema; Stevens-Johnson syndrome

TICARCILLIN — See Penicillins

TICARCILLIN/CLAVULANIC ACID — See Penicillins

TIGECYCLINE (*Tygacil*) — See also Tetracyclines
Frequent: GI disturbance; permanent discoloration of teeth when given during tooth develop-ment (last half of pregnancy, infancy, and childhood to age 8 yrs)
Occasional: photosensitivity; pseudotumor cerebri; pancreatitis; injection site reactions; increased aminotransferases and bilirubin
Rare: hepatic failure; CDAD

TINIDAZOLE (*Tindamax*)
Occasional: metallic taste; GI symptoms; rash
Rare: weakness

TIPRANAVIR (*Aptivus*)/**RITONAVIR** — See also Ritonavir
Frequent: diarrhea; nausea; elevated serum triglycerides, cholesterol; increased aminotransferases
Occasional: fatigue; vomiting; abdominal pain; dyspepsia; anorexia; hyperglycemia; rash; abnormal fat distribution; increased bleeding in hemophiliacs
Rare: hepatitis and hepatic failure; nephrotoxicity; intracranial hemorrhage

TOBRAMYCIN (*Nebcin*, others) — Similar to gentamicin
Rare: delirium

TRIFLURIDINE (*Viroptic*)
Occasional: burning or stinging; palpebral edema
Rare: epithelial keratopathy; hypersensitivity reactions

TRIMETHOPRIM (*Proloprim*, others)
Frequent: nausea, vomiting with high doses
Occasional: megaloblastic anemia; thrombocytopenia; neutropenia; rash; fixed drug eruption
Rare: pancytopenia; hyperkalemia

TRIMETHOPRIM/SULFAMETHOXA-ZOLE (*Bactrim, Septra*, others)
Frequent: hypersensitivity reactions (rash, photosensitivity, fever); nausea; vomiting; anorexia
Occasional: hemolysis in G6PD deficiency; hematologic abnormalities; CDAD; kernicterus in newborn; hyperkalemia
Rare: hepatotoxicity; pancreatitis; Stevens-Johnson syndrome; aseptic meningitis; fever; confusion; depression; hallucinations; intrahepatic cholestasis; methemoglobinemia; ataxia; CNS toxicity in patients with AIDS; deterioration in renal disease; renal tubular acidosis

VALACYCLOVIR (*Valtrex*) — Generally same as acyclovir
Rare: thrombotic thrombocytopenic purpura/hemolytic uremic syndrome in severely immunocompromised patients treated with high doses

VALGANCICLOVIR (*Valcyte*) — Generally same as ganciclovir

VANCOMYCIN (*Vancocin*, others)
Frequent: thrombophlebitis; fever, chills
Occasional: eighth-nerve damage (mainly hearing) especially with large or

continued doses (> than 10 days), in presence of renal damage, and in the elderly; neutropenia; renal damage; hypersensitivity reactions; rash; "redman" syndrome
Rare: peripheral neuropathy; hypotension with rapid IV administration; exfoliative dermatitis; thrombocytopenia

VORICONAZOLE *(Vfend)*
Frequent: transient visual disturbances
Occasional: nausea; vomiting; rash; increased aminotransferases; tachycardia; hallucinations; anaphylactoid infusion reactions; QTc prolongation
Rare: photosensitivity with prolonged use; Stevens-Johnson syndrome; hepatitis; optic neuritis; papilledema; torsades de pointes

ZALCITABINE (ddC; *Hivid*)
Frequent: peripheral neuropathy
Occasional: stomatitis; esophageal ulceration; nausea; abdominal pain; diarrhea; headache; fever; fatigue; rash
Rare: pancreatitis; hypersensitivity reactions

ZANAMIVIR *(Relenza)*
Occasional: nasal and throat discomfort; headache; cough
Rare: bronchospasm and decreased lung function

ZIDOVUDINE *(Retrovir)*
Frequent: anemia; neutropenia; granulocytopenia; nail pigment changes; nausea; vomiting; fatigue
Occasional: headache; insomnia; confusion; diarrhea; rash; fever; myalgias; myopathy; light-headedness; syndrome of lactic acidosis with hepatomegaly and steatosis; abnormal fat distribution; hyperlipidemia
Rare: seizures; Wernicke's encephalopathy; cholestatic hepatitis; transient ataxia and nystagmus with acute large overdosage

ZIDOVUDINE — LAMIVUDINE *(Combivir)* — See individual drugs

ZIDOVUDINE — LAMIVUDINE — ABACAVIR *(Trizivir)* — See individual drugs

SAFETY OF ANTIMICROBIAL DRUGS IN PREGNANCY

Drug	Toxicity in Pregnancy	Recommendation	FDA†
Abacavir (*Ziagen*, and others)	Teratogenic in animals	Caution*	C
Acyclovir (*Zovirax*, and others)	None known	Caution	B
Adefovir (*Hepsera*)	Embryotoxic in rats	Caution*	C
Albendazole (*Albenza*)	Teratogenic and embryotoxic in animals	Caution*	C
Amantadine	Teratogenic and embryotoxic in rats	Caution*; contraindicated in 1st trimester	C
Amikacin	Possible 8th-nerve toxicity in fetus	Caution*	D
Amoxicillin	None known	Probably safe	B
Amoxicillin/ clavulanic acid (*Augmentin*)	None known	Probably safe	B
Ampicillin (*Principen*, and others)	None known	Probably safe	B
Ampicillin/ sulbactam (*Unasyn*)	None known	Probably safe	B
Amphotericin B deoxycholate (*Fungizone*, and others)	None known	Caution*	B

* Use only for strong clinical indication in the absence of suitable alternative.
N/A = FDA pregnancy category not available

Continued on next page.

Drug	Toxicity in Pregnancy	Recommendation	FDA†
Amphotericin B cholesteryl sulfate (*Amphotec*)	Unknown	Caution*	B
Amphotericin B lipid complex (*Abelcet*)	Unknown	Caution*	B
Liposomal Amphotericin B (*AmBisome*)	Higher rate of spontaneous abortion in rabbits	Caution*	B
Anidulafungin (*Eraxis*)	Skeletal abnormalities in rats; reduced fetal weight in rabbits	Caution*	C
Artemether/ lumefantrine[1] (*Coartem, Riamet*)	Embryo-fetal loss in rats and rabbits	Contraindicated during 1st trimester; caution 2nd and 3rd trimesters*	C

1. The artemisinin-derivatives, artemether and artesunate, are both frequently used globally in combination regimens to treat malaria. Both are available in oral, parenteral and rectal formulations, but manufacturing standards are not consistent (HA Karunajeewa et al, JAMA 2007; 297:2381; EA Ashley and NJ White, Curr Opin Infect Dis 2005; 18:531). Oral artesunate is not available in the US; the IV formulation is available through the CDC Malaria branch (M-F, 8am-4:30pm ET, 770-488-7788, or after hours, 770-488-7100) under an IND for patients with severe disease who do not have timely access, cannot tolerate, or fail to respond to IV quinidine (Med Lett Drugs Ther 2008; 50:37). To avoid development of resistance, monotherapy should be avoided (PE Duffy and CH Sibley, Lancet 2005; 366:1908). Reduced susceptibility to artesunate characterized by slow parasitic clearance has been reported in Cambodia (WO Rogers et al, Malaria J 2009; 8:10; AM Dundorp et al, N Engl J Med 2009; 361:455). Based on the few studies available, artemesin have been relatively safe during pregnancy (I Adam et al, Am Trop Med Parisitol 2009; 103; 205), but some experts would not prescribe them in the 1st trimester (RL Clark, Reprod Toxicol 2009; 28:285). Artemether/lumefantrine is available as a fixed-dose combination tablet (*Coartem* in the US and in countries with endemic malaria, *Riamet* in Europe and countries without endemic malaria); each tablet contains artemether 20 mg and lumefantrine 120 mg. It is FDA-approved for treatment of uncomplicated malaria and should not be used for severe infection or for prophylaxis. It is contraindicated during the 1st trimester of pregnancy; safety during the 2nd and 3rd trimester is not known. The tablets should be taken with fatty food (tablets may be crushed and mixed with 1-2 tsp water, and taken with milk). Artemether/lumefantrine should not be used in patients with cardiac arrhythmias, bradycardia, severe cardiac disease or QT prolongation. Concomitant use of drugs that prolong the QT interval or are metabolized by CYP2D6 is contraindicated (Med Lett Drugs Ther 2009; 51:75).

Continued on next page.

Drug	Toxicity in Pregnancy	Recommendation	FDA†
Artesunate[2]	Embryocidal and teratogenic in rats	Contraindicated during 1st trimester; caution 2nd and 3rd trimesters*	N/A
Atazanavir (*Reyataz*)	None known	Caution	B
Atovaquone (*Mepron*)	Maternal and fetal toxicity in animals	Caution*	C
Atovaquone/ proguanil (*Malarone*, and others)	Maternal and fetal toxicity in animals	Caution*	C
Azithromycin (*Zithromax*, and others)	None known	Probably safe	B
Aztreonam (*Azactam*, and others)	None known	Probably safe	B
Benznidazole (*Rochagan*)	Unknown	Contraindicated	N/A
Benzyl alcohol lotion (*Ulesfia Lotion*)	Unknown	Probably safe	B
Capreomycin (*Capastat*)	Teratogenic in animals	Caution*	C
Caspofungin (*Cancidas*)	Embryotoxic in animals	Caution*	C

* Use only for strong clinical indication in the absence of suitable alternative.
N/A = FDA pregnancy category not available
2. The artemisinin-derivatives, artemether and artesunate, are both frequently used globally in combination regimens to treat malaria. Both are available in oral, parenteral and rectal formulations, but manufacturing standards are not consistent (HA Karunajeewa et al, JAMA 2007; 297:2381; EA Ashley and NJ White, Curr Opin Infect Dis 2005; 18:531). Oral artesunate is not available in the US; the IV formulation is available through the CDC Malaria branch (M-F, 8am-4:30pm ET, 770-488-7788, or after hours, 770-488-7100) under an IND for patients with severe disease who do not have timely access, cannot tolerate, or fail to respond to IV quinidine (Med Lett Drugs Ther 2008; 50:37). To avoid development of resistance, monotherapy should be avoided (PE Duffy and CH Sibley, Lancet 2005; 366:1908). Reduced susceptibility to artesunate characterized by slow parasitic clearance has been reported in Cambodia (WO Rogers et al, Malaria J 2009; 8:10; AM Dundorp et al, N Engl J Med 2009; 361:455). Based on the few studies available, artemesin have been relatively safe during pregnancy (I Adam et al, Am Trop Med Parisitol 2009; 103; 205), but some experts would not prescribe them in the 1st trimester (RL Clark, Reprod Toxicol 2009; 28:285).

Continued on next page.

Drug	Toxicity in Pregnancy	Recommendation	FDA†
Cephalosporins[3]	None known	Probably safe	B
Chloramphenicol	Unknown – gray syndrome in newborn	Caution,* especially at term	C
Chloroquine (*Aralen*, and others)	None known with doses recommended for malaria prophylaxis; embryotoxic and teratogenic in rats	Probably safe in low doses	C
Cidofovir (*Vistide*)	Embryotoxic and teratogenic in rats and rabbits	Caution*	C
Ciprofloxacin (*Cipro*, and others)	Arthropathy in immature animals; available data suggest teratogenic risk unlikely	Probably safe	C
Clarithromycin (*Biaxin*, and others)	Teratogenic in animals	Contraindicated	C
Clindamycin[4] (*Cleocin*, and others)	None known	Caution*	B
Crotamiton (*Eurax*, and others)	Unknown	Caution*	C
Cycloserine (*Seromycin*)	Unknown	Caution*	C
Dapsone (*Aczone*)	None known; carcinogenic in rats and mice; hemolytic reactions in neonates	Caution,* especially at term	C
Daptomycin (*Cubicin*)	None known	Caution	B
Darunavir (*Prezista*)	None known	Caution*	C

3. Cefaclor (*Raniclor*), cefadroxil (*Duricef*), cefazolin (*Ancef, others*), cefepime (*Maxipime*), cefdinir (*Omnicef*), cefditoren (*Spectracef*), cefixime (*Suprax*), cefoperazone (*Cefobid*), cefotaxime (*Claforan*), cefotetan (*Cefotan*), cefoxitin (*Mefoxin*), cefpodoxime (*Vantin*), cefprozil (*Cefzil*), ceftazadime (*Fortaz*), ceftaroline (*Teflaro*), ceftibuten (*Cedax*), ceftizoxime (*Cefizox*), ceftriaxone (*Rocephin*), cefuroxime (*Zinacef*), cefuroxime axetil (*Ceftin*), cephalexin (*Keflex*). Experience with newer agents is limited.
4. For use in pregnancy and in children <8 yrs.

Continued on next page.

Drug	Toxicity in Pregnancy	Recommendation	FDA†
Delavirdine (*Rescriptor*)	Teratogenic in rats	Caution*	C
Demeclocycline (*Declomycin*, and others)	Tooth discoloration and dysplasia, inhibition of bone growth in fetus; hepatic toxicity and azotemia with IV use in pregnant patients with decreased renal function or with overdosage	Contraindicated	D
Dicloxacillin (*Dycill*, and others)	None known	Probably safe	B
Didanosine (ddI; *Videx*, and others)	None known	Caution	B
Diethylcarbamazine (DEC; *Hetrazan*)	None known; abortifacient in one study in rabbits	Contraindicated	N/A
Diloxanide	Safety not established	Caution*	N/A
Doripenem (*Doribax*)	Unknown	Caution	B
Doxycycline (*Vibramycin*, and others)	Tooth discoloration and dysplasia, inhibition of bone growth in fetus; hepatic toxicity and azotemia with IV use in pregnant patients with decreased renal function or with overdosage	Contraindicated	D
Efavirenz (*Sustiva*, and others)	Neural tube defects	Caution,* contraindicated in 1st trimester	D
Eflornithine (*Ornidyl*, and others)	Embryocidal in animals	Contraindicated	C

* Use only for strong clinical indication in the absence of suitable alternative.
N/A = FDA pregnancy category not available

Continued on next page.

Drug	Toxicity in Pregnancy	Recommendation	FDA†
Emtricitabine (*Emtriva*, and others)	None known	Caution	B
Enfuvirtide (*Fuzeon*)	None known	Caution	B
Entecavir (*Baraclude*)	Skeletal abnormalities in rats at very large doses	Caution	C
Ertapenem (*Invanz*)	Decreased total weight in animals	Caution	B
Erythromycin (*Ery-Tab*, and others)	None known; neonatal use has been associated with pyloric stenosis	Probably safe	B
Ethambutol (*Myambutol*, and others)	Teratogenic in animals	Caution*	C
Ethionamide (*Trecator-SC*)	Teratogenic in animals	Caution*	C
Etravirine (*Intelence*)	No evidence of fetal harm in rats or rabbits	Caution	B
Famciclovir (*Famvir*, and others)	Carcinogenic in animals	Caution	B
Fluconazole (*Diflucan*, and others)	Teratogenic	Contraindicated for high dose; caution* for single dose	C
Flucytosine (*Ancobon*)	Teratogenic in rats	Contraindicated	C
Fosamprenavir (*Lexiva*)	Increased rate of abortion and skeletal abnormalities in rabbits	Caution*	C
Foscarnet (*Foscavir*, and others)	Animal toxicity	Caution*	C
Fosfomycin (*Monurol*)	Fetal toxicity in rabbits with maternally toxic doses	Caution	B

Continued on next page.

Drug	Toxicity in Pregnancy	Recommendation	FDA†
Furazolidone (*Furoxone*)	None known; carcinogenic in rodents; hemolysis with G-6-PD deficiency in newborn	Caution*; contraindicated at term	N/A
Ganciclovir (*Cytovene*; *Vitrasert*, and others)	Teratogenic and embryotoxic in animals	Caution*	C
Gemifloxacin (*Factive*)	Arthropathy in immature animals	Caution*	C
Gentamicin	Possible 8th-nerve toxicity in fetus	Caution*	D
Griseofulvin (*Fulvicin U/F*, and others)	Embryotoxic and teratogenic in animals; carcinogenic in rodents	Contraindicated	C
Hydroxychloroquine (*Plaquenil*, and others)	None known with doses recommended for malaria prophylaxis	Probably safe in low doses	C
Imipenemcilastatin (*Primaxin*)	Toxic in some pregnant animals	Caution*	C
Indinavir (*Crixivan*)	None known	Caution*	C
Interferon alfa (*Intron A*, and others)	Large doses cause abortions in animals	Caution*	C
Pegylated interferon (*PEG-Intron*, *Pegasys*)	As above	As above	C
Iodoquinol (*Yodoxin*, and others)	Unknown	Caution*	C
Isoniazid (*Nydrazid*, others)	Embryocidal in some animals	Probably safe	C

* Use only for strong clinical indication in the absence of suitable alternative.
N/A = FDA pregnancy category not available

Continued on next page.

Drug	Toxicity in Pregnancy	Recommendation	FDA†
Itraconazole (*Sporanox*, and others)	Teratogenic and embryotoxic in rats	Caution*	C
Ivermectin (*Stromectol*)[5]	Teratogenic in animals	Contraindicated	C
Kanamycin (*Kantrex*)	Possible 8th-nerve toxicity in fetus	Caution*	D
Ketoconazole (*Nizoral*, and others)	Teratogenic and embryotoxic in rats	Contraindicated; topical probably safe	C
Lamivudine (3TC; *Epivir*, and others)	Unknown	Caution*	C
Levofloxacin (*Levaquin*, and others)	Arthropathy in immature animals	Caution*	C
Lindane	Absorbed from the skin; potential CNS toxicity in fetus	Contraindicated	C
Linezolid (*Zyvox*)	Decreased fetal survival in rats	Caution*	C
Lopinavir/ ritonavir (*Kaletra*)	Animal toxicity	Caution*	C
Malathion, topical (*Ovide*, and others)	None known	Probably safe	B
Maraviroc (*Selzentry*)	Unknown	Caution	B

5. Diethylcarbamazine should not be used for treatment of this disease because rapid killing of the worms can lead to blindness. Periodic treatment with ivermectin (every 3-12 months), 150 mcg/kg PO, can prevent blindness due to ocular onchocerciasis (DN Udall, Clin Infect Dis 2007; 44:53). Skin reactions after ivermectin treatment are often reported in persons with high microfilarial skin densities. Ivermectin has been inadvertently given to pregnant women during mass treatment programs; the rates of congenital abnormalities were similar in treated and untreated women. Because of the high risk of blindness from onchocerciasis, the use of ivermectin after the first trimester is considered acceptable according to the WHO. Addition of 6-8 weeks of doxycycline to ivermectin is increasingly common. Doxycycline (100 mg/day PO for 6 weeks), followed by a single 150 mcg/kg PO dose of ivermectin, resulted in up to 19 months of amicrofilaridermia and 100% elimination of *Wolbachia* species (A Hoerauf et al, Lancet 2001; 357:1415).

Continued on next page.

Drug	Toxicity in Pregnancy	Recommendation	FDA†
Mebendazole (*Vermox*, and others)	Teratogenic and embryo-toxic in rats	Caution*	C
Mefloquine (*Lariam*)[6]	Teratogenic in animals	Caution*	C
Meglumine (*Glucantime*)	Not known	Caution*	N/A
Meropenem (*Merrem*, and others)	Unknown	Caution	B
Methenamine mandelate	Unknown	Probably safe	C
Metronidazole (*Flagyl*, and others)	None known – carcinogenic in rats and mice	Caution*	B
Micafungin (*Mycamine*)	Teratogenic and embryocidal in rabbits	Caution*	C
Miconazole (*Monistat i.v.*, and others)	None known	Caution*; topical probably safe	C
Miltefosine (*Impavido*)	Teratogenic in rats and induces abortions in animals	Contraindicated; effective contraception must be used for 2 months after the last dose	N/A

* Use only for strong clinical indication in the absence of suitable alternative.

N/A = FDA pregnancy category not available

6. Mefloquine should not be used for treatment of malaria during pregnancy unless there is no other treatment option (F Nosten et al, Curr Drug Saf 2006; 1:1). Mefloquine has not been approved for use during pregnancy. However, it has been reported to be safe for prophylactic use during the second or third trimester of pregnancy and possibly during early pregnancy as well (CDC Health Information for International Travel, 2010, page 141.). It should be avoided for treatment of malaria in persons with active depression or with a history of psychosis or seizures and should be used with caution in persons with any psychiatric illness. Mefloquine should not be used in patients with conduction abnormalities; it can be given to patients taking b-blockers if they do not have an underlying arrhythmia. Mefloquine should not be given together with quinine or quinidine, and caution is required in using quinine or quinidine to treat patients with malaria who have taken mefloquine for prophylaxis. Mefloquine should not be taken on an empty stomach; it should be taken with at least 8 oz of water. Not recommended for use in travelers with active depression or with a history of psychosis or seizures and should be used with caution in persons with psychiatric illness. Mefloquine should not be used in patients with conduction abnormalities; it can be given to patients taking b-blockers if they do not have an underlying arrhythmia.

Continued on next page.

Drug	Toxicity in Pregnancy	Recommendation	FDA†
Minocycline (*Minocin,* and others)	Tooth discoloration and dysplasia, inhibition of bone growth in fetus; hepatic toxicity and azotemia with IV use in pregnant patients with decreased renal function or with overdosage	Contraindicated	D
Moxifloxacin (*Avelox*)	Arthropathy in immature animals	Caution*	C
Nafcillin (*Nafcil*)	None known	Probably safe	B
Nalidixic acid (*NegGram*)	Arthropathy in immature animals; increased intracranial pressure in newborn, teratogenic and embryocidal in rats	Contraindicated	C
Nelfinavir (*Viracept*)	None known	Caution	B
Nevirapine (*Viramune,* and others)	Decrease in fetal weight in rats	Caution*, 7	C
Niclosamide (*Niclocide*)	Not absorbed; no known toxicity in fetus	Probably safe	B
Nitazoxanide (*Alinia*)	None known	Probably safe	B
Nitrofurantoin (*Macrodantin,* and others)	Hemolytic anemia in newborn	Caution*; contraindicated at term	B
Norfloxacin (*Noroxin*)	Arthropathy in immature animals	Probably safe	C
Nystatin (*Mycostatin,* and others)	None known	Probably safe	C
Ofloxacin (*Floxin,* and others)	Arthropathy in immature animals	Probably safe	C

7. Shown to be safe and effective for HIV-infected women at a single 200mg PO dose at start of labor.

Continued on next page.

Drug	Toxicity in Pregnancy	Recommendation	FDA†
Oseltamivir (*Tamiflu*)	Some minor skeletal abnormalities in animals	Caution*	C
Oxacillin	None known	Probably safe	B
Oxamniquine (*Vansil*)	Embryocidal in animals	Contraindicated	N/A
Oxytetracycline	Tooth discoloration and dysplasia, inhibition of bone growth in fetus; hepatic toxicity and azotemia with IV use in pregnant patients with decreased renal function or with overdosage	Contraindicated	D
Paromomycin	Poorly absorbed; toxicity in fetus unknown	Oral capsules probably safe	C
Penicillin	None known	Probably safe	B
Pentamidine (*Pentam 300*, *NebuPent*, and others)	Safety not established	Caution*	C
Permethrin (*Nix*, and others)	Poorly absorbed; no known toxicity in fetus	Probably safe	B
Piperacillin (*Pipracil*, and others)	None known	Probably safe	B
Piperacillin/ tazobactam (*Zosyn*, and others)	None known	Probably safe	B
Posaconazole (*Noxafil*)	Teratogenic in animals	Caution*	C
Praziquantel (*Biltricide*)	Increased abortion rate in rats	Caution	B
Primaquine	Hemolysis in G-6-PD deficiency	Contraindicated	C

* Use only for strong clinical indication in the absence of suitable alternative.
N/A = FDA pregnancy category not available

Continued on next page.

Drug	Toxicity in Pregnancy	Recommendation	FDA†
Pyrantel pamoate (*Antiminth*, and others)	Absorbed in small amounts; no known toxicity in fetus	Probably safe	C
Pyrazinamide	Unknown	Caution*	C
Pyrethrins and piperonyl butoxide (*A-200*, and others)	Poorly absorbed; no known toxicity in fetus	Probably safe	C
Pyrimethamine[8] (*Daraprim*)	Teratogenic in animals	Caution*; contra-indicated during 1st trimester	C
Quinacrine (*Atabrine*)	Safety not established	Caution*	N/A
Quinidine	Large doses can cause abortion	Probably safe	C
Quinine (*Qualaquin*)	Large doses can cause abortion; auditory nerve hypoplasia, deafness in fetus; visual changes, limb anomalies, visceral defects also reported	Caution*	C
Quinupristin/ dalfopristin (*Synercid*)	Unknown	Caution	B
Raltegravir (*Isentress*)	Fetal plasma concentrations are up to 2.5 times higher than maternal serum concentrations in animals	Caution*	C

8. Women who develop toxoplasmosis during the first trimester of pregnancy should be treated with spiramycin (3-4 g/d). After the first trimester, if there is no documented transmission to the fetus, spiramycin can be continued until term. Spiramycin is not currently available in the US but can be obtained at no cost from Palo Alto Medical Foundation Toxoplasma Serology Laboratory (PAMF-TSL, 650-853-4828), US National Collaborative Treatment Trials Study (773-834-4152), or the FDA (301-796-1600). If transmission has occurred *in utero*, therapy with pyrimethamine and sulfadiazine should be started. Pyrimethamine is a potential teratogen and should be used only after the first trimester (JG Montoya and JS Remington, Clin Infect Dis 2008; 47:554). Congenitally infected new borns should be treated with pyrimethamine every 2 or 3 days and a sulfonamide daily for about one year (JS Remington and G Desmonts in JS Remington and JO Klein, eds, *Infectious Disease of the Fetus and Newborn Infant*, 6th ed, Philadelphia:Saunders, 2006, page 1038).

Continued on next page.

Drug	Toxicity in Pregnancy	Recommendation	FDA†
Ribavirin (*Virazole*, *Rebetol*, and others)	Mutagenic, teratogenic, embryocidal in nearly all species, and possibly carcinogenic in animals	Contraindicated	X
Rifabutin (*Mycobutin*)	Unknown	Caution	B
Rifampin (*Rifadin*, *Rimactane*, and others)	Teratogenic in animals	Caution*	C
Rifapentine (*Priftin*)	Teratogenic in animals	Caution*	C
Rifaximin (*Xifaxan*)	Teratogenic in animals	Caution*	C
Rimantadine (*Flumadine*, and others)	Embryotoxic in rats	Caution*	C
Ritonavir (*Norvir*, and others)	Animal toxicity	Caution	B
Saquinavir (*Invirase*)	None known	Caution	B
Sodium stibogluconate (*Pentostam*)	Not known	Caution*	N/A
Spectinomycin (*Trobicin*)	Unknown	Probably safe	B
Spiramycin[8] (*Rovamycine*)	None known	Probably safe	N/A
Stavudine (d4T; *Zerit*, and others)	Animal toxicity with high doses	Caution*	C
Streptomycin	Possible 8th-nerve toxicity in fetus; a few cases of ototoxicity reported	Contraindicated	D

* Use only for strong clinical indication in the absence of suitable alternative.
N/A = FDA pregnancy category not available

Continued on next page.

Drug	Toxicity in Pregnancy	Recommendation	FDA†
Sulfonamides	Teratogenic in some animal studies; hemolysis in newborn with G-6-PD deficiency; increased risk of kernicterus in newborn	Caution*; contraindicated at term	C
Suramin sodium (*Germanin*)	Teratogenic in mice	Caution*	N/A
Telavancin (*Vibativ*)	Decreased fetal weight and limb and digit malformities in animals	Caution*	C
Telbivudine (*Tyzeka*)	None known	Caution*	B
Telithromycin (*Ketek*)	None known	Caution*	C
Tenofovir (*Viread*, and others)	None known	Caution	B
Tetracycline hydrochloride (*Sumycin*, and others)	Tooth discoloration and dysplasia, inhibition of bone growth in fetus; hepatic toxicity and azotemia with IV use in pregnant patients with decreased renal function or with overdosage	Contraindicated	D
Thiabendazole (*Mintezol*)	None known	Caution*	C
Ticarcillin/ clavulanic acid (*Timentin*)	None known	Probably safe	B
Tigecycline (*Tygacil*)	Decreased fetal weight and delays in bone ossification in animals	Caution*	D
Tinidazole (*Tindamax*)	Increased fetal mortality in rats	Caution*; contraindicated during 1st trimester	C
Tobramycin	Possible 8th-nerve toxicity in fetus	Caution*	D

Continued on next page.

Drug	Toxicity in Pregnancy	Recommendation	FDA†
Trimethoprim	Folate antagonism; teratogenic in rats	Caution*	C
Trimethoprim-sulfamethoxazole (*Bactrim*, and others)	Same as sulfonamides and trimethoprim	Caution*; contraindicated at term	C
Valacyclovir (*Valtrex*, and others)	None known	Caution	B
Valganciclovir (*Valcyte*)	Teratogenic and embryotoxic in animals	Caution*	C
Vancomycin (*Vancocin*, and others)	Unknown – possible auditory and renal toxicity in fetus	Caution*	C[9]
Voriconazole (*Vfend*, and others)	Teratogenic and embryotoxic in animals	Contraindicated	D
Zalcitabine (ddC; *Hivid*)	Teratogenic and embryotoxic in mice	Caution*	C
Zanamivir (*Relenza*)	None known	Caution*	C
Zidovudine (AZT; *Retrovir*, and others)	Mutagenic *in vitro*	Caution*, [10]	C

* Use only for strong clinical indication in the absence of suitable alternative.
N/A = FDA pregnancy category not available
9. Oral vancomycin capsules are poorly absorbed and are classified as category B for use in pregnancy.
10. Indicated to prevent HIV infection of fetus.

†FDA PREGNANCY CATEGORIES

Category	Interpretation
A	**Controlled studies show no risk** *Adequate, well-controlled studies in pregnant women have not shown an increased risk of fetal abnormalities*
B	**No evidence of risk in humans** *Animal studies have revealed no evidence of harm to the fetus. However, there are no adequate and well-controlled studies in pregnant women.* *or* *Animal studies have shown an adverse effect, but adequate and well-controlled studies in pregnant women have failed to demonstrate a risk to the fetus.*
C	**Risk cannot be ruled out** *Animal studies have shown an adverse effect and there are no adequate and well-controlled studies in pregnant women.* *or* *No animal studies have been conducted and there are no adequate and well-controlled studies in pregnant women.*
D	**Positive evidence of risk** *Studies, adequate well-controlled or observational, in pregnant women have demonstrated a risk to the fetus. However, the benefits of therapy may outweigh the potential risk.*
X	**Contraindicated in pregnancy** *Studies, adequate well-controlled or observational, in animals or pregnant women have demonstrated positive evidence of fetal abnormalities. The use of the product is contraindicated in women who are or may become pregnant.*

* Use only for strong clinical indication in the absence of suitable alternative.
N/A = FDA pregnancy category not available

DOSAGE OF ANTIMICROBIAL DRUGS

In choosing the dosage of an antimicrobial drug, the prescriber must consider the site of infection, the identity and antimicrobial susceptibility of the infecting organism, the possible toxicity of the drug of choice, and the condition of the patient, with special attention to renal function. This article and the table that follows on page 420 offer some guidelines for determining antimicrobial dosage, but dosage recommendations taken out of context of the clinical situation may be misleading.

RENAL INSUFFICIENCY — Antimicrobial drugs excreted through the urinary tract may be toxic for patients with renal insufficiency if they are given in usual therapeutic doses, because serum concentrations in these patients may become dangerously high. Nephrotoxic and ototoxic drugs such as gentamicin or other aminoglycosides may damage the kidney, further decreasing the excretion of these drugs, leading to higher serum concentrations that may be ototoxic and may cause additional renal damage. In patients with renal insufficiency, therefore, an antimicrobial drug with minimal nephrotoxicity, such as a beta-lactam, is preferred. When nephrotoxic drugs must be used, renal function should be monitored. Measurements of serum creatinine or blood urea nitrogen (BUN) concentrations are useful as indices of renal function, but are not as accurate as measurements of creatinine clearance; serum creatinine and BUN concentrations may be normal even with significant loss of renal function.

In renal insufficiency, control of serum concentrations of potentially toxic drugs can be achieved either by varying the dose or by varying the interval between doses. Serum antimicrobial concentrations should be measured whenever possible; rigid adherence to any dosage regimen can result in either inadequate or toxic serum concentrations in patients with renal insufficiency, particularly when renal function is changing rapidly.

Continuous renal replacement therapies (CRRTs) are increasingly being used to treat critically ill patients with acute or chronic renal failure.

There are several methods, including continuous arteriovenous hemofiltration (CAVH), continuous venovenous hemofiltration (CVVH), continuous venovenous hemodialysis (CVVHD), and continuous venovenous hemodialfiltration (CVVHDF). Dosing for CRRT depends on the method of renal replacement therapy used, flow rate and filter type.

PEDIATRIC DOSAGE — Many antimicrobial drugs have such a broad therapeutic index that it makes no difference in practice if children's dosage is based on weight or on surface area. Where dosage considerations are important in preventing severe toxic effects, as with the aminoglycosides, recommendations for safe usage are derived primarily from experience with dosage based on weight.

ONCE-DAILY AMINOGLYCOSIDES — In certain categories of patients, once-daily doses of gentamicin, tobramycin and amikacin are as effective for many indications as multiple daily doses and are equally or less nephrotoxic. Monitoring 24-hour trough drug levels is recommended to minimize the risk of toxicity. Once-daily dosing of aminoglycosides is not recommended for treatment of endocarditis and should be used cautiously in the elderly, immunocompromised patients and those with renal insufficiency.

THE TABLE — Dosage – The recommendations in the table that follows are based on the judgment of Medical Letter consultants. In some cases they differ from the manufacturer's recommendations, partly because clinical experience reported after the labeling is approved is not always reflected by an appropriate change in the manufacturer's recommendations. The range of dosage specified for some drugs may not include relatively rare indications. In general, lower doses are sufficient for treatment of urinary tract infection, and higher doses are recommended for such severe infections as meningitis, endocarditis osteomyelitis and the sepsis syndrome.

Interval – More than one interval between doses is recommended for some drugs. In general, the longer intervals should be used for infections of the urinary tract and for intramuscular administration. Recommendations are made in hours, but many oral drugs can be given three or four times during the daytime for convenience. For maximum absorption, which is often not necessary, most oral antibiotics should be given at least 30 minutes before or two hours after a meal.

ANTIMICROBIAL DRUG DOSAGE†

	Adults		Children	
	Oral	**Parenteral**	**Oral**	**Parenteral**
Abacavir	300 mg q12h or 600 mg q24h		8 mg/kg q12h	
Abacavir/ lamivudine	600 mg/300 mg q24h			
Abacavir/ lamivudine/ zidovudine	300 mg/150 mg/ 300 mg q12h			
Acyclovir	200 mg 5x/d or 400 mg q8h[1]	5-15 mg/kg q8h	20 mg/kg q6h	5-20 mg/kg q8h
Adefovir	10 mg q24h		≥12 yrs: 10 mg q24h	
Albendazole	400 mg q12-24h		10-15 mg/kg q24h	
Amantadine	100 mg q12h or 200 mg q24h		5 mg/kg div q12h[5]	
Amikacin		5 mg/kg q8h, 7.5 mg/kg q12h or 15-20 mg/kg q24h[6]		5 mg/kg q8h or 7.5 mg/kg q12h[6]
Aminosalicylic acid	8-12 g div q12-8h		200-300 mg/kg div q12-6h (max 10 g)	
Amoxicillin	250-500 mg q8h or 500-875 mg q12h[7]		20-50 mg/kg/d div q8-12h	
Amoxicillin/ clavulanic acid	250-500 mg[8] q8h or 875 mg[8] q12h or 2000 mg[8] q12h		6.6-13.3 mg/kg[8] q8h or 12.5-45 mg/kg[8] q12h	
Amphotericin B		0.3-1.0 mg/kg[9] q24h		0.3-1.0 mg/kg[9] q24h

† Dosage recommendations are also included in some articles within this handbook. Certain factors, such as site of infection, susceptibility of infecting organism and concomitant use of interacting drugs, need to be considered when dosing antimicrobial drugs. For dosing in patients receiving continuous renal replacement therapy, please refer to BH Heintz et al. Pharmacology 2009; 29:562.
1. For initial treatment of genital herpes. For suppression of genital herpes, 400 mg q12h is used. For treatment of varicella, 800 mg q6h and for zoster, 800 mg 5 times daily every 4 hours are recommended.
2. For CrCl 10-25 mL/min if normal dosing regimen is 800 mg q4h.
3. If normal dosing regimen is 200 mg q4h or 400 mg q12h.
4. For patients on hemodialysis, dose is 10 mg q7 days, given after hemodialysis.
5. In children ≥10 years and ≥40 kg dose is 100 mg q12h.

Usual Maximum Dose/Day	Adult Dosage Based on Creatinine Clearance (mL/min)			Extra Dose After Hemodialysis
	80-50	50-10	<10	
600 mg	Change not required			no
600 mg/ 300 mg	No change	Not recommended for CrCl <50 mL/min		
600 mg/ 300 mg/	No change	Not recommended for CrCl <50 mL/min		no
4 g oral 60 mg/kg IV	No change	PO: 800 mg q8h[1] IV: q12-24h	PO: 200 mg q12h[3] IV: 50% of dose q24h	yes
10 mg	10 mg q24h	10 mg q48-72h	Unknown	yes[4]
800 mg	Change not required			no
200 mg	100 mg q12-24h	100 mg q24-48h	200 mg q7d	no
1.5 g	5-7.5 mg/kg q12h	5-7.5 mg/kg q24-36h	see footnote 6	yes
12 g		50-75% of dose	50% of dose	yes (50% of dose)
3 g[7]	250-500 mg q8h	250-500 mg q12h	250-500 mg q24h	yes
4 g	No change	250-500 mg[8] q12h	250-500 mg[8] q24h	yes
1 mg/kg[9]	Change not required[10]			no

6. For information on once-daily dosing, see page 398. For renal failure give full dose once, then monitor levels.
7. Doses up to 4 g/d (80-100 mg/kg/d, divided q8-12h in children) are sometimes used for infections with intermediately-resistant pneumococcus. 1000 mg twice daily is used for *Helicobacter pylori*. An extended-release formulation *(Moxatag* 775 mg q24h) is approved for treatment of pharyngitis or tonsillitis caused by *Streptococcus pyogenes.*
8. Dosage based on amoxicillin content. In order to ensure the proper amount of clavulanic acid, the use of half or multiple tablets is not recommended (unless using *Augmentin XR*).
9. 1.5 mg/kg/day may be needed for some infections. Given IV, over a period of two to four hours.
10. A pre- and post-dose IV bolus of 500 mL normal saline may decrease renal toxicity.

Continued on next page.

ANTIMICROBIAL DRUG DOSAGE† (continued)

	Adults		Children	
	Oral	Parenteral	Oral	Parenteral
Ampho B cholesteryl sulfate complex (Amphotec)		3-4 mg/kg q24h		3-4 mg/kg q24h
Ampho B lipid complex (Abelcet)		5 mg/kg q24h		5 mg/kg q24h
Ampho B liposomal (AmBisome)		3-5 mg/kg q24h		3-5 mg/kg q24h
Ampicillin	250-500 mg q6h	1-2 g q4-6h	12.5-25 mg/kg q6h	25-50 mg/kg q6h[11]
Ampicillin/ sulbactam		1.5-3 g[12] q6h		50-100 mg/kg[12] q6h
Anidulafungin		100-200 mg day 1, then 50-100 mg q24h		0.75-1.5 mg/kg q24h[13]
Atazanavir	300 mg q24h[14]		See package insert	
Atovaquone	750 mg q12h[15]		30 mg/kg q24h[16]	
Atovaquone/ proguanil	1000 mg/400 mg q24h[17]		See foot- note 18	
Azithromycin	250-1000 mg[19] q24h or 2 g once[19]	500 mg q24h	5-12 mg/kg q24h[19]	
Aztreonam[20]		1-2 g q6-8h		30-50 mg/kg q6-8h
Capreomycin		15 mg/kg q24h		15-30 mg/kg q24h

11. For severe infections, such as meningitis caused by ampicillin-sensitive *H. influenzae* type b, Medical Letter consultants recommend up to 400 mg/kg/d. Meningitis should be treated q4h.
12. Combination formulation: 1.5-g vial contains 1 g ampicillin/500 mg sulbactam; 3-g vial contains 2 g ampicillin/1 g sulbactam. In children, dose based on ampicillin component.
13. Safety and effectiveness not established in children. Concentrations and exposures following administration of these maintenance doses in children 2-17 yrs old were similar to those observed in adults receiving maintenance doses of 50 and 100 mg/d.
14. With ritonavir 100 mg once daily. Treatment-naïve patients can take 400 mg once daily if they cannot tolerate ritonavir. For treatment-naïve patients taking efavirenz, the recommended dose is 400 mg taken once daily with 100 mg of ritonavir.
15. For treatment of *Pneumocystis jiroveci* pneumonia (PCP). The dose for prevention of PCP is 1500 mg once daily.

Usual Maximum Dose/Day	Adult Dosage Based on Creatinine Clearance (mL/min)			Extra Dose After Hemodialysis
	80-50	50-10	<10	
7.5 mg/kg		Unknown		
5 mg/kg		Unknown		no
6 mg/kg		Unknown		no
12 g	0.5-2 g q6h	0.5-2 g q6-12h	0.5-2 g q12-24h	yes
12 g	No change	1.5-3 g q8-12h	1.5-3 g q12-24h	yes
100 mg		Change not required		no
400 mg		Change not required		
1500 mg		Change not required		
1000 mg/ 400 mg	No change	Not recommended for CrCl <30 mL/min		no
500 mg		Change not required		
8 g	No change	500-1000 mg q8h	250-500 mg q8h	yes
1 g		See package insert		

16. For infants 1-3 months and children older than 24 months of age. The recommended dose for children 4-24 months of age is up to 45 mg/kg once daily.
17. Dosage for treatment of malaria. For prevention of malaria, dose is 250 mg/100 mg once daily. Each adult tablet contains 250 mg atovaquone/100 mg proguanil.
18. For pediatric dosing, see Drugs for Parasitic Infections (Malaria) page 244.
19. For adults: 500 mg on day 1 and 250 mg/d on days 2-5; urethritis and cervicitis: 1 g once for *C. trachomatis*, 2 g once for *N. gonorrhoeae;* MAC prophylaxis: 1200 mg once/week; MAC treatment: 600 mg once daily (with ethambutol); For children: pharyngitis/tonsillitis: 12 mg/kg once a day for 5 days; acute otitis media: 10 mg/kg on day 1 and 5 mg/kg on days 2 to 5 or single-dose 30 mg/kg or 10 mg/kg once daily for 3 days (max = 1500mg). Extended-release oral suspension *(Zmax)* is given as 2 g once for treatment of adults with acute bacterial sinusitis or mild-moderate community acquired pneumonia.
20. Dosage adjustment may be necessary in patients with hepatic dysfunction.

Continued on next page.

Dosage of Antimicrobial Drugs

ANTIMICROBIAL DRUG DOSAGE† (continued)

	Adults		Children	
	Oral	Parenteral	Oral	Parenteral
Caspofungin[20]		70 mg day 1, then 50 mg q24h[21,22]		See footnote 23
Cefaclor	250-500 mg q8h		20-40 mg/kg/d div q8-12h	
Cefadroxil	0.5-1 g q12h		15 mg/kg q12h	
Cefazolin		500 mg-2 g q6-8h		25-100 mg/kg/d, div q6-8h
Cefdinir	300 mg q12h or 600 mg q24h		7 mg/kg q12h or 14 mg/kg q24h	
Cefditoren	200-400 mg q12h		See footnote 24	
Cefepime		1-2 g q8-12h		50 mg/kg q8-12h
Cefixime	200 mg q12h or 400 mg q24h		4 mg/kg q12h or 8 mg/kg q24h	
Cefotaxime		1-2 g q4-12h		50-200 mg/kg/d, div q4-6h
Cefotetan		500 mg-3 g q12h		20-40 mg/kg q12h[25]
Cefoxitin		1-2 g q4-6h		80-160 mg/kg/d, div q4-6h
Cefpodoxime	100-400 mg q12h		5 mg/kg q12h	

21. Loading dose not needed for treatment of esophageal candidiasis.
22. For patients with moderate hepatic insufficiency (Child-Pugh score 7-9) the daily dose should be reduced to 35 mg following the standard 70 mg loading dose on day 1.
23. Not approved for use in children. Limited experience in clinical trials with children 2-11 yrs: 70 mg/m² on day 1 (max 70 mg), then 50 mg/m²/day (max 50 mg).

Usual Maximum Dose/Day	Adult Dosage Based on Creatinine Clearance (mL/min)			Extra Dose After Hemodialysis
	80-50	50-10	<10	
50 mg	Change not required			no
2 g	No change	50-100% of dose	50% of dose	yes
2 g	500 mg q12h	500 mg q12-24h	500 mg q36h	yes
6 g	No change	1 g q8-12h	1 g q18-24h	yes
600 mg	No change	CrCl <30mL/min 300 mg q24h		yes
800 mg	No change	200 mg q12-24h	Unknown	yes
6 g	1-2 g q8-12h	500 mg-2 g q12-24h	250 mg-1 g q24h	yes
400 mg	200-400 mg q24h	200-400 mg q24h	200 mg q24h	no
12 g	No change	1-2 g q8-12h	1-2 g q12-24h	yes
6 g	0.5-3g q12h	0.5-3g q12-24h	0.5-3g q48h	yes
12 g	No change	1-2 g q8-24h	0.5-1 g q12-48h	yes
800 mg	No change	CrCl <30 mL/min 200-400 mg q24h		yes

24. Has not been studied in children. Use adult dosage in adolescents ≥12 years of age.
25. Not approved for use in children. Dosage recommended by the Committee on Infectious Diseases of the American Academy of Pediatrics.

Continued on next page.

ANTIMICROBIAL DRUG DOSAGE† (continued)

	Adults		Children	
	Oral	Parenteral	Oral	Parenteral
Cefprozil	500 mg q12-24h		15 mg/kg q12h	
Ceftaroline		600 mg IV q12h		
Ceftazidime		500 mg-2 g q8-12h		30-50 mg/kg q8h
Ceftibuten	400 mg q24h		9 mg/kg q24h	
Ceftriaxone		1-2 g q12-24h		50-100 mg/kg/d, div q12-24h
Cefuroxime		750 mg-1.5 g q6-8h		50-150 mg/kg/d, div q6-8h
Cefuroxime axetil	125-500 mg q12h		10-15 mg/kg q12h	
Cephalexin	250 mg-1 g q6h or 500 mg q12h (for minor infections)		6.25-25 mg/kg q6h	
Chloram-phenicol[20]		12.5-25 mg/kg[26] q6h		12.5-25 mg/kg[26] q6h
Chloroquine	See foot-note 27		See foot-note 27	
Cidofovir		5 mg/kg once/wk x2, then 5 mg/kg every other wk[28]		
Ciprofloxacin	250-750 mg q12h or 1000 mg q24h[29]	200-400 mg q8-12h	10-20 mg/kg[30] q12h	6-10 mg/kg[30] q8-12h

26. IV administration; dosage should be adjusted according to serum concentration.
27. For specific dosing information, see Drugs for Parasitic Infections (Malaria), page 240.
28. For CMV. Initiation of therapy contraindicated in patients with serum creatinine >1.5 mg/dL, creatinine clearance ≤55 mL/min or urine protein ≥100 mg/dL. If serum creatinine increases by 0.3-0.4 mg/dL above baseline, decrease dose to 3 mg/kg. Discontinue for increases ≥0.5 mg/dL. Administer with probenecid and hydration before and after infusion.

Usual Maximum Dose/Day	Adult Dosage Based on Creatinine Clearance (mL/min)			Extra Dose After Hemodialysis
	80-50	50-10	<10	
1000 mg	No change	CrCl <30 mL/min: 250-500 mg q24h		yes
	No change	CrCl 31-50 mL/min: 400 mg q12h CrCl 15-30 mL/min: 300 mg q12h	200 mg q12h	no*
6 g	0.5-2 g q8-12h	0.5-2 g q12-24h	0.5-2 g q24-48h	yes
400 mg	No change	100-200 mg q24h	100 mg q24h	no*
4 g	Change not required			no
9 g	0.75-1.5 g q8h	0.75-1.5 g q8-12h	0.75-1.5 g q24h	yes
1 g	Change not required		250 mg q24h	yes
4 g	No change	0.25-1 g q8-12h	0.25-1 g q12-24h	yes
4 g	Change not required			no*
	No change	No change	50% of usual dose	no
	See footnote 28			
1.5 g	No change	CrCl <30 mL/min 200-400 mg IV or 250-500 mg PO q18-24h		no*

* But give usual dose after dialysis.
29. Extended-release formulation for treatment of UTI.
30. For PEP of inhalation anthrax oral dose is 15 mg/kg (max 500 mg) and IV dose is 10 mg/kg (max 400 mg).

Continued on next page.

ANTIMICROBIAL DRUG DOSAGE† (continued)

	Adults		Children	
	Oral	Parenteral	Oral	Parenteral
Clarithromycin	250-500 mg q12h or 1000 mg q24h[31]		7.5 mg/kg q12h	
Clindamycin[20]	300-450 mg q6h-8h	600-900 mg q6-8h	2-8 mg/kg q6-8h	2.5-10 mg/kg q6h
Colistin (colistimethate sodium)		2.5-5 mg/kg/d, div in 2-4 doses		2.5-5 mg/kg/d, div in 2-4 doses
Cycloserine[34]	250-500 mg q12h		5-10 mg/kg q12h	
Dapsone[35]	100 mg q24h		2 mg/kg q24h	
Daptomycin		4-6 mg/kg q24h[36]		
Darunavir/ ritonavir	600 mg/100 mg q12h[37]			
Delavirdine	400 mg tid			
Dicloxacillin	125-500 mg q6h		3.125-12.5 mg/kg q6h	
Didanosine	≥60 kg: 400 mg q24h[38] <60 kg: 250 mg q24h[38]		2 wks-≤8 mos: 100 mg/m² >8 mos: 120 mg/m² q12h[38]	
Doripenem		500 mg q8h		
Doxycycline	100 mg q12h	100-200 mg q12-24h	2.2 mg/kg[39] q12-24h	2.2 mg/kg[39] q12-24h
Efavirenz	600 mg q24h		200-600 mg q24h	

31. Extended-release formulation.
32. For patients taking a concomitant protease inhibitor: CrCl 30-60 mL/min reduce dose by 50% and CrCl <30 mL/min consider reducing dose by 75%.
33. Based on serum creatinine: 1.3-1.5 mg/dL, dose 2.5-3.8 mg/kg/d divided q12h; 1.6-2.5 mg/dL, dose 2.5 mg/kg/d q24h; 2.6-4 mg/dL, dose 1.5 mg/kg q36h.
34. Monitor concentrations, toxicity increases markedly above 30 mcg/mL. ATS/CDC/IDSA recommend not using in patients with CrCl <50 mL/min unless on HD. Dose in patients on HD: 250 mg once daily or 500 mg three times per week. Pyridoxine 100 mg PO q8h may help to prevent seizures.
35. Dosage for prophylaxis of *Pneumocystis jiroveci* pneumonia (PCP). Adult dosage can be changed to 50 mg daily or 200 mg weekly if given with weekly pyrimethamine and leucovorin.

Usual Maximum Dose/Day	Adult Dosage Based on Creatinine Clearance (mL/min)			Extra Dose After Hemodialysis
	80-50	50-10	<10	
1 g	No change	CrCl 30-60 mL/min: No change required[32] CrCl <30 mL/min: 50% of dose once daily[32]	Unknown	
4.8 g		Change not required		no
5 mg/kg		See footnote 33		
1 g	No change	See footnote 34		
100 mg	No change	No change	Unknown	
	No change	CrCl<30 mL/min 4-6 mg/kg q48h[36]		no*
1200 mg		Change not required		
1.2 g		Change not required		no
4 g		Change not required		no
400 mg	No change	50% of usual dose	25% of usual dose	no
1.5 g	No change	250 mg q8-12h	Unknown	no*
200 mg		Change not required		no
600 mg		Change not required		no

* But give usual dose after dialysis.
36. Higher doses (up to 10 mg/kg) have been used for severe infections such as endocarditis (DA Figueroa et al. Clin Infect Dis 2009; 49:177).
37. Dose for therapy-experienced patients with at least one darunavir resistance-associated mutation. Patients who are therapy-naïve or experienced but without resistance substitutions: 800 mg/100 mg once daily.
38. Refers to delayed-release capsules for adults and pediatric powder for oral solution for children.
39. Not recommended for children <8 years old.

Continued on next page.

ANTIMICROBIAL DRUG DOSAGE† (continued)

	Adults		Children	
	Oral	Parenteral	Oral	Parenteral
Efavirenz/ emtricitabine/ tenofovir	600 mg/200 mg/ 300 mg q24h			
Emtricitabine	200 mg q24h[40]		3-6 mg/kg (solution) q24h	
Emtricitabine/ tenofovir	200 mg/300 mg q24h			
Enfuvirtide		90 mg SC q12h		≥6 yrs: 2 mg/kg SC q12h
Entecavir	0.5 mg q24h[41]			
Ertapenem		1 g q24h		15 mg/kg q12h[25]
Erythromycin	250-500 mg q6h	0.5-1 g IV q6h[43]	7.5-12.5 mg/kg q6h	3.75-12.5 mg/kg IV q6h[43]
Ethambutol	15-25 mg/kg q24h or 50 mg/kg 2x/wk		15-25 mg/kg q24h[44] or 50 mg/kg 2x/wk	
Ethionamide	250-500 mg q12h		7.5-10 mg/kg q12h	
Famciclovir	500 mg q8h[45]			
Fluconazole	50-800 mg q24h	100-800 mg q24h	3-12 mg/kg q24h	3-12 mg/kg q24h
Flucytosine	25 mg/kg q6h		12.5-37.5 mg/kg q6h	

40. Dosage for capsules. For solution dosage is: 240 mg q24h; for CrCl 50-10 mL/min 80-120 mg q24h; for CrCl <10mL/min 60 mg q24h.
41. Dose for nucleoside-naive patients ≥16 years old. For patients refractory to lamivudine, regular dosage is 1 mg once daily and dosage in renal failure is CrCl 50-10: 0.3-0.5 mg q24h; CrCl <10: 0.1 mg q24h.
42. If the dose is given within 6 hours prior to HD, a supplemental dose of 150 mg is recommended after HD. If the dose is given >6 hours before HD, no supplemental dose is needed.
43. By slow infusion to minimize thrombophlebitis.

Usual Maximum Dose/Day	Adult Dosage Based on Creatinine Clearance (mL/min)			Extra Dose After Hemodialysis
	80-50	50-10	<10	
600 mg/ 200 mg/ 300 mg	No change	Not recommended		
200 mg	No change	200 mg q48-72h[40]	200 mg q96h[40]	no*
200 mg/ 300 mg	No change	CrCl 30-49 mL/min: q48h CrCl <30 mL/min: not recommended		
180 mg	No change	CrCl ≥35 mL/min: No change CrCl <35 mL/min: Unknown		
1 mg	No change	0.15-0.25 mg q24h[41]	0.05 mg q24h[41]	no*
1 g	No change	CrCl <30 mL/ min: 500 mg q24h	500 mg q24h	yes[42]
4 g	Change not required			no
2.5 g	CrCl <70 mL/ min: 15 mg/kg q24h	15 mg/kg q24-36h	15 mg/kg q48h	no*
1 g	No change	CrCl <30 mL/ min: 250-500 mg q24h	250-500 mg q24h	no
2 g	500 mg q12h	500 mg q24h	125-250 mg q24h	yes
800 mg[46]	No change	50-800 mg q48h	50-800 mg q72h	yes
150 mg/kg	No change	25 mg/kg q12-24h	25 mg/kg q24-48h	no*

* But give usual dose after dialysis.
44. Not recommended in children whose visual acuity cannot be monitored (<6 years old).
45. In immunocompetent patients, for herpes zoster. For first episode genital herpes, the dosage is 250 mg q8h for 5-10 days. For genital herpes recurrence, it is 1000 mg twice daily for 1 day or 125 mg q12h for 5 days. For suppression of genital herpes, it is 250 mg q12h. For treatment of recurrent herpes labialis the dose is 1500 mg once.
46. Doses of 1200 mg daily are used for initial treatment of cryptococcal meningitis.

Continued on next page.

ANTIMICROBIAL DRUG DOSAGE† (continued)

	Adults		Children	
	Oral	Parenteral	Oral	Parenteral
Fosampren-avir[20]	700 mg q12h[47]		30 mg/kg[48] q12h	
Foscarnet		60 mg/kg q8h or 90 mg/kg q12h[49]		600 mg/kg q8h
Fosfomycin	3 g once			
Furazolidone	100 mg q6h		5-8 mg/kg/d div q6h	
Ganciclovir	1 g q8h	5 mg/kg[50] q12h		5 mg/kg[50] q12h
Gemifloxacin	320 mg q24h		See foot-note 51	
Gentamicin		1-2.5 mg/kg q8h or 5-7 mg/kg q24h[6]		1-2.5 mg/kg q8h[6]
Griseofulvin micronized ultramicro-nized	500-1000 mg q24h 375-750 mg q24h		10-20 mg/kg/d div q12-24h 5-15 mg/kg/d div q12-24h	
Imipenem/cilastatin		250 mg-1 g q6-8h		15-25 mg/kg q6h
Indinavir	800 mg q8h[52]		500 mg/m² q8h	

47. With ritonavir 100 mg twice daily; may also be given as 1400 mg twice daily or 1400 mg once daily with ritonavir 100-200 mg once daily. Once daily and unboosted regimens are for protease inhibitor naïve patients only.
48. For therapy-naive patients ≥ 2 years old. A dose of 18 mg/kg q12h with ritonavir 3 mg/kg q12h is recommended for therapy-experienced patients ≥ 6 years old and is an alternative for therapy-naive patients > 6 years old.
49. For induction therapy of CMV, given over at least one hour; for maintenance, 90-120 mg/kg daily over two hours. For acyclovir-resistant HSV or VZV, 40-60 mg/kg q8h.
50. Dosage for CMV induction (give IV at constant rate over one hour); for IV maintenance without renal failure: 5 mg/kg once daily 7 days/week or 6 mg/kg once daily 5 days/week; for IV maintenance with renal failure: induction dose is reduced by half.

| Usual Maximum Dose/Day | Adult Dosage Based on Creatinine Clearance (mL/min) | | | Extra Dose After Hemodialysis |
	80-50	50-10	<10	
2.8 g		Change not required		no*
		See package insert		
3 g	Change not required		no data	yes
400 mg		Unknown		
10 mg/kg IV	2.5 mg/kg[50] IV q12h	1.25-2.5 IV mg/kg[50] q24h	1.25 mg/kg[50] IV 3x/wk	no*
3 g PO	0.5-1 g PO tid	0.5-1 g PO q24h	500 mg PO 3x/wk	no*
320 mg	No change	CrCl <40 mL/ min: 160 mg q24h	160 mg q24h	no*
	1.5 mg/kg q8-12h	1.5 mg/kg q12-24h	See footnote 6	yes
1 g		Change not required		
750 mg		Change not required		
4 g	250-500 mg q6-8h	250-500 mg q8-12h	250-500 mg q12h	yes
		Change not required		

* But give usual dose after dialysis.
51. According to The American Academy of Pediatrics, although fluoroquinolones are generally contra-indicated in children <18 years old, their use may be justified in special circumstances, such as when no other agent is available.
52. Or 800 mg twice daily with ritonavir 100 mg twice daily or 400 mg twice daily with ritonavir 400 mg twice daily. Dose adjustment is necessary when administered with other drugs including delavirdine, efavirenz, and lopinavir/ritonavir.

Continued on next page.

ANTIMICROBIAL DRUG DOSAGE† (continued)

	Adults		Children	
	Oral	**Parenteral**	**Oral**	**Parenteral**
Interferon alfa-2a, 2b alfacon-1 pegylated alfa-2a pegylated alfa-2b		3 MIU 3x/wk SC[53] 9 mcg 3x/wk SC 180 mcg SC qwk 1.5 mcg/kg SC qwk		See foot-note 53
Isoniazid[20]	300 mg q24h or DOT: 15 mg/kg 2-3x/wk	IM: same dose as PO	10-20 mg/kg q24h or DOT: 20-40 mg/kg 2-3x/wk	IM: same dose as PO
Itraconazole	200 mg q12-24h		5 mg/kg q24h	
Ivermectin	150-200 mcg/kg q24h		150-200 mcg/kg q24h	
Kanamycin		5 mg/kg q8h or 7.5 mg/kg q12h		5 mg/kg q8h or 7.5 mg/kg q12h
Ketoconazole	200-400 mg q12-24h		3.3-6.6 mg/kg q24h	
Lamivudine[54]	150 mg q12h or 300 mg q24h		4 mg/kg q12h	
Levofloxacin	250-750 mg q24h	250-750 mg q24h	See foot-note 51	
Lincomycin		600 mg-1g[56] IV q8-12h		10-20 mg/kg, IV div q8-12h

53. For chronic hepatitis C in adults. Interferon alfa-2b may also be given IM. For acute hepatitis C in adults the dosage is 5 MIU q24h x 3 weeks, then TIW. For chronic hepatitis B the dosage of interferon alfa-2b is 5 MIU q24h or 10 MIU TIW for adults and for children it is 3-6 MIU/m² TIW.
54. For treatment of HIV. For treatment of hepatitis B, the dose of lamivudine is 100 mg/d in adult patients with normal renal function and dosage in renal failure is CrCl 50-15 mL/min: 100 mg x 1, then 25-50 mg/d; CrCl <15 mL/min: 35 mg x 1, then 10-15 mg/d. The dose for children with hepatitis B is 3 mg/kg once daily.

Usual Maximum Dose/Day	Adult Dosage Based on Creatinine Clearance (mL/min)			Extra Dose After Hemodialysis
	80-50	50-10	<10	
3 MIU		Change not required		
9 mcg		Change not required		
1.5 mcg/kg		No change	Use caution	
180 mcg		No change	Use caution	
300 mg (900 mg DOT)		Change not required		no*
400 mg		Change not required		
		Unknown		
1.5 g	5-7.5 mg/kg q12-24h	5-7.5 mg/kg q24-48h	q48-72h	yes
400 mg		Change not required		
300 mg	No change	CrCl 30-49 mL/min: 150 mg q24h CrCl 15-29 mL/min: 150 mg x1, then 100 mg q24h	150 mg x1, then 25-50 mg q24h	no*
750 mg	No change	See footnote 55	500-750 mg x1, then 250-500 mg q48h	no
8 g	No change	Severe renal impairment: 25%-30% usual dose		

* But give usual dose after dialysis.
55. CrCl 20-49 mL/min: 500 mg once, then 250 mg q24h or 750 mg q48h; CrCl 10-19 mL/min: 500-750 mg once, then 250-500 mg q48h.
56. For life-threatening infections, dosage may be increased to a maximum of 8 g/d.

Continued on next page.

ANTIMICROBIAL DRUG DOSAGE† (continued)

	Adults		Children	
	Oral	Parenteral	Oral	Parenteral
Linezolid	400-600 mg q12h	600 mg q12h	10 mg/kg[57] q8h	10 mg/kg[57] q8h
Lopinavir/ ritonavir	400 mg/ 100 mg q12h[58] or 800 mg/ 200 mg q24h[59]		7-15 kg: 12/3 mg/kg q12h[58] 15-40 kg: 10/2.5 mg/kg q12h[58]	
Maraviroc	300 mg q12h[60]			
Mebendazole	100-200 mg q12h		100-200 mg q12h	
Mefloquine	1250 mg once[61]		15 mg/kg once[61]	
Meropenem		1-2 g q8h		20-40 mg/kg q8h
Methenamine hippurate	1 g q12h		6-12 yrs: 0.5-1 g q12h	
Methenamine mandelate	1 g q6h		12.5-18.75 mg/kg q6h	
Metroni- dazole[20]	500 mg q6-8h[62]	500 mg q6-8h[62]	7.5 mg/kg q6-8h[62]	7.5 mg/kg q6-8h[62]
Micafungin		150 mg q24h[63]		
Minocycline	200 mg x1, then 100 mg q12h	200 mg x1, then 100 mg q12h	4 mg/kg x1, 2 mg/kg q12h[39]	4 mg/kg x1, 2 mg/kg q12h[39]
Moxifloxacin[20]	400 mg q24h	400 mg q24h	See footnote 51	

57. For children up to 11 years of age. Pediatric patients ≥12 years should receive 600 mg q12h. Preterm neonates <1 week old should receive 10 mg/kg q12h initially.
58. A dose increase is necessary if coadministered with nevirapine or efavirenz in treatment-experienced patients when reduced susceptibility to lopinavir is suspected.
59. For treatment-naive patients. Should not be administered as once/d regimen in combination with efavirenz, nevirapine, amprenavir or nelfinavir.
60. The dose should be reduced to 150 mg twice daily in patients also taking a strong CYP3A4 inhibitor, including all protease inhibitors other than tipranavir. Concurrent use of maraviroc and strong CYP3A4 inhibitors is not recommended in patients with CrCl <30 mL/min. The dose should be increased to 600 mg twice daily if taken with a strong inducer of CYP3A4, such as rifampin.

Usual Maximum Dose/Day	Adult Dosage Based on Creatinine Clearance (mL/min)			Extra Dose After Hemodialysis
	80-50	50-10	<10	
1200 mg	Change not required			no*
800 mg/ 200 mg	Change not required			
600 mg	No change			
400 mg	Unknown			
1250 mg	Unknown			
6 g	No change	CrCl 26-50 mL/ min: 1 g q8-12h CrCl 10-25 mL/ min: 0.5-1 g q12h	0.5-1 g q24h	no*
4 g	No change	Not recommended		
4 g	No change	Not recommended		
4 g	Change not required			no*
	Change not required			no
400 mg	Change not required; consider doxycycline instead			
400 mg	Change not required			

* But give usual dose after dialysis.
61. Dosage for treatment of malaria; given as 750 mg followed 12 hrs later by 500 mg for adults and as 15 mg/kg followed 12 hrs later by 10 mg/kg for children. Dosage for once/wk prophylaxis of malaria; adults, 250 mg; children, 5 mg/kg (≤9 kg), 1/8 tab (5-10 kg), 1/4 tab (10-19 kg), 1/2 tab (20-30 kg), 3/4 tab (31-45 kg), 1 tab (>45 kg).
62. Dosage for anaerobic bacterial infections. Doses of 0.5-1 g q12h PO or IV may also be considered. For antiparasitic dosages, see Drugs for Parasitic Infections, page 221.
63. For treatment of invasive or esophageal candidiasis. The dose for prophylaxis of Candida infections in HSCT is 50 mg/d.

Continued on next page.

ANTIMICROBIAL DRUG DOSAGE† (continued)

	Adults		Children	
	Oral	**Parenteral**	**Oral**	**Parenteral**
Nafcillin		1-2 g q4-6h		25-50 mg/kg q6h
Nelfinavir[20]	1250 mg q12h		45-55 mg/kg q12h or 25-35 mg/kg q8h	
Nevirapine	200 mg/d x14 d, followed by 200 mg bid		<8 yrs: 4 mg/kg/d x14 d, followed by 7 mg/kg bid ≥8 yrs: 4 mg/kg/d x14 d, followed by 4 mg/kg bid	
Nitazoxanide	500 mg q12h		1-3 yrs: 100 mg q12h 4-11 yrs: 200 mg q12h	
Nitrofurantoin	50-100 mg q6h[64]		1.25-1.75 mg/kg q6h	
Norfloxacin	400 mg q12h		See foot- note 51	
Ofloxacin	200-400 mg q12h		See foot- note 51	
Oseltamivir	75 mg q12h[65]		≤15 kg: 30 mg q12h 16-23 kg: 45 mg q12h 24-40 kg: 60 mg q12h >40 kg: 75 mg q12h	
Oxacillin		1-2 g q4-6h		25-50 mg/kg q6h
Paromomycin	25-35 mg/kg/d div q8h		25-35 mg/kg/d div q8h	
Penicillin G potassium		2-4 million units q4h[66]		100,000- 250,000 U/d, div q2-12h[66]
Penicillin V	250-500 mg q6-8h		6.25-12.5 mg/kg q6h	
Pentamidine		3-4 mg/kg[68] q24h		3-4 mg/kg[68] q24h

64. Or 100 mg bid with *Macrobid.* The dose for prophylaxis of UTI is 50-100 mg once daily.
65. For treatment of influenza. For influenza prophylaxis dosage is 75 mg q24h for patients with normal renal function and 75 mg q48h or 30 mg q24h for patients with CrCl 10-30 mL/min.
66. The interval between parenteral doses can be as short as 2 hours for initial intravenous treatment of meningococcemia. The usual adult dose of penicillin G benzathine is 1.2-2.4 million units given as a single dose.

Usual Maximum Dose/Day	Adult Dosage Based on Creatinine Clearance (mL/min)			Extra Dose After Hemodialysis
	80-50	50-10	<10	
12 g	Change not required			no
2.5 g	Change not required			no*
400 mg	Change not required			no*
1 g	Unknown			
400 mg	No change	Not recommended for CrCl <60 mL/min		
800 mg	No change	CrCl <30 mL/min: 400 mg q24h		no
800 mg	No change	200-400 mg q24h	100-200 mg q24h	no
150 mg	No change	CrCl 10-30 mL/min: 75 mg q24h[65]	Unknown	
12 g	Change not required			no
	Unknown			
30 million units	Change not required		See footnote 67	yes
3 g	Change not required			
	4 mg/kg q24h	4 mg/kg q24-36h	4 mg/kg q48h	no

* But give usual dose after dialysis.
67. Patients with severe renal insufficiency should be given no more than one third to one half the maximum daily dosage, i.e., instead of giving 30 million units per day, 10-15 million units could be given. Patients on lower doses usually tolerate full dosage even with severe renal insufficiency.
68. For treatment of PCP. For prophylaxis of PCP, the dosage for adults and children ≥5 years is 300 mg inhaled monthly via nebulizer.

Continued on next page.

ANTIMICROBIAL DRUG DOSAGE† (continued)

| | Adults | | Children | |
	Oral	Parenteral	Oral	Parenteral
Piperacillin		3-4 g q4-6h		200-300 mg/kg/d, div q4-6h
Piperacillin/ tazobactam[69]		3.375 g q4-6h or 4.5 g q6-8h		240 mg/kg/d piperacillin div q8h
Polymyxin B		1.5-3 mg/kg/d div q12h[70]		≥ 2 yrs: 2.5-3 mg/kg/d < 2 yrs: 2.5-4 mg/kg/d q24h or div q12h
Posaconazole	200 mg q8h (prophylaxis) 200 mg q6h or 400 mg q12h (treatment)			
Praziquantel	20-25 mg/kg q8-12h		20-25 mg/kg q8-12h	
Primaquine	30 mg base q24h		0.5 mg base/kg q24h	
Pyrantel pamoate	11 mg/kg		11 mg/kg	
Pyrazinamide	15-30 mg/kg q24h		15-30 mg/kg q24h	
Pyrimethamine	25-100 mg q24h[71]		0.5-1 mg/kg q12h[71]	
Pyrimethamine/ sulfadoxine	75/1500 mg once		See footnote 72	
Quinidine gluconate		10 mg/kg then 0.02 mg/kg/min[73]		10 mg/kg then 0.02 mg/kg/min[73]
Quinine sulfate	650 mg q8h		10 mg/kg q8h	
Quinupristin/ dalfopristin		7.5 mg/kg q8-12h		7.5 mg/kg q8-12h

69. Combination formulation: A 2.25-g vial contains 2 g piperacillin/250 mg tazobactam; a 3.375-g vial contains 3 g piperacillin/375 mg tazobactam; a 4.5-g vial contains 4 g piperacillin/500 mg tazobactam.
70. 1 mg = 10,000 U.
71. For treatment of toxoplasmosis. Leucovorin should be administered with pyrimethamine.
72. Each tablet contains 25 mg pyrimethamine/500 mg sulfadoxine. Pediatric dose: <1 yr: 1/4 tab; 1-3 yrs: 1/2 tab; 4-8 yrs: 1 tab; 9-14 yrs: 2 tabs.

Usual Maximum Dose/Day	Adult Dosage Based on Creatinine Clearance (mL/min)			Extra Dose After Hemodialysis
	80-50	50-10	<10	
24 g	No change	3-4 g q6-8h	2-4 g q8-12h	yes
18 g	No change	2.25-3.375 g q6h	2.25 g q6-8h	yes
3 mg/kg	2.5-3 mg/kg once, then 1-1.5 mg/kg q24h (CrCl 30-50 mL/min) or q48h-72 (CrCl <30 mL/min)		anuric patients 1 mg/kg q5-7 days	no*
800 mg	Change not required			
	Change not required			
30 mg base	Change not required			
1 g	Unknown			
2 g	Change not required			
100 mg	Change not required			no
75/1500 mg	Unknown			
600 mg	No change	No change	75% of usual dose	yes
	No change	650 mg q8-12h	650 mg q24h	no*
Unknown	Change not required			

* But give usual dose after dialysis.
73. Loading dose should be decreased or omitted in patients who have received quinine or mefloquine. If >48 hours IV treatment required, dose should be reduced by 30-50%.

Continued on next page.

ANTIMICROBIAL DRUG DOSAGE† (continued)

	Adults		Children	
	Oral	Parenteral	Oral	Parenteral
Raltegravir	400 mg q12h			
Ribavirin	<75 kg: 400 mg q AM and 600 mg q PM >75 kg: 600 mg bid		≥3 yrs: 15 mg/kg/d div q12h	
Rifabutin	150 mg q12h or 300 mg q24h		<6 yrs: 5 mg/kg/d	
Rifampin[20]	600 mg q24h[74]	600 mg q24h	10-20 mg/kg q24h[74]	10-20 mg/kg q24h
Rifampin/ isoniazid[75]	600/300 mg[75] q24h			
Rifampin/ isoniazid/pyra- zinamide[75]	≤44 kg: 4 tabs[76] 45-54 kg: 5 tabs 55-90 kg: 6 tabs			
Rifapentine	600 mg once wkly			
Rifaximin	200 mg q8h[77]		≥12 yrs: 200 mg q8h[77]	
Rimantadine[20]	100 mg q12h		5 mg/kg once	
Ritonavir[20]	600 mg q12h[78]		400 mg/m² q12h	
Saquinavir/ ritonavir	1000 mg/100 mg q12h			
Spectinomycin		2 g once		< 45 kg: 40 mg/kg once
Stavudine[20]	≥60 kg: 40 mg q12h[79] <60 kg: 30 mg q12h		≥30 kg: 30 mg q12h <30 kg: 1 mg/kg q12h	
Streptomycin		15 mg/kg q24h[80] or 25-30 mg/kg 2-3x/wk		20-40 mg/kg q24h[80]

74. DOT: 600 mg 2-3x/week. For meningococcal carriers, dosage is 600 mg bid x 2 days for adults, 10 mg/kg q12h x 2 days for children more than one month old, and 5 mg/kg q12h x 2 days for infants less than one month old.
75. Pyridoxine 10-25 mg should be added to prevent neuropathy in malnourished or pregnant patients and those with HIV infection, alcoholism or diabetes.
76. Each tablet contains rifampin 120 mg, isoniazid 50 mg, and pyrazinamide 300 mg. For patients >90 kg - 6 tabs plus additional pyrazinamide to achieve total of 20-25 mg/kg/d.

Usual Maximum Dose/Day	Adult Dosage Based on Creatinine Clearance (mL/min)			Extra Dose After Hemodialysis
	80-50	50-10	<10	
800 mg	Change not required			
1200 mg	No change	Not recommended per manufacturer		
300 mg	CrCl <30 mL/min: 50% of dose once daily			no
600 mg	Change not required			
600/300 mg	Change not required			
	Change not required			
600 mg	Change not required			
600 mg	Change not required			
200 mg	No change	No change	100 mg q24h	no
1200 mg	No change	No change	100 mg q24h	no
2000 mg/ 200 mg	Change not required			
	No change	Change not required		no*
80 mg	No change	20 mg q12-24h 15 mg q12-24h	20 mg q24h 15 mg q24h	
1-2 g	q24-72h	q24-72h	q72-96h	yes

*But give usual dose after dialysis.
77. For travelers diarrhea. Doses of 400 mg q12h have also been used in *Clostridium difficile* infections.
78. When used in combination with other protease inhibitors the ritonavir dose is 100-400 mg PO twice daily.
79. Doses of 30 mg q12h may be effective and less toxic.
80. Given IM for tuberculosis. Dose for endocarditis: 500 mg-1 g q12h.
81. Given in conjunction with pyrimethamine for toxoplasmosis.

Continued on next page.

ANTIMICROBIAL DRUG DOSAGE† (continued)

	Adults		Children	
	Oral	**Parenteral**	**Oral**	**Parenteral**
Sulfadiazine[81]	1-1.5 g q6h		25-50 mg/kg q6h	
Sulfisoxazole	1 g q6h	25 mg/kg q6h	150 mg/kg/d div q4-6h	100 mg/kg/d div q6-8h
Telavancin		10 mg/kg q24h		
Telbivudine	600 mg q24h			
Telithromycin	800 mg q24h			
Tenofovir	300 mg q24h		2-8 yrs: 8 mg/kg q 24h >8 yrs: 210 mg/m² q24h	
Terbinafine	250 mg q24h			
Tetracy-cline[83]	250-500 mg q6h		6.25-12.5 mg/kg q6h[39]	
Ticarcillin/ clavulanic acid[84]		3.1 g q4-6h		200-300 mg/kg/d div q4-6h
Tigecycline[20]		100 mg x1, then 50 mg q12h		See foot-note 39
Tinidazole	2 g q24h[85]		50 mg/kg q24h[85]	
Tipranavir/ ritonavir	500/200 mg q12h			
Tobramycin		1-2.5 mg/kg q8h or 5-7 mg/kg q24h[6]		1-2.5 mg/kg q8h[6]

82. For patients with CrCl <30 mL/min and coexisting hepatic impairment the dose should be 400 mg once daily. Patients on hemodialysis: 600 mg should be given after dialysis on dialysis days.
83. Tetracycline or oxytetracycline. The oral dose of demeclocycline for adults is 600 mg daily in two to four divided doses.

Usual Maximum Dose/Day	Adult Dosage Based on Creatinine Clearance (mL/min)			Extra Dose After Hemodialysis
	80-50	50-10	<10	
8 g		Unknown		
8 g	1 g q6h	1 g q8h	1 g q12h	yes
		CrCl 30-50 mL/min: 7.5 mg/kg q24h CrCl 10-29 mL/min: 10 mg/kg q48h		
600 mg	No change	600 mg q48-72h	600 mg q72-96h	no*
800 mg	No change	CrCl < 30 mL/min: 600 mg q24h[82]		no[82]
300 mg	No change	CrCl 30-49 mL/min: 300 mg q48h CrCl 10-29 mL/min: 300 mg 2x/wk	300 mg q7days	
250 mg	No change	Not recommended		
2 g	250-500 mg q8-12h	250-500 mg q12-24h	250-500 mg q24h	no
24 g	No change	2 g q4-8h	2 g q12h	yes
100 mg		Change not required		
2 g		Change not required		yes
1 g/400 mg		Change not required		
	1.5 mg/kg q8-12h	1.5 mg/kg q12-24h	See footnote 6	yes

*But give usual dose after dialysis.
84. Combination formulation: a 3.1-g vial contains 3 g ticarcillin/100 mg clavulanic acid.
85. For 3-5 days for amebiasis. For treatment of giardiasis and trichomoniasis, the dose is 2 g once.

Continued on next page.

ANTIMICROBIAL DRUG DOSAGE† (continued)

	Adults		Children	
	Oral	Parenteral	Oral	Parenteral
Trimethoprim	100 mg q12h or 200 mg q24h		2 mg/kg q12h	
Trimethoprim-sulfamethoxazole (TMP-SMX)	1 SS tab[86] q6h or 2 SS tabs q12h[86]	4-5 mg/kg (TMP) q6-12h	4-5 mg/kg (TMP) q6h	4-5 mg/kg (TMP) q6-12h
Valacyclovir	1 g q8h[88]		20 mg/kg q8h	
Valganciclovir	Induction: 900 mg q12h Maintenance: 900 mg q24h		See footnote 24	
Vancomycin	125 mg q6h[89]	15-20 mg/kg IV q8-12h[90]	12.5 mg/kg q6h[89]	10-15 mg/kg IV q6h[90,91]
Voriconazole	≥40 kg: 200 mg bid[92] <40 kg: 100 mg bid[92]	Loading: 6 mg/kg q12h x2 Maintenance: 4 mg/kg q12h[93]	See footnote 94	
Zanamivir	10 mg q12h by inhalation[96]		>7 yrs: 10 mg q12h by inhalation[96]	
Zidovudine[20] (AZT)	200 mg q8h or 300 mg q12h		160 mg/m^2 q8h or 180-240 mg/m^2 q12h	
Zidovudine/ lamivudine	300/150 mg q12h		>12 yrs: 300/ 150 mg q12h	

86. Each SS tablet contains 80 mg trimethoprim and 400 mg sulfamethoxazole. Double-strength tablets are also available; the usual dosage of these is 1 tablet q12h. Suspension contains 40 mg trimethoprim and 200 mg sulfamethoxazole per 5 mL.
87. The usual maximum daily dose is 4 tablets orally or 1200 mg trimethoprim with 6000 mg sulfamethoxazole IV.
88. For herpes zoster. For a first episode of genital herpes, the dosage is 1 g q12h. For recurrence of genital herpes, it is 500 mg q12h. For suppression of genital herpes, it is 1 g q24h.
89. Only for treatment of *Clostridium difficile* infection. Doses up to 500 mg q6h can be used for fulminant infection or ileus.
90. Dose based on actual body weight. In seriously ill patients, a loading dose of 25-30 mg/kg can be considered to rapidly achieve target concentrations. Vancomycin should be infused over a period of at least 60 minutes.

Usual Maximum Dose/Day	Adult Dosage Based on Creatinine Clearance (mL/min)			Extra Dose After Hemodialysis
	80-50	50-10	<10	
200 mg	No change	CrCl 15-30 mL/min: 100 mg q18h or 50 mg q12h	CrCl <15 mL/min: 100 mg q24h	yes
See footnote 87	No change	CrCl 15-30 mL/min: 50% of dose PO and 5 mg/kg (TMP) q12h IV	Not recommended by manufacturer	yes
3 g	1 g q8h	1 g q12-24h	500 mg q24h	no*
1800 mg	Induction: No change Maintenance: No change	450 mg q12-48h 450 mg q24h-2x/wk	Not recommended Not recommended	
	No change	q24-48h	Full dose x1, then per levels	yes
	Change not required	Change not required for oral voriconazole[95]		
20 mg	Change not required			
600 mg	No change	No change	300 mg once daily	no*
600/300 mg	No change	Not recommended		

* But give usual dose after dialysis.
91. 60 mg/kg/d may be needed for staphylococcal central-nervous-system infections.
92. IV loading dose of 6 mg/kg q12h x 2 doses is recommended prior to oral maintenance. Dose may be increased to 300 mg q12h (if ≥40 kg) and 150 mg q12h (if <40 kg).
93. In patients also taking phenytoin, maintenance dose should be increased to 5 mg/kg q12h IV or 400 mg q12h PO.
94. Not approved for use in children <12 yrs. Adult dosage has been effective in children (TJ Walsh et al, Pediatr Infect Dis J 2002; 21:240).
95. Cyclodextrin (IV vehicle) accumulates in patients with CrCl <50 mL/min. Oral voriconazole is recommended in these patients.
96. For treatment of influenza. The dose for prophylaxis is 5 mg once daily.

A

abacavir – *Ziagen* (Viiv)

abacavir/lamivudine – *Epzicom* (Viiv)

abacavir/lamivudine/zidovudine – *Trizivir* (GlaxoSmithKline)

Abelcet (Sigma-Tau) – amphotericin B lipid complex

acyclovir – *Zovirax* (GlaxoSmithKline), others

adefovir – *Hepsera* (Gilead)

• *Agenerase* (GlaxoSmithKline) – amprenavir

• alatrofloxacin – *Trovan IV* (Pfizer)

albendazole – *Albenza* (GlaxoSmithKline)

Albenza (GlaxoSmithKline) – albendazole

* *Aldara* (Graceway) – imiquimod

Alferon N (Hemispherx) – interferon alfa-n3

Alinia (Romark) – nitazoxanide

Altabax (GlaxoSmithKline) – retapamulin

‡ amantadine – *Symmetrel* (Endo), others

AmBisome (Astellas) – amphotericin B liposomal

‡ amikacin – *Amikin* (Bristol-Myers Squibb), others

‡ *Amikin* (Bristol-Myers Squibb) – amikacin

aminosalicylic acid – *Paser* (Jacobus)

‡ amoxicillin – A*moxil* (GlaxoSmithKline), others

amoxicillin/clavulanic acid – *Augmentin* (GlaxoSmithKline), others

‡ *Amoxil* (GlaxoSmithKline) – amoxicillin

Amphotec (Three Rivers) – amphotericin B cholesteryl sulfate
     complex

---

* Also available generically.

• Drug has been discontinued in the US.

‡ Only available generically.

§ Not commercially available. It may be obtained through compounding pharmacies. See footnote 4 on page 223.

† Available from the Centers for Disease Control and Prevention (CDC) Drug Service. See footnote on page 274.

amphotericin B – *Fungizone* (Apothecon), others
amphotericin B cholesteryl sulfate complex – *Amphotec* (Three Rivers)
amphotericin B lipid complex – *Abelcet* (Sigma-Tau)
amphotericin B liposomal – *AmBisome* (Astellas)
ampicillin – *Principen* (Bristol-Myers Squibb), others
ampicillin/sulbactam – *Unasyn* (Pfizer), others
• amprenavir – *Agenerase* (GlaxoSmithKline)
* *Ancef* (GlaxoSmithKline) – cefazolin
Ancobon (Valeant) – flucytosine
anidulafungin – *Eraxis* (Pfizer)
§ *Antiminth* (Pfizer) – pyrantel pamoate
Aptivus (Boehringer Ingelheim) – tipranavir
* *Aralen* (Sanofi) – chloroquine
† artemether – *Artenam* (Arenco, Belgium)
artemether/lumefantrine – *CoArtem* (Novartis)
† *Artenam* (Arenco, Belgium) – artemether
† artesunate – (Walter Reed Army Institute of Research)
atazanavir – *Reyataz* (Bristol-Myers Squibb)
atovaquone – *Mepron* (GlaxoSmithKline)
atovaquone/proguanil – *Malarone* (GlaxoSmithKline)
Atripla (Gilead/BMS) – efavirenz/emtricitabine/tenofovir
* *Augmentin* (GlaxoSmithKline) – amoxicillin/clavulanic acid
Avelox (Bayer) – moxifloxacin
* *Azactam* (Bristol-Myers Squibb) – aztreonam
AZT – see zidovudine
azithromycin – *Zithromax*, *Zmax* (Pfizer), others

---

* Also available generically.
• Drug has been discontinued in the US.
‡ Only available generically.
§ Not commercially available. It may be obtained through compounding pharmacies. See footnote 4 on page 223.
† Available from the Centers for Disease Control and Prevention (CDC) Drug Service. See footnote on page 274.

aztreonam – *Azactam* (Bristol-Myers Squibb), others

B

* *Bactrim* (AR Scientific) – trimethoprim/sulfamethoxazole
Baraclude (Bristol-Myers Squibb) – entecavir
Beepen-VK (GlaxoSmithKline) – penicillin V
§ benznidazole – *Rochagan* (Roche, Brazil)
benzyl alcohol lotion – *Ulesfia Lotion* (Shionogi)
* *Biaxin* (Abbott) – clarithromycin
Bicillin L-A (King) – penicillin G benzathine
Biltricide (Bayer) – praziquantel
† bithionol – *Bitin* (Tanabe, Japan)
† *Bitin* – bithionol (Tanabe, Japan)
butoconazole – *Femstat* (Bayer), *Gynazole* (Ther-Rx)

C

Cancidas (Merck) – caspofungin
Capastat (Akorn) – capreomycin
capreomycin – *Capastat* (Akorn)
• carbenicillin – *Geocillin* (Pfizer)
caspofungin – *Cancidas* (Merck)
‡ *Ceclor* (Lilly) – cefaclor
Cedax (Pernix) – ceftibuten
‡ cefaclor – *Ceclor* (Lilly), others; *Raniclor* (Ranbaxy)

---

* Also available generically.
• Drug has been discontinued in the US.
‡ Only available generically.
§ Not commercially available. It may be obtained through compounding pharmacies. See footnote 4 on page 223.
† Available from the Centers for Disease Control and Prevention (CDC) Drug Service. See footnote on page 274.

cefadroxil – *Duricef* (Warner Chilcott), others
• *Cefadyl* (Bristol-Myers Squibb) – cephapirin
‡ cefazolin – *Ancef* (GlaxoSmithKline), *Kefzol* (ACS Dobfar) others
cefdinir – *Omnicef* (Abbott), others
cefditoren – *Spectracef* (Cornerstone Therapeutics)
cefepime – *Maxipime* (Elan), others
cefixime – *Suprax* (Lupin)
• *Cefizox* (Fujisawa) – ceftizoxime
• *Cefobid* (Pfizer) – cefoperazone
• cefoperazone – *Cefobid* (Pfizer)
‡ *Cefotan* (AstraZeneca) – cefotetan
ceftaroline – *Teflaro* (Forest)
cefotaxime – *Claforan* (Aventis), others
‡ cefotetan – *Cefotan* (AstraZeneca), others
‡ cefoxitin – *Mefoxin* (Merck), others
cefpodoxime – *Vantin* (Pfizer), others
cefprozil – *Cefzil* (Bristol-Myers Squibb), others
ceftazidime – *Fortaz* (GlaxoSmithKline), *Tazicef* (Hospira), others
ceftibuten – *Cedax* (Pernix)
* *Ceftin* (GlaxoSmithKline) – cefuroxime axetil
• ceftizoxime – *Cefizox* (Fujisawa)
ceftriaxone – *Rocephin* (Roche), others
cefuroxime – *Zinacef* (GlaxoSmithKline), others
cefuroxime axetil – *Ceftin* (GlaxoSmithKline), others
* *Cefzil* (Bristol-Myers Squibb) – cefprozil

---

* Also available generically.
• Drug has been discontinued in the US.
‡ Only available generically.
§ Not commercially available. It may be obtained through compounding pharmacies. See footnote 4 on page 223.
† Available from the Centers for Disease Control and Prevention (CDC) Drug Service. See footnote on page 274.

cephalexin – *Keflex* (Middle Brook), others
• cephapirin – *Cefadyl* (Bristol-Myers Squibb), others
• cephradine – *Velosef* (Bristol-Myers Squibb), others
chloramphenicol – *Chloromycetin* (Pfizer), others
* *Chloromycetin* (Pfizer) – chloramphenicol
chloroquine – *Aralen* (Sanofi), others
cidofovir – *Vistide* (Gilead)
* *Cipro* (Bayer) – ciprofloxacin
ciprofloxacin – *Cipro* (Bayer), others
* *Claforan* (Aventis) – cefotaxime
clarithromycin – *Biaxin* (Abbott), others
* *Cleocin* (Pfizer) – clindamycin
clindamycin – *Cleocin* (Pfizer), others
clofazimine – *Lamprene* (Novartis)
clotrimazole – *Mycelex* (Bayer), others
• cloxacillin – generic
* *Coartem* (Novartis) – artemether/lumefantrine
colistimethate – *Coly-Mycin M* (JHP), others
* *Coly-Mycin M* (JHP) – colistimethate
Combivir (Viiv) – lamivudine/zidovudine
* *Copegus* (Roche) – ribavirin
crotamiton – *Eurax* (Ranbaxy), others
Crixivan (Merck) – indinavir
Cubicin (Cubist) – daptomycin
cycloserine – *Seromycin* (The Chao Center)
* *Cytovene* (Roche) – ganciclovir

---

* Also available generically.
• Drug has been discontinued in the US.
‡ Only available generically.
§ Not commercially available. It may be obtained through compounding pharmacies. See footnote 4 on page 223.
† Available from the Centers for Disease Control and Prevention (CDC) Drug Service. See footnote on page 274.

D

dapsone – generic
daptomycin – *Cubicin* (Cubist)
Daraprim (GlaxoSmithKline) – pyrimethamine
darunavir – *Prezista* (Tibotec)
* *Declomycin* (Pfizer) – demeclocycline
delavirdine – *Rescriptor* (Viiv)
demeclocycline – *Declomycin* (Pfizer), others
Denavir (New American Therapeutics) – penciclovir
‡ dicloxacillin – *Dycill* (GlaxoSmithKline), others
didanosine – *Videx* (Bristol-Myers Squibb), others
† diethylcarbamazine – *Hetrazan* (Lederle)
* *Diflucan* (Pfizer) – fluconazole
§ diloxanide furoate – *Furamide* (Boots, U.K.)
Doripenem – *Doribax* (Ortho McNeil)
Doribax (Ortho-McNeil) – doripenem
Doryx (Warner Chilcott) – doxycycline
doxycycline – *Vibramycin, Vibra-Tabs* (Pfizer), others
* *Duricef* (Warner-Chilcott) – cefadroxil
‡ *Dycill* (GlaxoSmithKline) – dicloxacillin

E

E.E.S. (Abbott) – erythromycin
efavirenz – *Sustiva* (Bristol-Myers Squibb)

---

* Also available generically.
• Drug has been discontinued in the US.
‡ Only available generically.
§ Not commercially available. It may be obtained through compounding pharmacies. See footnote 4 on page 223.
† Available from the Centers for Disease Control and Prevention (CDC) Drug Service. See footnote on page 274.

efavirenz/emtricitabine/tenofovir – *Atripla* (Gilead/BMS)
§ *Egaten* (Novartis) – triclabendazole
† eflornithine – *Ornidyl* (Aventis)
* *Elimite* (Allergan) – permethrin
emitricitabine – *Emtriva* (Gilead)
emitricitabine/tenofovir – *Truvada* (Gilead)
Emtriva (Gilead) – emitricitabine
enfuvirtide – *Fuzeon* (Roche)
entecavir – *Baraclude* (Bristol-Myers Squibb)
Epivir (Viiv) – lamivudine
Epivir HBV (GlaxoSmithKline) – lamivudine
Epzicom (Viiv) – abacavir/lamivudine
Eraxis (Pfizer) – anidulafungin
Ertaczo – sertaconazole (Ortho Neutrogena)
ertapenem – *Invanz* (Merck)
* *ERYC* (Warner Chilcott) – erythromycin
* *Ery-Tab* (Abbott) – erythromycin
* *Erythrocin* (Abbott) – erythromycin
erythromycin – *Erythrocin, E.E.S.* (Abbott), others
‡ erythromycin/sulfisoxazole – *Pediazole* (Ross/Abbott),
    others
ethambutol – *Myambutol* (X-Gen), others
ethionamide – *Trecator* (Pfizer)
etravirine – *Intelence* (Tibotec)
* *Eurax* (Ranbaxy) – crotamiton
Exelderm (Ranbaxy) – sulconazole

---

* Also available generically.
• Drug has been discontinued in the US.
‡ Only available generically.
§ Not commercially available. It may be obtained through compounding pharmacies. See footnote 4 on page 223.
† Available from the Centers for Disease Control and Prevention (CDC) Drug Service. See footnote on page 274.

F

Factive (Cornerstone Therapeutics) – gemifloxacin
famciclovir – *Famvir* (Novartis), others
* *Famvir* (Novartis) – famciclovir
Fansidar (Roche) – pyrimethamine/sulfadoxine
Femstat (Bayer) – butoconazole
* *Flagyl* (Pfizer) – metronidazole
* *Floxin* (Ortho-McNeil) – ofloxacin
fluconazole – *Diflucan* (Pfizer), others
flucytosine – *Ancobon* (Valeant)
* *Flumadine* (Forest) – rimantadine
• fomivirsen – *Vitravene* (Novartis)
* *Fortaz* (GlaxoSmithKline) – ceftazidime
fosamprenavir – *Lexiva* (Viiv)
foscarnet – *Foscavir* (AstraZeneca), others
* *Foscavir* (AstraZeneca) – foscarnet
fosfomycin – *Monurol* (Forest)
* *Fungizone* (Apothecon) – amphotericin B
* *Furacin* (Shire) – nitrofurazone
Furadantin (Shionogi) – nitrofurantoin
§ *Furamide* (Boots, U.K.) – diloxanide furoate
§ furazolidone – *Furoxone* (Roberts)
§ *Furoxone* (Roberts) – furazolidone
Fuzeon (Roche) – enfuvirtide

---

* Also available generically.
• Drug has been discontinued in the US.
‡ Only available generically.
§ Not commercially available. It may be obtained through compounding pharmacies. See footnote 4 on page 223.
† Available from the Centers for Disease Control and Prevention (CDC) Drug Service. See footnote on page 274.

G

ganciclovir – *Cytovene* (Roche), others; *Vitrasert* (Bausch & Lomb)
* *Gantrisin* (Roche) – sulfisoxazole
‡ *Garamycin* (Schering) – gentamicin
gemifloxacin – *Factive* (Cornerstone Pharmaceuticals)
‡ gentamicin – *Garamycin* (Schering), others
• *Geocillin* (Pfizer) – carbenicillin
§ *Glucantime* (Aventis, France) – meglumine antimoniate
* *Grifulvin V* (Ortho) – griseofulvin
griseofulvin – *Girifulvin V* (Ortho), others
* *Gris-PEG* (Allergan) – griseofulvin
Gynazole (Ther-Rx) – butoconazole

H

• *Halfan* (GlaxoSmithKline) – halofantrine
• halofantrine – *Halfan* (GlaxoSmithKline)
• *Hepsera* (Gilead) – adefovir
† *Hetrazan* (Lederle) – diethylcarbamazine
* *Hiprex* (Aventis) – methenamine hippurate
• *Hivid* (Roche) – zalcitabine
‡ *Humatin* (King) – paromomycin
hydroxychloroquine – *Plaquenil* (Sanofi-Aventis), others

---

* Also available generically.
• Drug has been discontinued in the US.
‡ Only available generically.
§ Not commercially available. It may be obtained through compounding pharmacies. See footnote 4 on page 223.
† Available from the Centers for Disease Control and Prevention (CDC) Drug Service. See footnote on page 274.

I

imipenem/cilastatin sodium – *Primaxin* (Merck)
imiquimod – *Aldara* (Graceway), others
‡ *Impavido* (Palatin, Montreal, Canada) – miltefosine
indinavir – *Crixivan* (Merck)
Infergen (Three Rivers) – interferon alfacon-1
Invanz (Merck) – ertapenem
Intelence (Tibotec) – etravirine
interferon alfa-2a – *Roferon-A* (Roche)
interferon alfa-2a, pegylated – *Pegasys* (Roche)
interferon alfa-2b – *Intron A* (Merck)
interferon alfa-2b, pegylated – *PEG-Intron* (Merck)
interferon alfa-n3 – *Alferon N* (Hemispherx)
interferon alfacon-1 – *Infergen* (Three Rivers)
Intron A (Merck) – interferon alfa-2b
Invirase (Roche) – saquinavir
iodoquinol – *Yodoxin* (Glenwood), others
Isentress (Merck) – raltegravir
‡ isoniazid – *Nydrazid* (Bristol-Myers Squibb), others
itraconazole – *Sporanox* (Janssen), others
ivermectin – *Stromectol* (Merck)

K

Kaletra (Abbott) – lopinavir/ritonavir

---

* Also available generically.
• Drug has been discontinued in the US.
‡ Only available generically.
§ Not commercially available. It may be obtained through compounding pharmacies. See footnote 4 on page 223.
† Available from the Centers for Disease Control and Prevention (CDC) Drug Service. See footnote on page 274.

‡ kanamycin – *Kantrex* (Bristol-Myers Squibb), others
‡ *Kantrex* (Bristol-Myers Squibb) – kanamycin
* *Keflex* (Middle Brook) – cephalexin
* *Kefzol* (ACS Dobfar) – cefazolin
Ketek (Aventis) – telithromycin
ketoconazole – *Nizoral* (Janssen), others

L

lamivudine – *Epivir* (Viiv), *Epivir HBV*
    (GlaxoSmithKline)
lamivudine/zidovudine – *Combivir* (Viiv)
lamivudine/zidovudine/abacavir – *Trizivir* (Viiv)
† *Lampit* (Bayer, Germany) – nifurtimox
Lamprene (Novartis) – clofazimine
‡ *Lariam* (Roche) – mefloquine
Levaquin (Ortho-McNeil) – levofloxacin
levofloxacin – *Levaquin* (Ortho-McNeil)
Lexiva (Viiv) – fosamprenavir
Lincocin (Pfizer) – lincomycin
lincomycin – *Lincocin* (Pfizer), others
linezolid – *Zyvox* (Pfizer)
lopinavir/ritonavir – *Kaletra* (Abbott)
• *Lorabid* (Lilly) – loracarbef
• loracarbef – *Lorabid* (Lilly)

---

* Also available generically.
• Drug has been discontinued in the US.
‡ Only available generically.
§ Not commercially available. It may be obtained through compounding phar-
    macies. See footnote 4 on page 223.
† Available from the Centers for Disease Control and Prevention (CDC) Drug
    Service. See footnote on page 274.

M

* *Macrobid* (Procter & Gamble) – nitrofurantoin
* *Macrodantin* (Procter & Gamble) – nitrofurantoin
Malarone (GlaxoSmithKline) – atovaquone/proguanil
malathion – *Ovide* (Taro), others
* *Mandelamine* (Warner Chilcott) – methenamine mandelate
maraviroc – *Selzentry* (Viiv)
* *Maxipime* (Elan) – cefepime
‡ mebendazole – *Vermox* (Janssen), others
‡ mefloquine – *Lariam* (Roche), others
‡ *Mefoxin* (Merck) – cefoxitin
§ meglumine antimoniate – *Glucantime* (Aventis, France)
† *Mel-B* (Aventis) – melorsoprol
† melarsoprol – *Mel-B* (Aventis)
Mepron (GlaxoSmithKline) – atovaquone
meropenem – *Merrem IV* (AstraZeneca)
Merrem IV (AstraZeneca) – meropenem
methenamine hippurate – *Hiprex* (Aventis), *Urex* (Vatring),
　　others
methenamine mandelate – *Mandelamine* (Warner Chilcott),
　　others
metronidazole – *Flagyl* (Pfizer), others
micafungin – *Mycamine* (Astellas)
miconazole – *Monistat* (Ortho-McNeil), others; *Oravig* (Strativa)
§ miltefosine – *Impavido* (Paladin, Montreal, Canada)

---

* Also available generically.
• Drug has been discontinued in the US.
‡ Only available generically.
§ Not commercially available. It may be obtained through compounding pharmacies. See footnote 4 on page 223.
† Available from the Centers for Disease Control and Prevention (CDC) Drug Service. See footnote on page 274.

* *Minocin* (Wyeth) – minocycline
minocycline – *Minocin* (Wyeth), others
• *Mintezol* (Merck) – thiabendazole
* *Monistat* (Ortho-McNeil) – miconazole
Monodox (Watson) – doxycycline, others
Monurol (Forest) – fosfomycin
moxifloxacin – *Avelox* (Bayer)
* *Myambutol* (X-Gen) – ethambutol
Mycamine (Astellas) – micafungin
* *Mycelex* (Bayer) – clotrimazole
Mycobutin (Pfizer) – rifabutin
* *Mycostatin* (Bristol-Myers Squibb) – nystatin

N

‡ nafcillin – *Nallpen* (Baxter), others
• nalidixic acid – *NegGram* (Sanofi), others
‡ *Nallpen* (Baxter) – nafcillin
Natacyn (Alcon) – natamycin
natamycin – *Natacyn* (Alcon)
‡ *Nebcin* (Lilly) – tobramycin
NebuPent (APP) – pentamidine isethionate
• *NegGram* (Sanofi) – nalidixic acid
nelfinavir – *Viracept* (Viiv)
neomycin – generic
nevirapine – *Viramune* (Boehringer Ingelheim)

---

* Also available generically.
• Drug has been discontinued in the US.
‡ Only available generically.
§ Not commercially available. It may be obtained through compounding pharmacies. See footnote 4 on page 223.
† Available from the Centers for Disease Control and Prevention (CDC) Drug Service. See footnote on page 274.

§ niclosamide – *Yomesan* (Bayer, Germany)

† nifurtimox – *Lampit* (Bayer, Germany)

nitazoxanide – *Alinia* (Romark)

nitrofurantoin – *Macrodantin*, *Macrobid* (Procter & Gamble), others; *Furadantin* (Shionogi)

nitrofurazone – *Furacin* (Shire), others

* *Nix* (GlaxoSmithKline) – permethrin

* *Nizoral* (Janssen) – ketoconazole

norfloxacin – *Noroxin* (Merck)

Noroxin (Merck) – norfloxacin

Norvir (Abbott) – ritonavir

Noxafil (Merck) – posaconazole

* *Nydrazid* (Bristol-Myers Squibb) – isoniazid

nystatin – *Mycostatin* (Bristol-Myers Squibb); *Nystex* (Savage), others

* *Nystex* (Savage) – nystatin

O

ofloxacin – *Floxin* (Ortho-McNeil), others

* *Omnicef* (Abbott) – cefdinir

Oravig (Strativa) – miconazole

§ ornidazole – *Tiberal* (Roche, France)

† *Ornidyl* (Aventis) – eflornithine

oseltamivir – *Tamiflu* (Roche)

* *Ovide* (Medicis) – malathion

---

* Also available generically.

• Drug has been discontinued in the US.

‡ Only available generically.

§ Not commercially available. It may be obtained through compounding pharmacies. See footnote 4 on page 223.

† Available from the Centers for Disease Control and Prevention (CDC) Drug Service. See footnote on page 274.

oxacillin – generic
§ oxamniquine – *Vansil* (Pfizer)
• oxytetracycline – *Terramycin* (Pfizer)

P

§ *Paludrine* (Astra Zeneca, United Kingdom) – proguanil
‡ paromomycin – *Humatin* (Monarch)
Paser (Jacobus) – aminosalicylic acid
‡ *Pediazole* (Ross/Abbott) – erythromycin/sulfisoxazole
Pegasys (Roche) – pegylated interferon alfa 2a
PEG-Intron (Merck) – pegylated interferon alfa 2b
penciclovir – *Denavir* (New American Therapeutics)
penicillin G – generic, many manufacturers
penicillin G benzathine – *Bicillin L-A* (King), *Permapen* (Pfizer)
penicillin G procaine – generic, many manufacturers
penicillin V – generic, many manufacturers
* *Pentam 300* (APP) – pentamidine isethionate
* pentamidine isethionate – *Pentam 300* (Astellas), others; *NebuPent*
   (Astellas)
† *Pentostam* (GlaxoSmithKline, U.K.) – sodium stibogluconate
Permapen (Pfizer) – penicillin G benzathine
permethrin – *Elimite* (Allergan), *Nix* (GlaxoSmithKline), others
‡ piperacillin – *Pipracil* (Wyeth), others
piperacillin/tazobactam – *Zosyn* (Wyeth), others
‡ *Pipracil* (Wyeth) – piperacillin

---

* Also available generically.
• Drug has been discontinued in the US.
‡ Only available generically.
§ Not commercially available. It may be obtained through compounding pharmacies. See footnote 4 on page 223.
† Available from the Centers for Disease Control and Prevention (CDC) Drug Service. See footnote on page 274.

* *Plaquenil* (Sanofi-Aventis) – hydroxychloroquine
polymyxin B – generic
posaconacole – *Noxafil* (Merck)
praziquantel – *Biltricide* (Bayer)
Priftin (Aventis) – rifapentine
primaquine phosphate (Sanofi) – generic
Primaxin (Merck) – imipenem/cilastatin sodium
* *Principen* (Bristol-Myers Squibb) – ampicillin
Prezista (Tibotec) – darunavir
§ proguanil – *Paludrine* (Astra Zeneca, United Kingdom)
proguanil/atovaquone – *Malarone* (GlaxoSmithKline), others
‡ *Proloprim* (GlaxoSmithKline) – trimethoprim
Pronto Plus (Insight) – pyrethrins with piperonyl butoxide
§ pyrantel pamoate – *Antiminth* (Pfizer), others
pyrazinamide – generic
pyrethrins with piperonyl butoxide – *RID* (Bayer), others
pyrimethamine – *Daraprim* (GlaxoSmithKline)
pyrimethamine/sulfadoxine – *Fansidar* (Roche)

Q

Qualaquin (AR Scientific) – quinine sulfate
quinidine gluconate – generic
§ quinine dihydrochloride
quinine sulfate – *Qualaquin* (AR Scientific)
quinupristin/dalfopristin – *Synercid* (King)

---

* Also available generically.
• Drug has been discontinued in the US.
‡ Only available generically.
§ Not commercially available. It may be obtained through compounding pharmacies. See footnote 4 on page 223.
† Available from the Centers for Disease Control and Prevention (CDC) Drug Service. See footnote on page 274.

R

Raniclor (Ranbaxy) – cefaclor
raltegravir – *Isentress* (Merck)
* *Rebetol* (Merck) – ribavirin
Relenza (GlaxoSmithKline) – zanamivir
Rescriptor (Viiv) – delavirdine
retapamulin – *Altabax* (GlaxoSmithKline)
* *Retrovir* (Viiv) – zidovudine
Reyataz (Bristol-Myers Squibb) – atazanavir
ribavirin – *Rebetol* (Merck), *Copegus* (Roche), others; *Virazole*
    (Valeant)
* *RID* (Bayer) – pyrethrins with piperonyl butoxide
rifabutin – *Mycobutin* (Pfizer)
* *Rifadin* (Aventis) – rifampin
* *Rifamate* (Aventis) – rifampin/isoniazid
rifampin – *Rimactane* (Actavis), *Rifadin* (Aventis), others
rifampin/isoniazid – *Rifamate* (Aventis), others
rifampin/isoniazid/pyrazinamide – *Rifater* (Aventis)
rifapentine – *Priftin* (Aventis)
Rifater (Aventis) – rifampin/isoniazid/pyrazinamide
rifaximin – *Xifaxan* (Salix)
* *Rimactane* (Actavis) – rifampin
rimantadine – *Flumadine* (Forest), others
ritonavir – *Norvir* (Abbott)
ritonavir/lopinavir – *Kaletra* (Abbott)

---

* Also available generically.
• Drug has been discontinued in the US.
‡ Only available generically.
§ Not commercially available. It may be obtained through compounding pharmacies. See footnote 4 on page 223.
† Available from the Centers for Disease Control and Prevention (CDC) Drug Service. See footnote on page 274.

* *Rocephin* (Roche) – ceftriaxone
§ *Rochagan* (Roche, Brazil) – benznidazole
Roferon-A (Roche) – interferon alfa-2a
Rovamycine (Aventis) – spiramycin (available in the US from the
    manufacturer)

S

saquinavir – *Invirase* (Roche)
Selzentry (Viiv) – maraviroc
* *Septra* (King) – trimethoprim/sulfamethoxazole
Seromycin (The Chao Center) – cycloserine
Sertaconazole – *Ertaczo* (Ortho Neutrogena)
sinecatechins – *Veregen* (Medigene)
† sodium stibogluconate – *Pentostam* (GlaxoSmithKline, U.K.)
spectinomycin – *Trobicin* (Pfizer)
Spectracef (Cornerstone Therapeutics) – cefditoren
spiramycin – *Rovamycine* (Aventis; available in the US from the
    manufacturer)
* *Sporanox* (Janssen) – itraconazole
stavudine – *Zerit* (Bristol-Myers Squibb), others
streptomycin – generic
Stromectol (Merck) – ivermectin
sulconazole – *Exelderm* (Ranbaxy)
Sulfatrim (Actavis Mid Atlantic) – trimethoprim/sulfamethoxazole
sulfisoxazole – *Gantrisin* (Roche), others

---

* Also available generically.
• Drug has been discontinued in the US.
‡ Only available generically.
§ Not commercially available. It may be obtained through compounding pharmacies. See footnote 4 on page 223.
† Available from the Centers for Disease Control and Prevention (CDC) Drug Service. See footnote on page 274.

* *Sumycin* (Par) – tetracycline HCl
Suprax (Lupin) – cefixime
† suramin sodium – *Germanin* (Bayer, Germany)
Sustiva (Bristol-Myers Squibb) – efavirenz
‡ *Symmetrel* (Endo) – amantadine
Synercid (King) – quinupristin/dalfopristin

T

Tamiflu (Roche) – oseltamivir
* *Tazicef* (Hospira) – ceftazidime
Teflaro (Forest) – ceftaroline
telavancin – *Vibativ* (Astellas/Theravance)
telbivudine – *Tyzeka* (Novartis/Idenix)
telithromycin – *Ketek* (Aventis)
tenofovir – *Viread* (Gilead)
• *Terramycin* (Pfizer) – oxytetracycline
tetracycline HCl – *Sumycin* (Par), others
• thiabendazole – *Mintezol* (Merck)
§ *Tiberal* (Roche, France) – ornidazole
• *Ticar* (GlaxoSmithKline) – ticarcillin
• ticarcillin – *Ticar* (GlaxoSmithKline)
ticarcillin/clavulanic acid – *Timentin* (GlaxoSmithKline)
tigecycline – *Tygacil* (Wyeth)
Timentin (GlaxoSmithKline) – ticarcillin/clavulanic acid
Tindamax (Presutti) – tinidazole

---

* Also available generically.
• Drug has been discontinued in the US.
‡ Only available generically.
§ Not commercially available. It may be obtained through compounding pharmacies. See footnote 4 on page 223.
† Available from the Centers for Disease Control and Prevention (CDC) Drug Service. See footnote on page 274.

* *Tinactin* (Schering-Plough) – tolnaftate

tinidazole – *Tindamax* (Presutti)

tioconazole – *Vagistat* (Bristol-Myers Squibb), others

tipranavir – *Aptivus* (Boehringer Ingelheim)

‡ tobramycin – *Nebcin* (Lilly), others

tolnaftate – *Tinactin* (Schering-Plough), others

Trecator (Pfizer) – ethionamide

§ triclabendazole – *Egaten* (Novartis)

trifluridine – *Viroptic* (King), others

‡ trimethoprim – *Proloprim* (GlaxoSmithKline), *Trimpex* (Roche), others

trimethoprim/sulfamethoxazole – *Bactrim* (AR Scientific), *Septra* (King), others

‡ *Trimpex* (Roche) – trimethoprim

Trizivir (Viiv) – abacavir/lamivudine/zidovudine

Trobicin (Pfizer) – spectinomycin

• *Trovan* (Pfizer) – trovafloxacin

• trovafloxacin – *Trovan* (Pfizer)

Truvada (Gilead) – emitricitabine/tenofovir

Tygacil (Wyeth) – tigecycline

Tyzeka (Novartis/Idenix) – telbivudine

U

* *Unasyn* (Pfizer) – ampicillin/sulbactam

Ulesfia Lotion (Shionogi) – benzyl alcohol lotion

---

* Also available generically.

• Drug has been discontinued in the US.

‡ Only available generically.

§ Not commercially available. It may be obtained through compounding pharmacies. See footnote 4 on page 223.

† Available from the Centers for Disease Control and Prevention (CDC) Drug Service. See footnote on page 274.

* *Urex* (Vatring) – methenamine hippurate

V

* *Vagistat* (Bristol-Myers Squibb) – tioconazole
valacyclovir – *Valtrex* (GlaxoSmithKline), others
Valcyte (Roche) – valganciclovir
valganciclovir – *Valcyte* (Roche)
* *Valtrex* (GlaxoSmithKline) – valacyclovir
* *Vancocin* (Lilly) – vancomycin
vancomycin – *Vancocin* (Lilly), others
§ *Vansil* (Pfizer) – oxamniquine
* *Vantin* (Pfizer) – cefpodoxime
‡ *Veetids* (Bristol-Myers Squibb) – penicillin V
• *Velosef* (Bristol-Myers Squibb) – cephradine
Veregen (Medigene) – sinecatechins
‡ *Vermox* (Janssen) – mebendazole
* *Vfend* (Pfizer) – voriconazole
Vibativ (Astellas/Theravance) – telavancin
* *Vibramycin* (Pfizer) – doxycycline
* *Vibra-Tabs* (Pfizer) – doxycycline
vidarabine – *Vira-A* (King)
* *Videx* (Bristol-Myers Squibb) – didanosine
Vira-A (King) – vidarabine
Viracept (Viiv) – nelfinavir
Viramune (Boehringer Ingelheim) – nevirapine

---

* Also available generically.
• Drug has been discontinued in the US.
‡ Only available generically.
§ Not commercially available. It may be obtained through compounding pharmacies. See footnote 4 on page 223.
† Available from the Centers for Disease Control and Prevention (CDC) Drug Service. See footnote on page 274.

Virazole (Valeant) – ribavirin
Viread (Gilead) – tenofovir
Viroptic (King) – trifluridine
Vistide (Gilead) – cidofovir
Vitrasert (Bausch & Lomb) – ganciclovir
• *Vitravene* (Novartis) – fomivirsen
voriconazole – *Vfend* (Pfizer), others

X

Xifaxan (Salix) – rifaximin

Y

* *Yodoxin* (Glenwood) – iodoquinol
§ *Yomesan* (Bayer, Germany) – niclosamide

Z

• zalcitabine – *Hivid* (Roche)
zanamivir – *Relenza* (GlaxoSmithKline)
* *Zerit* (Bristol-Myers Squibb) – stavudine
Ziagen (GlaxoSmithKline) – abacavir
zidovudine – *Retrovir* (Viiv), others
zidovudine/lamivudine – *Combivir* (Viiv)
zidovudine/lamivudine/abacavir – *Trizivir* (Viiv)

---

* Also available generically.
• Drug has been discontinued in the US.
‡ Only available generically.
§ Not commercially available. It may be obtained through compounding pharmacies. See footnote 4 on page 223.
† Available from the Centers for Disease Control and Prevention (CDC) Drug Service. See footnote on page 274.

* *Zinacef* (GlaxoSmithKline) – cefuroxime
* *Zithromax* (Pfizer) – azithromycin
* *Zmax* (Pfizer) – azithromycin
* *Zosyn* (Wyeth) – piperacillin/tazobactam
* *Zovirax* (GlaxoSmithKline) – acyclovir
Zyvox (Pfizer) – linezolid

---

* Also available generically.
• Drug has been discontinued in the US.
‡ Only available generically.
§ Not commercially available. It may be obtained through compounding pharmacies. See footnote 4 on page 223.
† Available from the Centers for Disease Control and Prevention (CDC) Drug Service. See footnote on page 274.

INDEX

Note: Page numbers in bold type indicate major references

Index

Index

Index

Index

TABLE INDEX